Methadone Maintenance Treatment and Other Opioid Replacement Therapies

Methadone Maintenance Treatment and Other Opioid Replacement Therapies

Edited by
Jeff Ward
Division of Psychology, Faculty of Science,
Australian National University

Richard P. Mattick and Wayne Hall
National Drug and Alcohol Research Centre,
University of NSW, Australia

harwood academic publishers
Australia • Canada • China • France • Germany • India
Japan • Luxembourg • Malaysia • The Netherlands • Russia
Singapore • Switzerland • Thailand

Amsteldijk 166
1st Floor
1079 LH Amsterdam
The Netherlands

British Library Cataloguing in Publication Data

Methadone maintenance treatment and other opioid
    replacement therapies
    1. Methadone maintenance 2. Methadone – Therapeutic use
    3. Drug abuse – Treatment
    I. Ward, Jeff II. Mattick, Richard P. III. Hall, Wayne
    616.8'632'061

ISBN 90-5702-239-7 (Softcover)

Acknowledgement

This book arises out of a project funded by the Drug and Alcohol
Directorate of the New South Wales Department of Health,
Sydney.

Contents

IV CONCLUSION

LIST OF CONTRIBUTORS

James Bell, Director, Drug and Alcohol Unit, Prince of Wales Hospital, Sydney, Australia.

Shane Darke, Senior Lecturer, National Drug and Alcohol Research Centre, University of New South Wales, Sydney, Australia.

Kate Dolan, Research Officer, National Drug and Alcohol Research Centre, University of New South Wales, Sydney, Australia.

Wayne Hall, Executive Director, National Drug and Alcohol Research Centre, University of New South Wales, Sydney, Australia.

Richard P. Mattick, Director of Research, National Drug and Alcohol Research Centre, University of New South Wales, Sydney, Australia.

Dorothy Oliphant, Research Officer, National Drug and Alcohol Research Centre, University of New South Walls, Australia.

Matthew Sutton, Australian National Drug Strategy Fellow, National Drug and Alcohol Research Centre, University of New South Wales, Sydney, Australia (currently Research Fellow, Centre for Health Economics, York University, York, United Kingdom).

Jeff Ward, Research Officer, National Drug and Alcohol Research Centre, University of New South Wales, Sydney, Australia (currently Lecturer, Division of Psychology, School of Life Sciences, Faculty of Science, Australian National University, Canberra, ACT, Australia).

Pat Ward, Visiting Fellow, National Drug and Alcohol Research Centre, University of New South Wales, Sydney, Australia (currently Policy Analyst, Drug and Alcohol Directorate, New South Wales Department of Health, Sydney, Australia).

Alex Wodak, Director, Alcohol and Drug Service, St Vincent's Hospital, Sydney, Australia.

1

INTRODUCTION

WAYNE HALL, JEFF WARD AND RICHARD P. MATTICK

OPIOID REPLACEMENT THERAPY

Opioid replacement therapy involves the administration of a long-acting opioid drug to an opioid dependent person, usually by a nonparenteral route of administration, for the therapeutic purposes of preventing or substantially reducing the injection of illicit opioids, such as heroin. Its goal is to improve the health status and psychological and social well-being of the opioid-dependent person. Historically, methadone maintenance treatment was the earliest form and continues to be the most widely used form of opioid replacement therapy in the United States, Europe and Australia. We choose the more neutral phrase "opioid replacement therapy" to distinguish the general approach from the specific instance, motivated by a desire to broaden thinking about this approach to treating opioid dependence, and to take due account of recent work on alternative maintenance agents, such as, buprenorphine, as well as recent proposals for trials of opioid maintenance using injectable heroin (Bammer, 1995; Rihs, 1994). Most of the book will be concerned with methadone maintenance treatment because it has generated the greatest amount of research, and because the principles for the management of methadone treatment have general application to other forms of opioid replacement therapy.

THE ORIGINS, RATIONALE AND OBJECTIVES OF METHADONE MAINTENANCE

In the early 1960s, Dole and Nyswander introduced orally administered maintenance doses of the synthetic opioid drug methadone as a drug-substitution treatment for opioid dependence. According to Dole and Nyswander, opioid dependence was 'a physiological disease characterised by a permanent metabolic deficiency' which was best managed by administering to the opioid dependent patient 'a sufficient amount of drug to stabilise the metabolic deficiency' (Dole & Nyswander, 1965). The use of methadone as a substitute opioid provided a legal and controlled supply of an orally administered opioid drug which had to be taken only once a day because its long duration of action eliminated opiate withdrawal symptoms for 24 to 36 hours. It was claimed that high or 'blockade' daily doses of oral methadone removed the craving for heroin and blocked its euphoric effects, thereby providing an opportunity for the individual to improve his or her social functioning by taking advantage of the psychotherapeutic and rehabilitative services that were an integral part of the program (Dole & Nyswander, 1967).

Methadone maintenance treatment quickly became the most common form of drug replacement therapy for opioid dependence once it had been shown to reduce heroin use and criminal activity. In the process of this popularisation in the USA, methadone maintenance underwent a number of important changes in treatment goal, the dosage, and the extent of ancillary services that were provided in addition to the provision of methadone (Gerstein & Harwood, 1990). The treatment goal of many programs shifted from long-term maintenance towards achieving abstinence from all opioid drugs, including methadone, within a period of a few years. The average dose of methadone also declined from the high blockade doses favoured by Dole and Nyswander to the much lower doses that were required to avert withdrawal symptoms, and in some recent programs to doses that failed to avert withdrawal symptoms. Furthermore, under the exigencies of Federal funding cuts for methadone maintenance programs, the extent of ancillary services declined.

The proliferation of variations on the basic Dole and Nyswander model of methadone maintenance makes it difficult to draw strong conclusions about the effectiveness of methadone maintenance treatment from the research and clinical literature. As will become apparent, because these programs differ in effectiveness, conclusions can only be drawn about the 'average' effectiveness of methadone maintenance. The variability in the outcome of methadone maintenance treatment has been addressed by discussing the characteristics of programs that appear to affect treatment outcome, namely, methadone dose, duration of treatment, and ancillary services.

An additional complication in drawing conclusions about the effectiveness of methadone maintenance is the variety of goals that it may serve, the relative importance of which may depend upon which perspective is used – that of the individuals in treatment, or of the community that funds many of the programs. From the perspective of the community, the major treatment goals are reducing illicit drug use and the predatory criminal activity by which many users finance their drug use (Chaiken & Chaiken, 1990; Hall, 1996; Johnson *et al.,* 1985) and preventing the transmission of HIV and hepatitis by needle sharing. The community also has an interest in improving the users' health, employment status and personal relationships, and minimising the spread of drug addiction by reducing the recruitment of new users from the social networks of existing addicts who finance their own drug use by selling drugs to others. Opioid-dependent drug users may share some of the community's treatment goals but give them very different priorities. The prevention of HIV and improvement of health and social well-being, for example, may be given a higher priority by dependent opioid users than reducing drug use and criminal activity.

The focus of this book is unavoidably on the impact of methadone maintenance on illicit drug use and criminal acts. Since the reduction of these activities was the main aim of methadone treatment, and the major reason why it continues to be publicly supported, these outcomes have been most consistently assessed in studies of methadone maintenance treatment. The important role of methadone maintenance treatment in the containment of HIV transmission, which has been much less extensively investigated, will also be discussed. The focus on the goals of reducing injecting drug use and criminal activity does not mean that the patients' perspective on treatment should be ignored. Indeed, as we argue throughout the book, methadone maintenance should become more patient-centred. If this is to happen, future research on methadone maintenance will need to evaluate not only its effectiveness in reducing opioid drug use and involvement in criminal acts but also the extent to which it improves patients' personal health and social well-being. The recent development of multidimensional assessment instruments such as the Opiate Treatment Index (Darke *et al.*, 1992) should make this task easier to achieve.

HOW THIS BOOK CAME ABOUT

In 1990 the National Drug and Alcohol Research Centre was approached by the New South Wales (NSW) Drug and Alcohol Directorate to undertake a review of the research literature on methadone maintenance. The results of this review were to be used to revise methadone maintenance treatment guidelines. Nine key areas were identified:

- the effectiveness of methadone maintenance;
- methadone maintenance and HIV/AIDS;
- the duration of methadone maintenance;
- methadone dosage;
- assessment for methadone maintenance;
- the role of urinalysis;
- the role of counselling;
- methadone maintenance during pregnancy; and
- withdrawal regimens at the conclusion of treatment.

Jeff Ward worked full-time for over a year reviewing the research literature. The method used to review the literature was a modification of the procedure used in the quality assurance project (Mattick & Hall, 1993) which in turn was based upon a similar project in psychiatry (Andrews *et al.*, 1982). The review process for each of the nine topics went through three stages. First, the relevant literature was identified from a variety of sources: commercial computer data bases (Psychlit, Medline); a bibliography compiled by the library of the Australian Council on Alcohol and Other Drug Associations; bibliographies in papers collected from the literature; and in a few cases from papers provided by people working in the field. The literature so retrieved was critically read and a review drafted for each of the nine topic areas.

Secondly, the draft reviews were forwarded to an Australia-wide panel of commentators who had been selected for their clinical expertise in methadone maintenance treatment. These commentators not only represented a range of views on the practice and philosophy of methadone maintenance treatment, but many of them also had an active research interest in the field. They were asked to comment on three things: any important studies that were not included in the review; any errors in the interpretation of the research literature; and the extent to which the findings of the reviews conformed with their clinical experience. Thirdly, the draft reviews were revised to take account of the comments of the clinical experts although no attempt was made to arrive at a consensus of expert opinion in the process of revision.

The publication of *Key Issues in Methadone Maintenance Treatment* in 1992 generated much more interest than we had expected for a book that was written primarily to serve a local purpose, informing policy on the provision of methadone maintenance treatment in New South Wales. It was well received by researchers and practitioners, and widely read in Australia. It also sold well in Europe and generated considerable interest in the United States. Much to our surprise, the book sold out of its first edition.

In 1995 the NSW Drug and Alcohol Directorate approached NDARC to update the book. In the light of reflections upon the first edition, and the comments of colleagues and readers, we decided to broaden the second edition in a number of ways. First, we included the research literature on newer forms of opioid maintenance as alternatives to methadone. Second, we decided to better bridge the gap between a review of research literature and a guide to clinical practice in opioid replacement therapy by inviting contributions from practitioners and policy makers in the field. This decision prompted us to produce an edited collection of chapters rather than a book under our joint authorship, as was the case with the first edition. We hope that these choices will make the book more relevant to the field while retaining the comprehensive coverage of issues and a focus on evidence-based practice that was a feature of *Key Issues in Methadone Maintenance Treatment.*

OUR APPROACH

This book provides a perspective on key issues in opioid replacement therapy which is research-based where possible. The key issues that were addressed in the first edition were the following:

- Is methadone maintenance treatment effective in reducing drug use, criminality and rates of HIV transmission?
- If so, what is the best way to deliver the treatment?
- What sorts of persons are most appropriate for methadone maintenance treatment?
- How should patients' suitability for methadone maintenance be assessed?
- What dose range of opioids should be used?
- How long should treatment last?
- What role should urinalysis play in methadone maintenance programs?
- If so, how should the results of urinalyses be used?
- How should programs respond to continued drug use?
- What role should counselling play?
- How should special groups of patients, such as pregnant women, HIV positive people, and people with psychiatric comorbidity, be managed within methadone maintenance programs?

The following additional issues are discussed in the second edition:

- How effective are alternative opioid drugs in reducing heroin use and crime and improving the health and well-being of opioid-dependent people?
- What patient factors may moderate the effectiveness of methadone maintenance treatment?
- How cost-effective is methadone maintenance treatment compared to other forms of treatment for opioid dependence?
- What are the issues involved in delivering effective methadone maintenance treatment?
- How should staff be trained in delivering methadone maintenance treatment?

- How should methadone maintenance treatment be provided in prison?

A research perspective has been adopted throughout the book in that our conclusions are based on the best available research evidence. As with any therapeutic approach, there are issues which have not been adequately researched. When there is little or no research evidence, we have relied upon the plausibility and logic of the practitioners' views as expressed in the professional literature. What is meant by the 'best available research evidence' is outlined in Chapter 2.

ETHICAL ASPECTS OF OPIOID REPLACEMENT THERAPY

Not all the controversies surrounding opioid replacement therapy can be empirically resolved. There are critics, for example, who have strong moral reservations about opioid maintenance programs. The underlying basis for these moral reservations, and the bearing of research evidence and clinical opinion on them, needs to be briefly discussed because there remain many people in the general community and in the drug treatment community who are opposed on moral grounds to opioid replacement therapy.

We accept Hume's (1739/1888) argument that statements about what one ought to do cannot be inferred from statements about what is the case. Nonetheless we believe that empirical evidence has a bearing upon the evaluation of moral principles, as do many modern ethicists (e.g., Rachels, 1986). This is clearest in the case of the utilitarian moral justification offered for opioid replacement therapy by its proponents that its benefits to both the patients and the community outweigh its costs. They accordingly have an obligation to demonstrate that it achieves its aims of reducing injecting heroin use and crime, while improving the health and well-being of a substantial proportion of its patients, and without incurring greater social harms. Some opponents of opioid replacement therapy argue that it fails to achieve these goals in that substantial numbers of patients continue to inject illicit drugs and engage in criminal activity. Research evidence on the impact of opioid replacement therapy on illicit opioid use, crime and health status is clearly relevant to an evaluation of these competing claims.

A utilitarian appraisal of costs and benefits does not address all the moral objections to opioid replacement therapy. Some of its opponents, for example, argue that opioid replacement therapy is unacceptable because it simply "replaces one drug of dependence with another". These critics often insist that all opioid addicts should become abstinent from all opioid drugs, including methadone. Empirical evidence is relevant to the evaluation of this moral objection to opioid replacement therapy for the reason outlined by Kant in the late eighteenth century – namely, showing that a moral obligation is empirically impossible, or at least extremely difficult to meet, provides a good reason for modifying it. An appraisal of this moral objection to opioid replacement therapy is made difficult by the fact that the reasons why such critics find drug substitution so morally objectionable are rarely spelt out. Its appraisal requires a brief consideration of the possible underlying reasons for this moral objection.

The opposition to opioid replacement therapy is rarely based upon an objection in principle to the therapeutic use of opioid drugs (although one of the side-effects of the hostility to opioid drugs has been an aversion to their legitimate medical use on the part of both doctors and patients). If the objection to opioid replacement therapy was simply one consequence of a general opposition to the medical use of opioid drugs, then the use of opioid drugs to produce analgesia for childbirth and post-operative pain would also be morally objectionable.

If opioid replacement therapy is objectionable because long-term opioid use may maintain opioid dependence then similar objections would have to be made to the use of opioid drugs for analgesia in palliative care, and the management of chronic intractable pain of non-malignant origin. In cases of life-threatening illnesses and chronic painful conditions, patients may be maintained for months, sometimes years, on substantial daily doses of opioid drugs, with many of them developing the signs and symptoms of opioid dependence.

If the long-term medical use of opioid drugs is condoned, it is difficult to understand the basis for the moral objection to opioid replacement therapy. Is it because heroin addicts were not "ill" when they began to use opioid drugs for their intoxicating effects? Is it because they are in some sense "responsible" for becoming dependent upon non-medically prescribed opioid drugs? An exclusive focus on the original reasons why people become dependent, such as the pursuit of intoxication, ignores the real distress and adverse effects of opioid dependence on the user's health. It is also a moral appraisal that is rarely applied consistently. Our community, for example, provides expensive medical treatment to deal with the consequences of behaviour that was in some limited sense "voluntarily" entered into. These consequences include conditions as varied as: alcoholic liver disease, AIDS, lung cancer, heart disease, obesity, and sexually transmitted diseases. If treatment for these conditions is regarded as morally acceptable while opioid replacement therapy is not, the suspicion is that the objection to this form of therapy is based upon the prejudice that opioid drug users are "undeserving" of treatment.

Whatever the underlying rationale for the objection to opioid replacement therapy, research evidence is relevant to an evaluation of the moral claim that abstinence is the only acceptable treatment goal for opioid-dependent people. An insistence on abstinence from all opioids presupposes that abstinence is relatively easily achieved and sustained by those who have become dependent upon opioids. This assumption is contradicted by evidence on the results of opioid detoxification and drug-free treatment, and by the findings of the small number of studies of the careers of opioid-dependent persons (Gerstein & Harwood, 1990, chapter 4; Goldstein & Herrera, 1995; Hser *et al.*, 1993; Stimson & Oppenheimer, 1982; Thorley, 1980; Vaillant, 1973, 1988), all of which show that opioid dependence can become a chronic, relapsing condition with a high rate of premature mortality.

The evidence indicates that the majority of opioid addicts relapse to heroin use shortly after detoxification. Drug-free treatments attract fewer patients than methadone maintenance, have lower rates of retention in treatment, and lower rates of successful graduation to a sustained drug-free lifestyle, although they do reduce the frequency of injecting drug use and benefit their patients in other ways (Gerstein & Harwood, 1990).

The evidence on the heroin using careers of opioid-dependent persons shows that the proportion of people who become and remain abstinent is of the order of 10% within the first year after treatment, and that about 2% per annum achieve abstinence thereafter (Goldstein & Herrera, 1995; Hser *et al.*, 1993; Joe & Simpson, 1990; Vaillant, 1973). The small literature on the longer-term outcomes of methadone maintenance treatment, also indicates that over 5 years and longer the proportion of opioid-dependent persons who achieve enduring abstinence from all opioids (including methadone) does not differ between those receiving drug-free treatment and methadone maintenance treatment (Maddux & Desmond, 1992).

While people remain opioid dependent, their annual chances of becoming abstinent are not much higher than their risk of dying prematurely. Dependent heroin users have a substantially increased risk of premature death from various causes. These include: drug overdoses, violence, infectious diseases spread by sharing contaminated injecting equipment, and alcohol-related causes in a substantial minority of heroin users with concurrent alcohol problems (Goldstein & Herrera, 1995; Hser *et al.,* 1993; Joe & Simpson, 1990; Vaillant, 1973). Mortality studies among cohorts of treated heroin users before the advent of HIV/AIDS indicated that they were 13 times more likely to die prematurely than their age peers (English *et al.,* 1995). More recently, HIV/AIDS has been added to the causes of premature deaths among heroin users in the USA (Des Jarlais *et al.,* 1989) and Europe; emerging evidence suggests that this will become a more important cause of premature death among heroin users in Australia in the future, as will liver disease caused by infection with the prevalent hepatitis C virus (Crofts *et al.,* 1993).

The difficulty that many dependent opioid users experience in achieving abstinence does not exclude abstinence as a treatment goal for opioid-dependent people. Drug-free treatments which aim to achieve abstinence clearly have a place in the treatment response for those opioid-dependent people who want to become abstinent. Some opioid-dependent people also choose to enter drug-free treatment programs after a trial of methadone maintenance treatment. But it is clear from the high failure rate of abstinence-oriented programs and the mortality risks of chronic opioid dependence that there is no compelling moral reason for insisting that abstinence is the only acceptable treatment goal for everyone who is opioid dependent.

For all these reasons we believe that there is a strong utilitarian ethical justification for communities to provide opioid replacement therapy to opioid-dependent people. In the light of some misunderstandings of our view, it is necessary to say that a utilitarian rationale for opioid replacement therapy should not ignore the rights and interests of patients who participate in opioid replacement therapy programs. Opioid replacement therapy and other forms of treatment for dependent heroin users ought to be provided first and foremost for the benefit of those who seek them. But they will also benefit the rest of the community, which provides the utilitarian justification that is an important part of the case for public provision of opioid replacement therapy in these self-interested times. Opioid dependence should not disqualify persons from citizenship, nor is it a reason for their enjoying less than full civil rights. Opioid replacement therapy patients accordingly should enjoy the same rights as any other patients, including an opportunity to comment on the way that treatment is provided, and access to the same procedures as other patients for resolving grievances or addressing complaints about the way that their treatment is provided. Anything less than this risks making opioid replacement therapy the coercive form of social control that some critics accuse it of being.

THE PLAN OF THE BOOK

Section I of this book evaluates the safety and effectiveness of opioid replacement therapy as a treatment for opioid dependence. Given the preponderance of research on methadone maintenance treatment, this largely deals with research on the safety and effectiveness of methadone. Chapter 2 addresses the fundamental question: Do opioid-dependent people have a reasonable chance of benefiting from methadone maintenance treatment in that their heroin use and criminal activity will decrease? If the answer to this question is "no" then there is little point in considering how methadone maintenance is best provided. Chapter 2 reviews the results of the small number of randomised controlled trials and the best available observational research evidence on the effectiveness of methadone maintenance treatment.

Chapter 3 deals with the research literature which has evaluated the impact of methadone maintenance treatment on the transmission of HIV/AIDS among injecting drug users. With the advent of HIV in the early 1980s and the rapid increase in its prevalence among injecting drug users in Europe and parts of North America, its containment has become a relevant outcome on which to assess the effectiveness of methadone maintenance treatment. In Chapter 4 Shane Darke discusses patient characteristics that affect the outcome of methadone maintenance treatment. In chapter 5, Patricia Ward and Matthew Sutton review the available evidence on the cost-effectiveness of methadone maintenance treatment and address the question: does methadone maintenance treatment provide value for money as a form of treatment for opioid dependence? Chapter 6 reviews research evidence on the safety and effectiveness of alternative opioid maintenance agents, such as, buprenorphine, LAAM, naltrexone and injectable heroin and methadone.

Section II reviews evidence on the contribution that various components of methadone maintenance treatment make to its impact on illicit opioid use and crime. In Chapter 7, James Bell provides an overview of the issues involved in delivering effective methadone maintenance treatment. Chapter 8 reviews the research evidence on the assessment of patients for methadone maintenance treatment while Chapter 9 reviews the pharmacology of methadone, and the relationship between methadone dose, retention in treatment, and heroin use. Chapter 10 deals with the contentious issue of monitoring illicit opioid and other drug use in treatment. This includes the role that urinalysis should play in monitoring patients' drug use, and what might constitute an appropriate response to patients who continue to use illicit drugs. Chapter 11 considers the evidence on the role of counselling in methadone maintenance treatment. Chapter 12 considers the contentious but under-researched issue of the optimal duration of treatment. It reveals the fundamental division between two influential opposing philosophies of methadone maintenance treatment: the model of potentially indefinite maintenance on methadone originally espoused by Dole and Nyswander, and the more recent model of methadone as a step towards achieving abstinence from all opioid drugs, within a limited period of approximately two years. Chapter 13 deals with the question of how best to withdraw a patient from methadone when they have succeeded in stabilising their lives after some years of maintenance treatment, or when they decide to leave the program against staff advice.

Section III deals with a number of special issues. In Chapter 14, James Bell discusses how best to train staff in the delivery of effective methadone maintenance treatment. In Chapter 15 Kate Dolan and Alex Wodak discuss the special issues raised by the provision of methadone in the prison setting where many heroin users spend some part of their drug use careers. Chapter 16 reviews the research and clinical evidence on the role of methadone maintenance in managing the pregnancies of opioid-dependent women. In Chapter 17, the special issues raised by the high prevalence of psychiatric comorbidity among methadone patients are discussed. In the concluding chapter, we make some conjectures about the future of opioid replacement therapy and briefly discuss some of the high priority issues for research in this area.

REFERENCES

Andrews, G., Armstrong, M., Brodaty, H., Hall, W., Harvey, R., Tennant, C., & Weekes, P. (1982). A methodology for preparing 'ideal' treatment outlines in psychiatry. *Australian and New Zealand Journal of Psychiatry,* **16,** 153-158.

Bammer, G. (1995). *Report and recommendations of stage 2 feasibility research into the controlled availability of opioids.* Canberra, Australia: National Centre for Epidemiology and Population Health and Australian Institute of Criminology.

Bell, J., Batey, R.G., Farrell, G.C., Crewe, E.B., Cunningham, A.L., & Byth, K. (1990). Hepatitis C virus in intravenous drug users. *Medical Journal of Australia,* **153,** 274-276.

Chaiken, J.M., & Chaiken, M.R. (1990). Drugs and predatory crime. In M. Tonry and J.Q. Wilson (Eds.). *Drugs and crime: A review of research.* Chicago: University of Chicago Press.

Crofts, N., Hopper, J.L., Bowden, D.S., Beschkin, A.M., Milner, R., & Locarnini, S.A. (1993). Hepatitis C virus infection among a cohort of Victorian injecting drug users. *Medical Journal of Australia,* **159,** 237-241.

Darke, S., Hall, W., Heather, N., Ward, J., & Wodak, A. (1992). Development and validation of a multi-dimensional instrument for assessing outcome among opiate users: The Opiate Treatment Index. *British Journal of Addiction,* **87,** 773-742.

Des Jarlais, D.C., Friedman, S.R., Novick, D.M., Sotheran, J.L., Thomas, P., Yancovitz, S.R., Mildvan, D., Weber, J., Kreek, M.J., Maslansky, R., Bartelme, S., Spira, T., & Marmor, M. (1989). HIV-1 infection among intravenous drug users in Manhattan, New York City, from 1977 through 1987. *Journal of the American Medical Association,* **261,** 1008–1012.

Dole, V.P., & Nyswander, M. (1965). A medical treatment for diacetylmorphine (heroin) addiction. *Journal of the American Medical Association,* **193,** 80-84.

Dole, V.P., & Nyswander, M.E. (1967). Heroin addiction – a metabolic disease. *Archives of Internal Medicine,* **120,** 19-24.

English, D., Holman, C.D.J., Milne, E., Winter, M.G., Hulse, G.K., Codde, J.P., Corti, B., Dawes, V., de Klerk, N., Knuiman, M.W., Kurinczuk, J.J., Lewin, G.F., & Ryan, G.A. (1995). *The quantification of drug caused morbidity and mortality in Australia – 1995 edition.* Canberra, Australia: Commonwealth Department of Human Services and Health.

Gerstein, D.R., & Harwood, H.J. (1990). *Treating drug problems. Volume 1: A study of effectiveness and financing of public and private drug treatment systems.* Washington, D.C: National Academy Press.

Goldstein, A., & Herrera, J. (1995). Heroin addicts and methadone treatment in Alburquerque: A 22-year follow-up. *Drug and Alcohol Dependence, 40,* 139-150.

Hall, W. (1996). *Methadone maintenance treatment as a crime control measure* (Crime and Justice Bulletin, Number 29). Sydney, Australia: New South Wales Bureau of Crime Statistics and Research.

Hser, Y.I, Anglin, D., & Powers, K. (1993). A 24-year follow-up of California narcotics addicts. *Archives of General Psychiatry, 50,* 577-584.

Hume, D. (1888). *A treatise on human nature.* (L.A. Selby-Bigge, Ed.). Oxford, England: Oxford University Press. (Original work published 1739).

Joe, G.W., & Simpson, D.D. (1990). Death rates and risk factors. In D.D. Simpson, & S.B. Sells (Eds.). *Opioid addiction and treatment: A 12-year follow-up* (pp. 193-202). Malabar, FL: Robert E Krieger.

Johnson, B.D., Goldstein, P.J., Preble, E., Schmeidler, J., Lipton, D.S., Spunt, B., & Miller, T. (1985). *Taking care of business: The economics of crime by heroin users.* Lexington, MA: Lexington Books.

Maddux, J.F., & Desmond, D.P. (1992). Methadone maintenance and recovery from opioid dependence. *American Journal of Drug and Alcohol Abuse, 18,* 63-74.

Mattick, R.P., and Hall, W. (Eds.) (1993). *A treatment outline for approaches to opioid dependence: Quality assurance project* (National Drug Strategy Monograph No. 21). Canberra, Australia: Australian Government Publishing Service.

Rachels, J. (1986). *The elements of moral philosophy.* Philadelphia: Temple University Press.

Rihs, M. (1994). *The prescription of narcotics under medical supervision and research relating to drugs at the Federal Office of Public Health.* Bern, Switzerland: The Swiss Federal Office of Public Health.

Stimson, G.V., & Oppenheimer, E. (1982). *Heroin addiction: Treatment and control in Britain.* London: Tavistock.

Thorley, A. (1980). Longitudinal studies of drug dependence. In G. Edwards and C. Rush (Eds.). *Drug problems in Britain: A review of ten years* (pp. 118-169). London: Academic Press.

Vaillant, G. (1973). A 20-year follow-up of New York narcotic addicts. *Archives of General Psychiatry, 29,* 237-241.

Vaillant, G. (1988). What can long-term follow-up teach us about relapse and prevention of relapse in addiction. *British Journal of Addiction, 83,* 1147-1157.

Ward, J., Mattick, R., & Hall, W. (1992). *Key issues in methadone maintenance treatment.* Sydney, Australia: New South Wales University Press.

I OUTCOME

2

THE EFFECTIVENESS OF METHADONE MAINTENANCE TREATMENT 1: HEROIN USE AND CRIME

WAYNE HALL, JEFF WARD AND RICHARD P. MATTICK

ASSESSING TREATMENT EFFECTIVENESS

The gold standard for establishing the effectiveness of any treatment in modern medicine is a *reproducible* demonstration in a *randomised controlled trial* that the treatment produces a superior outcome to a relevant comparison treatment, such as no treatment or minimal treatment. The simplest type of randomised controlled trial is one in which people with a condition or disorder (e.g., opioid dependence) are randomly assigned to receive either the *active* treatment (e.g., methadone maintenance) or a comparison treatment (e.g., drug-free counselling). The evaluation of treatment effectiveness presupposes a comparison condition so that one can discover what would have happened if the patient had received a different treatment or no treatment at all. The aim of randomisation is to ensure that the subjects who are allocated to the treatment and the comparison conditions are equivalent in *the long run,* that is, over a large number of trials subjects who have been randomly assigned to the treatment and comparison condition should not differ in any systematic way. Only when the two groups have been assigned in this way can one be confident that a difference in treatment outcome is more likely to reflect the effects of treatment than any pre-existing characteristics of the subjects who were assigned to the two conditions.

In order to minimise bias in assessment, it is desirable that both the administration of treatment and the assessment of treatment outcome should be conducted in such a way that neither the person receiving the treatment, nor the person assessing its effects, are aware of which treatment the patient has received. When these conditions are met, the trial is said to be "double-blind". When a double-blind trial is not possible, as it may not be, the next most desirable practice is a "single-blind" trial in which the assessment of treatment outcome is conducted by an assessor who is unaware of which treatment the subject has received.

The measurement of treatment outcome should use instruments of demonstrated validity. In assessing the effectiveness of methadone maintenance treatment, this requires valid measures of opioid and other drug use, as well as other outcomes that methadone maintenance treatment may affect, such as, criminal activity, social adjustment, health status, and HIV risk behaviour. Drug use may be assessed by urinalysis to detect drug metabolites in urine. The broader range of outcomes can be assessed by multidimensional outcome instruments, such as the Addiction Severity Index (McLellan *et al.,* 1985) and the Opiate Treatment Index (Darke *et al.,* 1991), both of which have shown to provide valid assessments of the status of methadone maintenance patients.

Because the outcomes in the treatment and control groups can differ by chance evidence is required that chance is an unlikely explanation of any outcome differences. Such evidence may be provided when a statistical test indicates that any observed difference would have been unlikely to arise if there was no such difference in outcome in the population from which the treatment and control groups were sampled. The phrase "unlikely to arise by chance" is usually taken to mean that the event occurs less than once in twenty trials. Increasingly in the biomedical sciences, confidence intervals are preferred to statistical significance tests as the method of excluding chance (Gardner & Altman, 1989). Typically a 95% confidence interval is constructed around the difference in outcome between treatment and control conditions observed in the study. The upper limit of the confidence interval indicates the largest difference in the population which is consistent with the sample difference while its lower limit indicates the smallest value of the difference in the population that is consistent with the sample result. If the confidence interval does not include zero, then one infers with 95% confidence that there is a difference between the treatment and comparison conditions.

Confidence intervals have come to be preferred to significance tests for two main reasons. First, the width of the confidence interval indicates the degree of uncertainty surrounding the sample estimate of the difference in outcome. In general, the wider the confidence interval around the sample estimate, the greater the uncertainty about the size of the difference in outcome. Second, the upper limit of the confidence interval indicates the largest size of a difference in outcome that may have gone undetected in the sample (Gardner & Altman, 1989). If this value is substantial it would be unwise to conclude that the failure to observe a difference in the sample meant that there was no difference in outcome in the population.

The demonstration in a single study that a treatment produces a better outcome than a control condition is rarely decisive in evaluating therapeutic effectiveness. It is the ability to reliably reproduce or replicate such findings that establishes therapeutic effectiveness (Fisher, 1949). The successful *replication* of positive results is important because it reduces the likelihood that statistical errors have been made in comparing the outcomes of the treatments. When we use the conventional "significance level" of $p < 0.05$, we expect to mistakenly conclude that treatment is superior to the comparison condition in 5% of tests. The more reliably a result is reproduced in a series of separate studies, the greater our confidence in it, because the chance of making errors in all of the tests decreases dramatically as the number of replications increases. So, for example, if we always use a significance level of 5% (or conversely construct a 95% confidence interval) then the chances of finding a difference in five studies is $(0.05)^5 = 0.00000003125$.

False positive (or type I) errors are not the only type of decision errors that can be made. We can also incorrectly conclude that a treatment does not differ from its comparison condition in its effects on outcome. This type of error is a false negative error or type II error. The percentage of occasions in which a type II error is made depends upon the size of the difference we are trying to detect and the sample size we use in our attempts to detect it. In the past, a failure to use a large enough sample size has been a common reason for randomised controlled trials failing to detect differences in effectiveness between different treatments (Freiman *et al.,* 1978). As a consequence, it is now a standard requirement that controlled evaluations of medical treatments use sample sizes that have been determined by statistical power analyses (Cohen, 1992). Such analyses use the previous literature and informed opinion about the likely size of treatment effects to ensure that the study has a sufficiently large sample size to provide an adequate chance (e.g., greater than 90%) of detecting a difference in treatment outcome, if one exists.

The design characteristics listed (random assignment, double or single blind assessment, the use of valid assessment instruments, and the use of statistical methods of trial design and analysis) are all desirable for valid assessment of treatment outcome. However, they cannot be met for many forms of medical treatment which were introduced before the randomised controlled trial became a routine part of treatment evaluation (Cochrane, 1972). The modern randomised controlled trial was introduced into medicine after World War Two (e.g., Hill *et al.,* 1951) and did not become a standard part of treatment evaluation until much more recently. In its absence, evaluations of treatment effectiveness have depended upon the coherence and consistency of evidence from observational studies, in much the same way that knowledge about the causes of diseases and disorders has been derived (Hill, 1965). These principles will be used to answer the question: Does the average opioid-dependent person who enrols in methadone maintenance treatment have a reasonable chance of benefiting from the encounter in terms of reducing their illicit opioid use, reducing their involvement in criminal activity, and improving their health and well-being?

RANDOMISED CONTROLLED TRIALS
OF METHADONE MAINTENANCE

Only a small number of randomised controlled trials have compared the effectiveness of methadone maintenance with an appropriate control condition in reducing illicit opioid use. When methadone maintenance was first introduced (Dole & Nyswander, 1965), the randomised controlled trial was not part of the culture of treatment evaluation in the same way that it is today. Consequently, the opportunity to randomly assign opioid-dependent patients to methadone and minimal treatment was only rarely used before methadone maintenance became a widely available form of treatment. By the time that methadone maintenance had become an important part of the publicly-funded treatment system for opioid dependence in the early 1970s, it was difficult to deny the treatment to people who might have benefited from it. Although it was still ethically acceptable to randomly assign opioid addicts to methadone and other competing forms of treatment, in practice it became difficult in countries that provided methadone maintenance to do so for other than short periods of time. Patients who were randomly assigned to treatments of which they did not approve, could obtain their preferred treatment elsewhere (e.g., Bale *et al.*, 1980; Bell *et al.*, 1992).

Only three randomised controlled trials have been performed in which comprehensive methadone maintenance has been compared with a control condition over a substantial period of time (Dole *et al.*, 1969; Newman & Whitehill, 1979; Gunne & Grönbladh, 1981). All three studies were undertaken in a context in which methadone maintenance program places were strictly rationed – a fact that made it ethically acceptable to randomly assign patients to either methadone or a control condition. More recently, three randomised controlled trials have compared some form of methadone maintenance with an alternative treatment over short periods of time (30, 45 and 105 days). These trials will also be reviewed. Randomised controlled trials have also compared variations of methadone maintenance treatment with one another (e.g., high and low dose methadone maintenance), or methadone maintenance with other forms of opioid maintenance using other synthetic opioids such as LAAM. However, these studies do not bear as directly on the effectiveness of methadone as do the studies that have been included in this chapter. They are reviewed where relevant in subsequent chapters (for example, on methadone dose, and on alternative opioid maintenance agents).

Dole and Colleagues (1969)

Dole and colleagues conducted the first randomised controlled trial of methadone maintenance in New York using imprisoned, recidivist opioid addicts who had at least a four-year history of opioid use. Thirty-four men who became eligible for release over a four-month period were invited to participate in the trial, and 32 agreed to participate. Sixteen were randomly assigned to methadone maintenance of whom twelve entered treatment which commenced before they left prison and continued after their release. The other 16 addicts were randomly assigned to a no treatment waiting list.

Both groups were followed up 12 months after release from prison, and only one subject in each group was lost to follow-up. There were dramatic differences in favour of methadone maintenance when outcome was assessed by rates of imprisonment and return to daily heroin use. Six of the 12 men who entered methadone maintenance were employed or in school, and only three had been gaoled, whereas all 16 in the control condition had returned to gaol. Similarly, while all 16 men in the control condition had returned to daily heroin use, none of the men in methadone maintenance had done so, even though 10 out of 12 had used heroin since their release, and three continued to use intermittently.

Even a conservative analysis on the basis of "intention to treat" favoured methadone maintenance. That is, the outcomes of those in methadone maintenance remained superior to those in the control condition even when all 16 men who were originally assigned to methadone maintenance were included (rather than the 12 who entered treatment), and all subjects who were lost to follow-up were counted as treatment failures. The outcomes from an analysis by intention to treat are shown in Table 2.1 expressed in terms of relative risk ratios with their accompanying 95% confidence intervals. These express the relative risk of the control and methadone maintenance conditions returning to daily heroin use or being imprisoned in the year after treatment.

Table 2.1 shows that the risk of being imprisoned was 2.67 times higher, while the risk of returning to daily heroin use was 4 times higher, among those in the control condition than those in methadone maintenance treatment. The number of cases in each group are small which makes the estimates of the relative risk uncertain, as is reflected in the width of their 95% confidence intervals. In the case of daily heroin use, for example, the confidence interval ranges between a lower limit of 1.43 and an upper limit of 5.02. Contrary to popular prejudice, the fact that such differences are statistically significant with such small samples makes the size of the differences in favour of methadone all the more impressive.

Table 2.1

The one-year outcome of the Dole *et al.*, (1969) randomised controlled trial from an analysis by "intention to treat"

	Reincarcerated		Daily heroin use	
	yes	no	yes	no
Methadone	6	10	4	12
Control	16	0	16	0
RR*	2.67		4.00	
95% CI	1.43	5.02	1.72	9.35

*Relative risk of control versus methadone

Newman and Whitehill (1979)

Newman and Whitehill conducted a randomised controlled trial of methadone versus placebo maintenance among heroin addicts in Hong Kong. The trial was made possible by the late introduction of methadone maintenance treatment to the colony, which meant that people who were randomly assigned to the control condition were unable to obtain it elsewhere. The patients included in the trial were the first 100 male addicts who met the same criteria that had been used in the Dole *et al.*, (1969) study, namely, that they had at least a four-year history of opioid addiction, at least one failed attempt at rehabilitation by other means, and evidence on urinalysis of daily opioid use.

All who consented to participate in the trial were first admitted to the treatment unit for two weeks and stabilised on 60 mg of methadone. They were then randomly assigned to be placed on methadone maintenance or placebo maintenance after discharge. Both groups were offered extensive follow-up counselling and treatment. The methadone group received a high dose of methadone determined by the patient (average 97 mg per day) while those in the placebo condition were withdrawn from methadone under double-blind conditions. In the methadone condition, patients who continued to use heroin as monitored by urinalysis (more than six positive urines), and those who failed to comply with the requirement for daily dosing (by missing six consecutive doses) were discharged from the program.

Both groups were followed for three years and outcome was assessed in terms of the numbers retained in treatment. The differences in treatment retention were dramatic (Table 2.2). By the end of 32 weeks five of the 50 placebo controls and 38 of the 50 methadone treated group were still in treatment. By the end of three years the numbers still in treatment were one and 28 respectively (RR = 28.0, 95% CI: 3.96, 197.95). The reasons for discontinuing treatment also favoured the methadone group: 31 of the 49 patients from the placebo group were discharged for continued heroin use, compared with only eight of the 22 patients in the methadone group. There were three deaths in the study, all in the methadone group. In only one case was there any suspicion of an overdose. The other two deaths were from causes not related to continued heroin use (although both deaths were probably attributable in part to the adverse health effects of opioid use prior to entry to methadone maintenance).

Table 2.2
Results of Newman and Whitehill (1979) randomised controlled trial at three year follow up.

	Retained		Discharged for heroin use	
	yes	no	yes	no
Methadone	28	22	8	14
Control	1	49	31	18
RR*	28.00		0.58	
95% CI	3.96	198.00	0.32	1.04

*Relative risk of methadone versus control

Gunne and Grönbladh (1981)

These authors conducted a randomised controlled trial of the Swedish methadone maintenance program that was closely modelled on the original Dole and Nyswander (1965) approach. As with the Newman and Whitehill (1979) study, it was possible to undertake a randomised controlled trial because methadone maintenance treatment was only introduced into Sweden in the early 1970s, and the number of places in the program was strictly rationed because of political opposition to methadone maintenance as a form of treatment (Grönbladh & Gunne, 1989).

The criteria used to select persons who were eligible for inclusion in the study were substantially the same as those of Dole *et al.,* (1969), and Newman and Whitehill (1979), namely, at least a four-year history of opioid addiction, a previous failed attempt at rehabilitation, and evidence from urinalysis of daily opioid use. Those who were under the age of 20 were excluded, as were those who used other drugs, or who were facing criminal charges. The methadone maintenance program in this case involved substantial vocational rehabilitation during an inpatient admission of up to six months. All subjects who were assigned to the control condition refused drug-free treatment. The two conditions under comparison, then, were methadone maintenance in an inpatient setting with intensive vocational rehabilitation and referral to drug-free treatment which in fact meant no treatment because so few took up the referral.

This study used a sequential design. Instead of assigning a predetermined number of subjects to methadone or a control condition, the trial continued until a statistically significant difference emerged in favour of either condition. This occurred after 36 subjects had been recruited, 17 of whom were assigned to methadone, and 19 to the comparison treatment (with two subsequently being excluded because they enrolled in methadone elsewhere).

The outcomes were assessed at the end of two years when those who were initially assigned to the control condition became eligible for entry to methadone. Twelve of the 17 in the treatment condition were no longer regularly using opiates or other drugs, and were either employed (10) or undertaking further education (2). The remaining five treatment subjects continued to abuse opioids or hypnotics, and had been discharged from the program. Only one of the 17 subjects in the control condition had ceased drug abuse; 12 continued to abuse opioid drugs; two had died and two were in prison (RR = 3.2, 95% CI: 1.5, 6.75). The results reported by Gunne and Grönbladh among the treatment patients in their study were confirmed among 174 patients who were subsequently admitted to the methadone maintenance program over a 20-year period (Grönbladh & Gunne, 1989).

Vanichseni and Colleagues (1991)

Vanichseni *et al.*, conducted a randomised controlled trial comparing 45-day methadone detoxification with 45 days of methadone maintenance. The subjects of the trial were 240 heroin injectors in Bangkok, Thailand who applied for detoxification and who had at least six prior detoxifications. They were randomly assigned to methadone assisted withdrawal over 45 days (the standard detoxification regime in Thailand), or to methadone maintenance for the equivalent period (average dose 74 mg per day). Outcome was measured by the rate of continued illicit heroin use, as assessed by morphine positive urines during twice-weekly urinalysis, and by retention in treatment. There was no further description of the treatment program.

There were major differences between the withdrawal and maintenance groups on both outcome measures. The drop-out rates by the end of the 45-day period were 66% and 24% respectively (RR = 2.76 95% CI: 1.96, 3.88), with the withdrawal group dropping out of treatment earlier than the maintenance group. The percentages of morphine positive urines were 53% and 28% in the withdrawal and maintenance groups respectively (RR = 1.88, 95% CI: 1.44, 2.46). That is, the relative risk odds of dropping out of treatment was 2.76 times and that of providing a morphine positive urine was 1.88 times higher for those on the withdrawal program than among those on the maintenance regime.

The practical significance of these findings is uncertain. It is reassuring that Thai heroin addicts who enter methadone maintenance are more likely to remain in treatment, and less likely to continue to inject heroin while in treatment, than are those who are placed on the standard withdrawal regime. But this does not provide a rigorous test of the effectiveness of methadone maintenance in retaining patients in treatment and minimising their injection of heroin in the longer term measured in years rather than days.

Yancovitz and Colleagues (1991)

Yancovitz and colleagues reported a randomised controlled trial of "interim" methadone compared with limited contact while opioid dependent patients were on a waiting list to enter a comprehensive methadone maintenance treatment program in New York. "Interim" methadone involved the "provision of limited services to patients awaiting treatment positions in comprehensive methadone programs". It consisted of an initial medical examination, education about AIDS, and the daily receipt of oral methadone medication "to prevent narcotic withdrawal symptoms and to block the euphoric effects of heroin" (p. 1185). No vocational or other social rehabilitation or counselling was provided.

The subjects for the study were 301 heroin addicts recruited from the waiting lists of 23 methadone maintenance treatment programs in New York. Initially, patients were randomly assigned to one of three conditions: interim methadone; waiting list with frequent contact and urinalysis; and waiting list without contact. Once a treatment place became available they entered comprehensive treatment and left the study. Recruitment into the trial slowed dramatically when potential participants realised that they only had a one in three chance of receiving methadone. The protocol was subsequently simplified to a two-group design with interim methadone and frequent contact, and the duration of both conditions was limited to one month, after which all entered comprehensive methadone maintenance treatment.

Urinalyses showed that the proportion of patients in interim methadone who had used heroin declined from 63% to 29% while the proportion remained stationary in the frequent contact control group (62% and 60%) (RR = 1.88, 95% CI: 1.44, 2.46). There was no change in cocaine use in either group. The difference in favour of interim methadone persisted when the results of the patients with incomplete data were examined (by using the urinalysis result closest to the conclusion of the trial). In this case the proportions of patients with urines positive for morphine were 36% in the interim methadone group and 60% in the frequent contact control group.

Sixteen months after the trial the proportion of patients who had subsequently enrolled in comprehensive methadone maintenance treatment were 72% in the interim methadone condition and 56% in the frequent contact condition (RR = 1.28, 95% CI: 1.08, 1.53). A subsequent study of rates of retention in comprehensive methadone maintenance treatment (Friedmann *et al.*, 1994) found that patients who had first enrolled in interim methadone were as likely to be retained in comprehensive methadone treatment at one year (55%) as patients who had directly admitted to a comprehensive methadone program (61%).

The Yancovitz *et al.*, study illustrates the difficulties of conducting randomised controlled trials of methadone maintenance treatment. The need to entice participants into the trial, and to keep them in the trial, limited its duration and consequently the inferences that could be drawn about the effectiveness of interim methadone treatment. As was the case with the trial of Vanichseni *et al.*, the reduction in heroin use was reassuring but not compelling proof of the effectiveness of interim methadone over longer periods. The increase in the number of persons who subsequently entered comprehensive treatment was perhaps of greater clinical significance.

Strain, Stitzer, Liebson and Bigelow (1993)

Strain and colleagues conducted a double-blind randomised controlled trial comparing the effects on treatment retention and illicit opioid and cocaine use of three doses of methadone (0, 20 and 50 mg per day) over a period of 15 weeks. The methadone doses were selected to represent the range of low and medium doses used in many contemporary American methadone maintenance treatment programs. The patients consisted of 247 opioid-dependent persons, just under half of whom (47%) were also regular cocaine users. On entry they were given 25 mgs of methadone for a week and then randomly assigned to one of the three methadone doses which were achieved over the next 5 weeks. Patients were then maintained on the assigned dose for 15 weeks and given access to all the ancillary services, such as counselling, that are routinely provided in American methadone maintenance programs. The three conditions were compared on retention in treatment, patient compliance with treatment requirements, and the rate of illicit opioid and cocaine use monitored by urinalyses performed three times a week.

Survival analyses showed that the group receiving the 50 mgs of methadone were more likely to remain in treatment than the group receiving the placebo (0 mgs of methadone), although the differences between the 50 mg and the 20 mg groups and between the 20 mg and the 0 mgs groups in rates of survival were of borderline statistical significance. A comparison of the proportions retained at the end of 15 weeks showed a clear dose-response relationship (namely, 52% in the 50 mg group, 42% in the 20 mg group, and 21% in the 0 mg group), as did the number of days spent in treatment (100, 87 and 72 days respectively). The same was true of the proportion reporting one or more morphine positive urines during the follow up period, namely, 56% in the 50 mg group, 68% in the 20 mg group and 74% in the 0 mg group. The 50 mg group also showed a lower rate of cocaine positive urines (53%) than the other two groups which did not differ from each other (62% and 67%).

The findings of this study are broadly supportive of the effectiveness of methadone treatment despite some caveats. The differences in outcome between the groups receiving 0 and 50 mg of methadone support the earlier findings of Dole *et al.,* (1969) even though the fixed dose of 50 mgs was below the level regarded as required for optimal therapeutic response (namely, 60 mg or more a day, see Chapter 9). Although 15 weeks is considerably longer than 30 to 45 days, it is still considerably shorter than the period of years over which Dole and Nyswander argued that methadone maintenance had to be evaluated.

OBSERVATIONAL STUDIES OF TREATMENT EFFECTIVENESS

In the absence of a sufficient number of randomised controlled trials to draw strong inferences about treatment effectiveness, the assessment of the effectiveness of methadone maintenance depends upon the results of observational studies of patient outcome. In such studies the outcomes of treatment are observed among patients who have assigned themselves to different forms of treatment rather than being randomly assigned by a treatment researcher. Observational studies of treatment effectiveness comprise two major types. First, there are comparative studies in which the outcomes are compared in persons who selected themselves into different treatments (e.g., methadone maintenance, therapeutic communities, and drug-free counselling). Secondly, there are pre-post evaluations of treatment in which a group of people entering a single type of treatment are assessed at intake and at some time after treatment, with the effect of treatment being assessed by changes in outcomes such as drug use between pre-treatment and post-treatment.

Controlled Comparative Studies

The major problem with all observational studies is whether the people receiving different forms of treatment were comparable prior to treatment. As a consequence, it is difficult to rule out the possibility that apparent differences in treatment outcome arise because of differences in patient prognosis prior to treatment. The strategy of quasi-experimentation (Cook & Campbell, 1979) provides a way of making cautious inferences about treatment effectiveness from observational studies. This involves three processes. First, plausible rival hypotheses are generated which may explain any differences between treatments in outcome. Of these the most plausible is that the treatments differed in the number of patients who had a good or a poor prognosis regardless of treatment exposure. Secondly, patients are measured on variables that may predict a better or worse outcome, such as prior history of drug use, degree of criminal involvement, and severity of drug dependence. Thirdly, statistical methods (e.g., stratification and covariate adjustment) are used to decide whether these rival hypotheses explain the differences in outcomes between treatments. That is, do the differences in treatment outcome persist when account is taken of pre-existing patient differences? If the differences in outcome persist after statistical adjustment, one can be more confident that there is a treatment effect.

The inclusion of evidence from the quasi-experimental studies in a review of the effectiveness of any form of treatment is unavoidable, even when there is abundant evidence of effectiveness from randomised controlled trials. In order to conclude from the evidence of the randomised controlled trials that the treatment under investigation is effective, a quasi-experimental comparison is required to justify the inference that the people who have been included in the randomised controlled trials are comparable in all relevant respects to the patients who receive such treatments in clinical practice. Moreover, a refusal to accept anything other than the evidence from randomised controlled trials (e.g., McMaster Department of Clinical Epidemiology, 1981) would have the unintended effect of endorsing minimally evaluated treatments for opioid dependence. Given the serious individual and societal consequences of opioid dependence, the community will insist upon offering some form of treatment, and in the absence of evaluation by randomised controlled trials, the proponents of all therapeutic approaches have an equal claim for public support.

Comparative Studies of Methadone Maintenance Treatment

Bale and Colleagues (1980)

Bale and colleagues (1980) planned to conduct a randomised controlled trial in which the outcomes of methadone maintenance and therapeutic communities would be compared with detoxification; however, ethical and practical problems prevented random assignment of subjects to treatment. The result was a study that compared the outcomes of patients who selected methadone maintenance treatment, therapeutic communities and detoxification at 12 months post-treatment.

There were several distinctive features of this study. First, subjects who entered methadone and therapeutic communities were very nearly comparable, as indicated by a comprehensive pre-treatment assessment. The main reasons for this were that subjects were recruited from a common pool of potential patients (opioid-addicted veterans in the Veterans' Administration treatment system), and that staff from each of the treatment programs competed for the patients on conditions of near equality. All program staff had access to the potential subjects while they were in hospital, and subjects were encouraged to spend three weeks in the program to which they were assigned before they changed to the program of their choice.

Secondly, a number of different programs were represented within each treatment modality. There were three therapeutic communities with a variety of orientations, and two low-dose methadone maintenance programs that were compared with detoxification only, which was provided in the main treatment centre from which all subjects for the study were recruited. Thirdly, 93% of patients were followed up at six and 12 months. The results of treatment were therefore available for almost all who entered treatment, regardless of how long they stayed, and not just for the treatment successes. Fourthly, the 12-month outcome was assessed by an independent interviewer who was unaware of which treatment the subject had received, and efforts were made to validate self-reports of drug use and criminal activity.

The major results of relevance to this review are those that compared the outcomes of methadone maintenance with those of simple detoxification. The comparison between methadone maintenance treatment and therapeutic communities – which failed to find any difference between the two in average effectiveness – will not be discussed. The results indicated that the two methadone maintenance programs produced better outcomes than did detoxification when measured by reductions in opioid drug use during the past month, and the number of convictions recorded during the past year. Moreover, the differences in outcome between methadone maintenance and detoxification persisted after adjustment for 10 patient characteristics that had been shown to predict outcome.

A number of issues need to be considered in interpreting this study. First, the methadone maintenance programs provided in this study differed from that recommended by Dole and Nyswander. Both programs prescribed low doses of methadone and encouraged their patients to become abstinent from all opioids, including methadone. Secondly, the combination of a small sample size for methadone and the use of crude dichotomous measures of outcome reduced statistical power, and hence the sensitivity of the study to detect differences in outcome between treatment modalities. Thirdly, those who received detoxification only were entirely self-selected in that they consisted of people who had declined any other form of treatment.

Even allowing for these qualifications, the findings of the Bale *et al.,* study supported the results obtained in the three randomised controlled trials. The methadone maintenance programs produced better outcomes in terms of drug use and criminality than detoxification, and this difference in treatment outcome was not explained by the covariates that Bale *et al.,* measured. In terms of the quasi-experimental strategy outlined above, this study provides qualified support for the conclusion that the differences in outcome between methadone maintenance and detoxification were caused by the difference in treatment.

Anglin and Associates (1981, 1984, 1989)

Anglin and his colleagues conducted a series of studies in California to evaluate the impact of treatment on the behaviour of patients in a number of methadone clinics (Anglin & McGlothlin, 1984). In each study, retrospective data were collected using a time line technique in which the interviewer went over a detailed chart marked with the subject's criminal and treatment history. After establishing the date of first opioid use and the date of first dependence, the interviewer and subject filled in details of opioid use, criminal activity, and other relevant outcome measures up until the time of interview. The authors claim that this technique yielded reasonably accurate, retrospective information (Anglin *et al.,* 1993).

Methadone Versus No Methadone Treatment

The authors originally set out to study a group of opioid-dependent people who were committed for seven years to compulsory inpatient treatment as an alternative to imprisonment during 1962–64 as part of the California Civil Addict Program (CAP) (Anglin & McGlothin,

1984). Of the 439 subjects in this early study, 118 later entered methadone maintenance treatment when it was commenced in California in the early 1970s. By this time nearly all of the subjects in the CAP had finished their first commitment period (Anglin, 1988). Among the subjects who did not enter methadone maintenance treatment, two groups were defined on the basis of their opioid use post-CAP: a group of inactive recovered heroin users who gave up their addiction during CAP treatment; and a group of active users who relapsed to daily heroin use. For the purposes of evaluating the effectiveness of methadone maintenance treatment, the comparison group for the methadone patients was the active heroin-using group.

Using the time line technique developed by the authors, the three groups were compared before and after the commencement of methadone treatment by taking the date of admission for each of the methadone subjects as the commencement of the intervention and using the median admission date for the methadone group as a whole to establish a comparison point for the recovered and active heroin users. Heroin use and crime were compared one year before and one year after the commencement of methadone treatment and functioning in these two areas was recorded for the subsequent three years.

Entry into methadone maintenance brought about a marked reduction in daily heroin use which endured throughout the 3-year follow-up period (Anglin & McGlothlin, 1984). While daily heroin use was reduced from just over 60% in the year before treatment to around 10% during the year after treatment in the methadone group, 80% of the active heroin users continued daily use during this period. While a reduction was observed over the subsequent three years in this group of active users, the proportion of daily users only fell to just below 60%, whereas only 10% of the methadone treatment entrants continued to report daily use. A similar pattern of results was observed for crime.

Involuntary Termination of Methadone Treatment

In 1976 the only methadone program operating in Bakersfield, California was closed. The nearest clinic was 70 miles away in Tulare. The closing of the Bakersfield program provided McGlothlin and Anglin (1981) with the conditions for a natural experiment in which the Bakersfield patients could be compared to a group from nearby Tulare who were not involuntarily discharged from treatment.

Follow-up interviews were conducted two years after the closure of the Bakersfield clinic. Overall, the Tulare group spent 73% of non-incarcerated time during the follow-up period in methadone maintenance compared with 8% for the Bakersfield group.

There were substantial improvements in heroin use and criminal activity reported by both groups when the pre-treatment and treatment periods were compared. In terms of the effect of the closure of the Bakersfield program, 60% of the men and 56% of the women became dependent again (excluding eight patients who transferred to another clinic). At the time of interview, an unexpected urine sample was taken, and the rate of morphine-positive urines was higher for the Bakersfield group. Of the 14 subjects who tested positive in the Tulare group only two were still on methadone. The Bakersfield group also had about twice the percentage of individuals arrested during the follow-up period when compared with the Tulare group. The overall outcome for the Bakersfield group was poor: 54% became dependent on opioids again, 73% were arrested, 61% were imprisoned for more than 30 days, and two died from drug overdoses.

Anglin, Speckart, Booth and Ryan (1989) conducted a similar study after the closure of the San Diego public methadone program, using a similar comparison group. However, the study found few differences between people in the involuntarily terminated and continuing methadone maintenance programs, largely because a substantial proportion of the San Diego group transferred to private methadone programs. Even so, the patients who did not transfer had poorer outcomes than those who did.

Overall, the studies of Anglin and his colleagues include two reasonably powerful tests of methadone maintenance treatment: a comparison of the effects of the introduction of methadone maintenance treatment to a group of opioid-dependent patients with a no-treatment comparison group; and a study of the effects of involuntary cessation of methadone maintenance treatment with a comparison group of patients who remained in methadone maintenance treatment. The studies showed the expected effects of the introduction and removal of treatment. The fact that heroin use was measured by retrospective self-report over the period of a decade raises some concerns, but Anglin and colleagues have since shown that these reports have reasonable test-retest reliability when repeated at ten year intervals (Anglin *et al.*, 1993).

The Drug Abuse Reporting Program (1982)

The Drug Abuse Reporting Program was a large-scale treatment outcome study that collected data on approximately 44,000 clients who applied for treatment at 52 drug treatment agencies in the USA and Puerto Rico between 1969 and 1973 (Simpson & Sells, 1982). The treatment modalities represented in the study were methadone maintenance, residential therapeutic communities, outpatient drug-free treatment, and short-term detoxification programs. Another category was created to include those people who applied for, but never began treatment. Bi-monthly status reports were received over a year for those clients who entered treatment.

Follow-up interviews took place five to seven years after initial assessment for treatment. A total of 4,627 subjects were interviewed from each of three annual cohorts for the years 1969–71, 1971–72, and 1972–73. Treatment outcome was assessed retrospectively by interviews in which subjects were asked about their behaviour during each month between the end of treatment and the time of the interview. The outcomes assessed in these interviews were: drug use, crime, employment status, alcohol consumption, living situation, and further treatment episodes.

The findings from the Drug Abuse Reporting Program have been reported in a series of papers (e.g., Bracy & Simpson, 1982–83; Simpson, 1981; Simpson *et al.*, 1982; Simpson & Sells, 1982). In terms of comparisons between treatments, patients in methadone maintenance, therapeutic communities and outpatient drug-free programs had better outcomes than those who went through detoxification programs or had no treatment at all (Simpson & Sells, 1982). This finding was apparent in the year immediately following treatment, and was still evident, although the differences had diminished, at the five-year follow-up (Bracy & Simpson, 1982–83). One Drug Abuse Reporting Program study, however, found that these differences in treatment outcome did not persist for such long periods (Simpson *et al.*, 1982).

The finding of the Drug Abuse Reporting Program research that is most often quoted is the positive relationship between time spent in treatment and post-treatment performance (see Chapter 12 for an extensive discussion of this issue). Length of time spent in treatment was predictive of improved treatment outcome for treatment periods of at least one year for methadone maintenance. In general, there was a linear relationship between improvement and treatment duration between thee months and two years, the longest treatment period given the duration of the project (Simpson, 1981). The only other variable that predicted post-treatment performance was pre-treatment criminal history, in which case higher levels of criminal activity predicted poorer outcome in terms of opioid use, employment and crime (Simpson & Sells, 1982).

There are a number of problems with the Drug Abuse Reporting Program studies as evaluations of the effectiveness of methadone. The major problem was that the follow-up data on post-treatment outcome was collected retrospectively for the four years preceding follow-up. The credibility of month by month recollections of drug use over such a period is doubtful. Behaviour during periods closer to the follow-up period would be more reliable, but could be confounded by a number of unknown variables that may have nothing to do with treatment, as the authors acknowledge.

The Treatment Outcome Prospective Study (1989)

The Treatment Outcome Prospective Study (TOPS) (Hubbard *et al.,* 1984; Hubbard *et al.,* 1989) was a prospective study of over 11,000 illicit drug users who applied for treatment in 41 programs in the USA. The major drug treatment modalities represented by the participating programs were methadone maintenance treatment, residential therapeutic communities, and outpatient drug-free treatment. All the applicants for treatment in the participating treatment programs for the years 1979, 1980, and 1981 were interviewed about their drug use, criminality and other behaviour before treatment, and were then followed up during treatment.

The purposes of the study were to assess the effect of treatment on clients' behaviour, and to identify client and treatment factors that predicted different treatment outcomes. The key outcomes measured were illicit drug use, criminal activity, employment, depression and suicide. All outcomes were assessed by self-reports that were validated by a variety of procedures. Statistical techniques were used to control for the effects on outcomes of potential confounding variables such as sex, marital status, education level, age, race/ethnicity and number of prior admissions.

The study can be divided into two phases. In the first in-treatment phase all applicants for treatment were interviewed and followed up every three months while they remained in treatment. In the second phase, selected subgroups from each admission year were followed up at three months, one year, two years and at three to five years after treatment (with the length of the latter follow-up depending on their year of admission).

The results of the TOPS study confirmed those of previous studies in that patients in all three treatment modalities showed a reduction in illicit drug use. TOPS also confirmed the observation that length of time in treatment was an important predictor of post-treatment behaviour for some of the outcomes measured (see Chapter 12).

Methadone treatment had the best retention rates of the three treatment modalities in TOPS. Patients in methadone maintenance treatment were less likely to drop out of treatment than those in drug-free outpatient and therapeutic communities: after three months, 65% of methadone patients remained in treatment, compared with less than 40% of the outpatient drug-free clients and 44% of the residents in therapeutic communities. At the end of six months 50% of patients were still in methadone maintenance treatment.

Patients in methadone maintenance substantially reduced their heroin use while in treatment, with less than 10% regularly using heroin (weekly or daily) after three months. Table 2.3 summarises the results of a logistic regression analysis which examined the likelihood of regular heroin and predatory criminal activity in the year after leaving treatment (or the past year in the case of patients who remained in long-term methadone maintenance) for patients grouped by time in treatment. The comparison group consists of those patients who remained in methadone maintenance for less than one week. The numbers in the table are odds ratios which can be interpreted as follows. Odds ratios of less than one for each of the groups who spent more than one week in methadone maintenance represent a reduction in the likelihood of the outcome (e.g., heroin use) and odds ratios greater than one indicate that the outcome is more likely. When the decreases or increases in the likelihood of the behaviour become statistically significant this has been indicated. The logistic regression analysis controlled for a variety of potential confounding variables and its results can be understood as representing the patients' outcomes when these other potentially confounding variables have been controlled for.

As can be seen from Table 2.3, a significant reduction in regular heroin use was observed among patients who spent more than a year in methadone maintenance even when they left treatment before follow-up interviews took place. Patients who left treatment within one week of entry were twice as likely to be regular heroin users as those who stayed for a year or more. Similarly, compared with those patients who remained in methadone maintenance throughout the period to follow-up, the group that stayed less than a week were four times more likely to be regularly using heroin.

Table 2.3

Summary of TOPS findings on the relationship between time in methadone maintenance and outcome during first year after treatment expressed as odds ratios.

	Time in Methadone Maintenance				
Outcome	< 1 week# n=86	1-13 weeks n=161	14-52 weeks n=268	> 52 weeks n=137	Long-term maintenance n=183
Regular heroin use	1.00	1.16	0.83	0.47*	0.23*
Predatory crime	1.00	0.81	0.81	0.59	0.36*

(Source: Hubbard *et al.*, 1989)
comparison group for calculation of odds ratios.
* p<.05

Criminal activity was assessed by self-reported predatory crimes such as breaking and entering and robbery. Among patients in methadone maintenance, one-third reported committing a predatory crime in the year before treatment. This dropped to 10% during the first month of treatment. As Table 2.3 suggests, significant reductions in self-reported predatory crime were observed only while patients remained in methadone maintenance. Post-treatment criminal activity was predicted by level of pre-treatment involvement in crime but was unrelated to treatment. Methadone treatment, therefore, was associated with a reduction in criminal activity during treatment but did not permanently change the behaviour of the more criminally involved patients in the post-treatment period.

TOPS is the largest controlled prospective study of drug treatment to be conducted in recent times. It provides information on the behaviour of a large number of subjects before, during and after treatment in methadone maintenance, therapeutic communities, and outpatient drug-free programs. The use of statistical procedures to control for the influence of variables like client characteristics on treatment outcome lends more weight to the findings. The results of the study suggest that participating in methadone maintenance treatment is associated with marked and enduring reductions in heroin use and criminal activity.

Pre-Post Studies of Treatment Effectiveness

The interpretation of pre-post observational treatment studies is more problematic than the interpretation of comparative observational studies because they do not include a comparison treatment condition. Inferences about treatment effectiveness from pre-post studies are often made by examining the relationship between length of time in treatment and outcome. Such inferences are of uncertain value because of the existence of a plausible rival explanation – namely, that those with the best outcome (e.g., who were the least dependent on opioids, and the most motivated to discontinue drug use) were the most likely to be retained in treatment. This is a form of "selection" bias.

The quasi-experimental strategy can provide a limited evaluation of this alternative explanation. First, the hypothesis that patients with a good outcome were more likely to be retained in treatment can be tested by measuring the relevant characteristics (e.g., degree of dependence, previous treatment history, and motivation to change) of those who do and do not remain in treatment. Secondly, if selection bias is operating, statistical methods (e.g., covariate adjustment) can be used to discover whether the relationship between treatment duration and patient outcome persists when differences in patient characteristics are taken into account.

Gearing and Schweitzer (1974)

Gearing and Schweitzer (1974) provided an independent evaluation of 17,500 patients admitted to New York City methadone maintenance programs between January 1964 and December 1971. They identified four cohorts by date of admission, which defined changes in admission criteria over time, and a shift from inpatient to outpatient induction to the methadone program. Outcome was evaluated by changes in social productivity, arrests for predatory crime, and mortality rates.

The demographic characteristics of patients entering the program changed over the period of study. The average age declined from 33 to 29 years; the proportion of women increased from 15% to 23%; and the percentage of whites decreased from 40% to 32%, while the percentage of persons of Spanish origin increased from 19% to 26%. Despite these changes in patient characteristics, retention in treatment was high and relatively constant across the first three cohorts who had been enrolled sufficiently long enough for it to be assessed, namely, 90% after one year, 80% after two years, and 75% after three years.

Retention in treatment was associated with improved social productivity, reduced crime and a reduced mortality rate. The percentage who were employed, attending school or homemakers increased with treatment for all three cohorts, although less so for later cohorts. The three cohorts showed similar decreases in rates of arrest with increasing time in treatment, namely, 6.5% in the first year, 4.6% in the second year, 3.1% in the third year, and 2.9% in the fourth year.

The only comparative component of the study was a comparison of mortality rates among 3,000 patients while in treatment, 850 patients who left methadone, 100 patients entering detoxification in 1965, and the general New York population in 1969 to 1970 in the age range 20 to 54 years. The rates among patients while in treatment (7.6 per 1,000 population) were not substantially higher than those in the general population (5.6 per 1,000 population) which is impressive given that the mortality rate among opioid users is generally higher than that in the general population (English *et al.,* 1995). The mortality rate among those entering detoxification was almost 11 times higher than that of those in treatment (82.5 per 1,000 population), while those who had left treatment had a rate that was almost four times higher than that of those who remained in treatment (28.2 per 1,000 population). The percentage of deaths that were judged to be probably or possibly drug related was 50% among those in treatment, 80% among those who died after leaving treatment, and 100% among those who entered detoxification.

Gearing and Schweitzer's study was uncontrolled (with the exception of mortality), there was no comparison group with which to compare outcome in the absence of treatment, and there were no statistical methods used to exclude alternative explanations of the results. Nonetheless, their results are noteworthy in independently replicating the positive results for drug use and crime reported by Dole and Nyswander in their early reports, and in showing that these positive outcomes were sustained over four cohorts of 17,500 patients who were admitted to their program over a period of eight years. The outcomes assessed were relatively objective, and the advantage in favour of methadone maintenance was substantial in the case of mortality where comparative data were available.

Ball and Colleagues (1988, 1991)

Ball and his colleagues (Ball *et al.*, 1988; Ball & Ross, 1991) reported the results of a large-scale outcome study of methadone maintenance treatment involving six methadone maintenance programs, two each in Baltimore, Philadelphia and New York, over a three-year period between 1985 and 1987. During the winter of 1985–86, 633 male patients were interviewed, and 506 were re-interviewed a year later about their drug use history, their last period of injecting drug use, and their past and current criminal activity. The initial sample consisted of 113 new admissions and 520 patients who had been in treatment for at least six months. At follow-up 388 remained in treatment and 107 had left treatment at some time during the intervening year. The characteristics of the methadone maintenance programs were also extensively assessed to determine if there was any relationship between program characteristics and outcome.

The findings suggested that methadone maintenance had a dramatic impact on injecting drug use and crime among the 388 patients who remained in treatment during the follow-up year: 36% had not injected since the first month on methadone maintenance, 22% had not injected for a year or more, and 13% had not injected in the past one to 11 months. In all, 71% had not injected in the month prior to interview, and the rate of injection among the 29% who had injected in the past month was substantially less than before treatment.

The results also suggested that some programs were more effective at eliminating drug use than others: four of the programs reduced drug use by between 75% and 90%, whereas around 56% of patients in the other two programs were still injecting. Among the 107 patients who had left treatment by the time of follow-up, 68% had relapsed to injecting drug use. The relapse rate increased linearly over time, reaching a maximum of 82% among patients who had been out of treatment for more than 10 months. Those patients who had been in the less successful programs had higher relapse rates than those who had been in the more successful programs. Overall, these results suggest that methadone maintenance was effective at substantially reducing injecting drug use among the majority of patients, and that some methadone maintenance programs were more effective than others in achieving this goal.

The reduction of crime associated with retention in methadone maintenance was also impressive. The study sample had an extensive criminal history prior to entering methadone: a total of 4,723 arrests, with a mean of nine arrests for the 86% of the sample who had been arrested. Sixty-six per cent of the group had spent some time in gaol, 36% having been incarcerated for two years or more. Although these figures indicate extensive criminal involvement, they seriously underestimate criminal activity which is better estimated by self-reported crime.

The sample admitted to 293,308 offences per year during their last period of addiction, with each offender committing an average of 601 crimes per year (range 1 to 3,588), on an average of 304 days per year during their last addiction period. After entry to methadone, the number of self-reported offences declined to 50,103 crimes per year and the mean number of "crime days" per year decreased from 238 in the year prior to entry to 69 crime days during the early months of methadone maintenance. The number of crime days declined with the number of years spent in treatment. The reduction in the number of crimes committed during methadone maintenance was 192,000 offences per year. As Ball and Ross (1991) remark, such a substantial reduction in criminal activity among heroin users is usually only achieved during incarceration. As might be expected, given the relationship between drug use and crime, some programs were more successful than others in reducing crime.

According to Ball and Ross (1991) and Ball *et al.,* (1988), the more effective programs in their study were characterised by the following features: they prescribed higher doses of methadone and had maintenance rather than abstinence as their treatment goal (see Chapter 12); they offered better quality and more intensive counselling services (see Chapter 11) and provided more medical services; they retained their patients in treatment and managed to achieve compliance in terms of regular clinic attendance; they also had close, long-term relationships with their patients; and, they had low staff turnover rates.

Two important points emerge from this study. The first is that methadone maintenance treatment programs differ in effectiveness. The second is that, on average, methadone maintenance treatment is effective for the majority of patients while they are maintained on methadone; they relapse quickly once they leave treatment. The fact that the sample in this study was restricted to inner-city males with long histories of dependence (mean = 11.2 years), and long-standing criminal involvement, provided a stringent test of methadone maintenance treatment. It is reasonable to assume that if methadone maintenance treatment is effective in this difficult population, then it would also be effective with a less troubled group. As was the case with the DARP study, however, there is some concern about the reliance upon retrospective self-reports about drug use and crime. In the case of crime, the study may have over-estimated the impact of methadone maintenance in that it compared crime recalled during the last period of addiction with that reported during treatment. This comparison may have exaggerated the difference between the amount of crime reported before and during methadone maintenance.

Bell and Colleagues (1995)

Bell and colleagues (1995) replicated the Ball and Ross (1991) study by following a cohort of 304 methadone maintenance patients in three Sydney private methadone maintenance programs who were interviewed three times over a year about their heroin use, criminal activity and health and well-being. Urinalysis results were available for statistical analysis and police records were used to validate self-reported criminal activity.

The frequency of self-reported heroin use, and the average daily amount of heroin used, dropped promptly on admission to treatment, and it continued to decline with increasing time in treatment in two of the clinics. Just under half of the patients continued to inject heroin intermittently. As in Ball and Ross's study, there were marked differences between clinics in rates of heroin use, with the least effective clinic having nearly twice the rate of heroin use (59%) of the most effective clinic (34%). Methadone dose was correlated with heroin use. Reductions in heroin use were accompanied by improvements in social functioning and HIV risk-taking.

Methadone treatment had no effects on non-opioid drug use which was very common among the patients. Two-thirds had used cannabis, about a third had used benzodiazepines, a sixth had used amphetamine, and only 10% had used no other illicit drug in the month prior to interview. Forty-three percent were using psychoactive drugs other than methadone in a hazardous way. These drug use patterns remained stable during treatment, except for cannabis use which increased among a third of the patients. Continued cannabis use was associated with poorer social functioning and continued criminal activity.

Self-reported crime days in the last 30 days of active addiction were compared with the number in the last 30 days on methadone maintenance treatment (for those who had been in treatment longer than 30 days). There were substantial reductions in the self-reported rates of both property and drug offences, with the percentage reporting drug selling declining from 40% to 12%, and the percentage engaging in property crimes declining from 35% to 9%. The number of days in the last 30 on which they reported engaging in each type of offence declined from 21 to 11 days for drug selling, and from 18 to 9 days for other crime. The percentage engaging in any income generating crime in the previous 30 days declined from 59% to 20% (Bell *et al.*, 1995). Analyses of rates of convictions for property and drug offences confirmed the self-reported reductions, with rates of property offences declining from 0.75 per annum to 0.22, while those for drug offences declined from 0.30 to 0.06.

General Accounting Office Study (1990)

In 1989 the Chairman of the Select Committee on Narcotics Abuse and Control asked the General Accounting Office of the United States Congress to evaluate the effectiveness of methadone maintenance treatment programs in reducing heroin and other drug use. The General Accounting Office staff selected 24 methadone maintenance programs in California, Florida, Massachusetts, New Jersey, New York, Texas, and Washington State which had at least 200 patients enrolled, and had operated for at least five years. They obtained data on heroin and cocaine use by urine analysis from 5,600 patients who had been enrolled for at least six months in methadone maintenance treatment. This included all patients from 21 programs and a random sample of patients from the other three programs. The effectiveness of the programs was evaluated in terms of whether less than 20% of patients who had been enrolled for at least six months were still injecting heroin. By this standard 10 of the 24 programs were judged to be ineffective.

The General Accounting Office study confirms Ball and Ross's

(1991) findings that there was substantial variability between the programs' policies. The programs varied widely in the frequency with which urinalyses were conducted, in the consequences of continued drug use, and in the average dose of methadone. The majority of the programs (21 out of 24) provided sub-optimal doses of methadone, as defined by the minimum dose recommended by the National Institute for Drug Abuse, namely, 60 mg per day (Schuster, 1989). The mean dose in all 24 programs was 48 mg of methadone per day.

Given these differences in policies it is not surprising that there were also substantial differences in patient outcomes between programs. The proportion of patients in each program who had been retained in treatment at six months varied between 83% and 4%, with an average of 54%. The proportion that continued to inject heroin ranged between 13% and 67%, and the proportion who injected cocaine varied between 0% and 40%. Secondary analyses of the grouped data by Newman and Des Jarlais (1991) suggested that the mean dose of methadone in each program predicted both retention and continued illicit heroin use.

Overall, the results of the General Accounting Office study provide evidence that many methadone maintenance treatment programs in the United States are relatively ineffective in terms of reducing injecting drug use among those they retain in treatment. Nevertheless, the results also provided suggestive support for the Dole and Nyswander model of treatment in that the treatment programs that used adequate doses of methadone had the best outcomes in terms of patient retention and the frequency of injecting heroin use in treatment (Newman & Des Jarlais, 1991).

A COMPARISON OF RANDOMISED CONTROLLED TRIALS AND OBSERVATIONAL STUDIES

The observational studies of the effectiveness of methadone maintenance treatment generally support the results of the small number of randomised controlled trials in showing that heroin use and criminal activity decreased while opioid addicts remained in methadone maintenance treatment. These studies also revealed two other features of contemporary methadone maintenance treatment. The first was that there was substantial variation between different programs in outcomes as measured by treatment retention and continued heroin and other illicit drug use, which most clearly emerged in the studies by Ball and Ross and the General Accounting Office. The second was that the average results of methadone maintenance treatment in recent observational studies are not as impressive as those reported from the randomised controlled trials. For example, the retention rates from the randomised controlled trials are usually of the order of 70% or more after one year whereas the retention rate in the DARP and General Accounting Office studies was approximately 50% after six months. Similarly, the early randomised controlled trials reported very little continuing heroin use among those who remained in treatment whereas the proportion who continued to use heroin in the General Accounting Office study, for example, was as high as 67% in some programs.

There are a number of candidate explanations for the differences in the apparent effectiveness of methadone maintenance in randomised and observational studies. First, it is likely that randomised controlled trials have provided a somewhat optimistic estimate of treatment effectiveness. In order to produce clear results, such studies usually exclude some of the more difficult patients from entry, and they often have greater degree of control over the quality of the treatment that is provided than usually occurs under the ordinary exigencies of clinical practice. In addition, in many of the initial randomised controlled trials, patients who were denied access to methadone maintenance treatment were unlikely to receive it or any other form of treatment elsewhere. The comparison of methadone maintenance treatment with control treatment in such studies was not attenuated by the effects of treatment obtained elsewhere, as has more often been the case in recent observational studies, such as that of Bale and his colleagues.

Secondly, there is clear evidence that many current methadone maintenance treatment programs in the USA have departed from the original model of Dole and Nyswander in directions that are likely to reduce average effectiveness. As the data presented by D'Aunno and Vaughn (1992) and in the General Accounting Office report show, many programs have reduced average methadone dose and put pressure on patients to become abstinent from all opioids, including methadone. There has also been a wide variation in the practices that different programs follow, and an absence of any interest in evaluating their impact on treatment outcome.

Thirdly, there have been important historical changes in patterns of illicit drug use between the time when methadone was introduced and when the more recent observational studies were conducted. The most obvious of these has been the spread of poly drug use among people presenting for treatment. In the USA, cocaine use in particular has become widespread among methadone patients. Methadone has no specific effects on cocaine use, neither blocking the effects of cocaine nor preventing withdrawal symptoms, so it has had minimal impact on the use of non-opioid illicit drugs.

Fourthly, the context within which methadone maintenance treatment has been provided has changed dramatically in the past 20 years. The federal financial support for methadone maintenance treatment in the mid-1970s has given way in the USA to fiscal restraint on program budgets with consequent reductions in the quality of treatment services, and to a steady decline in the number of treatment places on methadone maintenance. This decline in the quantity and quality of treatment in the USA has been accompanied by an increase in Federal Government regulations that have encouraged the reduction in average methadone dose and the introduction of time limits (usually two years) on treatment.

AN OVERALL APPRAISAL OF EFFECTIVENESS

An overall evaluation of the effectiveness of methadone maintenance has been reached by examining the degree to which the observational and experimental evidence satisfies a set of criteria which were originally suggested by Hill (1965) as a way of making inferences about disease aetiology from observational data. These criteria can be readily adapted to the task of making causal inferences about treatment effectiveness. Although no single one of these criteria is necessary, the more of them that are satisfied, the greater our confidence that a causal relationship exists between treatment and outcome.

Strength of association: Relationships that are strong indicate that the outcome of treatment is highly predictable. They are generally more deserving of trust than those based on a weak relationship because stronger relationships are less open to alternative explanations, such as assessment or selection bias, than are weaker ones.

The relationship between methadone maintenance and a reduction in both illicit opioid use and criminal behaviour is, on average, a reasonably strong one. The rate of each approximately halves with each year that a patient remains in treatment. The relationship between methadone and outcome is strongest in the small number of randomised controlled trials that compare its effectiveness with little or no treatment.

Consistency: A relationship is consistent if it is observed in studies conducted by different investigators, using different study methods, in different populations. Relationships that are consistent are less likely to be due to sampling error and methods of study.

A relationship between methadone treatment and reduced drug use and criminal behaviour has been consistently observed in controlled trials, quasi-experimental studies, comparative studies, and pre-post studies in the USA, Sweden, Hong Kong, and Australia. This relationship is most consistent in studies of programs that use doses above 60 mg and which have maintenance as their treatment goal.

Specificity: Specificity exists when the relationship between treatment and outcome is such that if treatment is given, the outcome occurs, and if the outcome is observed, then one can confidently infer that treatment has been given. This criterion is desirable in that, if it exists, it suggests that there is a strong relationship between treatment and outcome. But it is not necessary in that its absence does not exclude the possibility that treatment makes a contribution to a good outcome.

A degree of specificity is evident in the relationship between methadone treatment and outcome. Its effects are most evident on those outcomes it has been designed to change: opioid use and criminal behaviour motivated by the need to finance illicit opioid use. Its effects are less marked on other outcomes such as non-opioid illicit drug use (e.g., cocaine and amphetamine) and vocational adjustment, unless this is specifically addressed in the program, as was the case in the Swedish methadone program.

A dose-response relationship: A dose-response relationship between exposure to treatment and outcome (e.g., the longer the time in treatment, the more intensive the treatment) is desirable. Such a relationship increases confidence that there are some specific treatment components that are responsible for the benefits of treatment.

A dose-response relationship between methadone maintenance and reduced opioid use and criminality is shown in three ways. First, there is a relationship between the dose of methadone received and treatment retention and outcome. Both within individual programs and between programs, the higher the dose of methadone, the longer the retention in treatment and the better the outcome in terms of reduced heroin use and criminal behaviour. Secondly, there is a relationship between treatment duration and benefit: the longer patients remain in treatment, the better the outcome. This relationship does not appear to be explained by a higher retention rate among patients who have a good prognosis. Thirdly, there is suggestive evidence that the strength of the relationship between methadone treatment and outcome also varies with the fidelity with which the Dole and Nyswander model of treatment has been implemented. That is, demonstrated effectiveness decreases to the degree that methadone moves away from the high-dose *maintenance* treatment with extensive ancillary services initiated by Dole and Nyswander towards low-dose programs which often aim to achieve abstinence within a period of several years.

Plausibility: A relationship is plausible if it is consistent with other relevant knowledge such as, for example, the mechanisms of addiction. The consonance of a relationship with such mechanisms enhances our confidence in it.

The rationale for the effectiveness of methadone maintenance is plausible. Opioid dependence is characterised by a persistent preoccupation with procuring and using illicit opioid drugs to the detriment of the user's health and well-being. The provision of a legal opioid drug (methadone), which is cross-tolerant to heroin, in doses which avert withdrawal and reduce the positive effects of illicit opioid use, reduces the salience of opioid use and the necessity for users to spend most of their daily existence in the pursuit of opioid drugs.

Coherence: A relationship is coherent if it makes sense of other information about the natural history of the condition.

The evidence on the effects of methadone maintenance is coherent with what is known about the natural history of opioid drug use: by the time patients present for treatment they have a long history of opioid use so it takes time for methadone maintenance to achieve its benefits; and opioid dependence is a chronic condition with a high relapse rate, so the effects of methadone maintenance treatment appear to last only while people remain in treatment.

Experiment: Although there is limited experimental evidence of the effectiveness of methadone maintenance, it is consistently positive.

There are only three controlled trials of comprehensive methadone maintenance over periods of a year or more (Dole *et al.,* 1969; Newman & Whitehill, 1979; Gunne & Grönbladh, 1981), all involving small numbers of patients and conducted in three very different cultural settings. All provide evidence of substantial differences in outcome on opioid drug use and crime that favours methadone maintenance treatment.

Some Caveats

Taken as a whole, the evidence provides good reasons for believing that methadone maintenance is an effective form of treatment for opioid dependence *on average.* The phrase "on average" implies a number of caveats that need to be spelt out.

First, methadone is not a "cure" for heroin dependence. On average, about half of those who enter treatment leave treatment or are discharged for continued illicit drug use within 12 months, and a substantial but variable proportion of those who stay in treatment continue to use heroin and other illicit drugs, albeit at much reduced rates.

These outcomes will be regarded as "poor" if judged by the unrealistic expectation that all patients should achieve enduring abstinence from all opioid drugs, a standard implicitly demanded of methadone maintenance by some of its critics (Hall, 1993). In evaluating the treatment of heroin dependence, we need to compare the outcome of methadone treatment with what is likely to have happened in its absence (Gerstein & Harwood, 1990). By this standard, methadone maintenance is the best of the available alternatives: other forms of treatment attract and retain fewer patients, and do not produce superior outcomes to methadone maintenance among those who complete treatment; and a failure to provide treatment carries a high risk of premature mortality and serious morbidity for users, and high social and economic costs for the community (Collins & Lapsley, 1991; English *et al.,* 1995; Gerstein & Harwood, 1990).

Secondly, methadone programs vary in their policies and in their effectiveness in reducing drug use and criminal acts. The factors responsible for this variability are not well understood, although the evidence strongly suggests that they include the dose of methadone given, the duration of treatment, and the characteristics of the patients in the programs. Other relevant factors probably include the quality of the therapeutic relationships between patients and staff, and the intensiveness of ancillary services.

Thirdly, the most effective methadone programs are those that resemble the model introduced by Dole and Nyswander, namely, higher doses of methadone in the context of a comprehensive treatment program with maintenance rather than abstinence as a treatment goal. The effectiveness is much less certain for programs that depart from this model by reducing methadone dose and imposing abstinence from methadone as a treatment goal. Indeed, there is no good evidence that such programs are effective at achieving the goal of abstinence among a substantial proportion of patients within one to two years. Uncertainty also exists about the effectiveness of the newer low-threshold and low-intervention programs (that lower the admission criteria, reduce ancillary services, and reduce the expectation that patients will decrease their heroin use) which are proposed as a way of preventing the transmission of HIV by needle sharing and unsafe sexual behaviour.

Fourthly, the benefits of methadone maintenance continue only as long as patients remain in treatment. Patients who discontinue treatment relapse to opioid use at a high rate. There have been too few studies of persons who successfully 'graduate' from methadone programs to say whether planned attempts at withdrawal and rehabilitation are more likely to succeed.

SUMMARY

The three controlled trials of comprehensive methadone maintenance over a period of a year or more produced similar results: all showed that methadone maintenance was more effective than either placebo or no treatment in retaining people in treatment, in reducing opioid use, and in reducing the rate of imprisonment. This is an impressive result for studies that have typically used small sample sizes that reduce the chances of finding differences, and which have been conducted in three different countries over a period of about 15 years.

The more recent controlled studies of time-limited methadone maintenance programs provide evidence of the short-term effectiveness of methadone maintenance in retaining patients in treatment and reducing their heroin use while they remain in treatment. Although the results of the randomised controlled trials are strongly supportive of the effectiveness of methadone, there are arguably too few replications to enable definitive conclusions to be drawn about the effectiveness of methadone. Our confidence in the results of the randomised controlled trials is enhanced to the degree that similar results have been reported in larger observational studies of effectiveness.

The findings of the comparative observational studies of methadone maintenance are consistent with the results of the small number of randomised controlled trials in showing that methadone maintenance retains patients in treatment and substantially reduces illicit opioid drug use and involvement in criminal activity in comparison with patients who do not enter treatment. The pre-post-studies generally agree with the results of the comparative studies in showing that the longer patients remain in treatment, the less likely they are to inject heroin or to engage in criminal activity. In those studies that have used a quasi-experimental strategy to evaluate rival explanations, these results have proved robust.

The observational studies also indicate that there is substantial variation between different programs in their effectiveness in retaining patients in treatment, and reducing their drug use and criminality while they are in treatment. Analyses of the characteristics that predict the variations between programs in retention, drug use and criminality have generally supported the original model of Dole and Nyswander in showing that programs with higher doses, a maintenance goal and ancillary services have better outcomes than programs that use lower doses and aim to achieve abstinence.

The *average* effects of methadone maintenance treatment in the observational studies have been lower than those observed in the randomised controlled trials. Among the more important reasons that can be identified for the decline in the average effectiveness of methadone maintenance have been: a systematic departure from the model of methadone maintenance proposed by Dole and Nyswander in the direction of lower dose and time-limited treatment; a decline in the quality of methadone maintenance programs in the face of fiscal restraint and federal regulations in the USA; and changes in the patient population of methadone maintenance treatment programs with the rise in poly drug use.

Comparison of the evidence on effectiveness of methadone maintenance with criteria for causal inference proposed by Hill indicate that methadone maintenance is well supported. There is strong evidence that there are substantial reductions in heroin use and crime while opioid addicts are enrolled in methadone maintenance; a finding that has been consistently obtained in randomised controlled trials and observational studies in a number of very different cultures over the past 30 years. There is a degree of specificity in the effect of methadone maintenance treatment in that clearest benefits are in reducing opioid use and criminal acts undertaken to finance drug use. A dose-response relationship is observed in: the strong relationship between methadone dose and treatment retention and opioid use; the relationship between reductions in drug use and crime and increasing time in treatment; and the relationship between effectiveness and the fidelity of programs to the high dose maintenance oriented program developed by Dole and Nyswander. The effectiveness of methadone maintenance treatment is plausible in the light of knowledge about opioid dependence, and coherent with what is known about the careers of opioid-dependent persons. It is supported by the consistently positive results in each of the small number of experimental studies of the effectiveness of methadone maintenance.

A number of caveats have to be entered to avoid unrealistic expectations of methadone maintenance treatment. First, methadone maintenance does not produce abstinence from all illicit opioids in all patients; nevertheless, it produces a substantial reduction in rates of heroin use and abstinence from illicit opioids in approximately half of those who receive it. Second, different programs differ in their effectiveness. Third, the best supported model of treatment is that developed by Dole and Nsywander, namely, opioid maintenance treatment. Fourth, accordingly, the benefits of methadone treatment continue only as long as patients remain in treatment.

REFERENCES

Anglin, M.D. (1988). The efficacy of civil commitment in treating narcotic drug addiction. In C.G. Leukefeld., & F.M. Tims (Eds.), *Compulsory treatment of drug abuse: Research and clinical practice* (NIDA Research Monograph 86, pp. 8-34). Rockville, MD: National Institute on Drug Abuse.

Anglin, M.D., & McGlothlin, W.H. (1984). Outcome of narcotic addict treatment in California. In F.M. Timms & J.P. Ludford (Eds.), *Drug abuse treatment evaluation: Strategies, progress and prospect* (NIDA Research Monograph 51, pp. 106-128). Rockville, MD: National Institute on Drug Abuse.

Anglin, M.D., Hser, Y-I., & Chou, C-P. (1993). Reliability and validity of retrospective behavioral self-report by narcotics addicts. *Evaluation Review,* **17,** 91-108.

Anglin, M.D., Speckart, G.R., Booth, M.W., & Ryan, T.M. (1989). Consequences and costs of shutting off methadone. *Addictive Behaviors,* **14,** 302-326.

Bale, R.N., Van Stone, W.W., Kuldau, J.M., Engelsing, T.M.J., Elashoff, R.M., & Zarcone, V.P. (1980). Therapeutic communities vs methadone maintenance. A prospective controlled study of narcotic addiction treatment: design and one-year follow-up. *Archives of General Psychiatry,* **37,** 179-193.

Ball, J.C. & Ross, A. (1991). *The effectiveness of methadone maintenance treatment: Patients, programs, services, and outcomes.* New York: Springer-Verlag.

Ball, J.C., Lange, W.R., Myers, C.P., & Friedman, S.R. (1988). Reducing the risk of AIDS through methadone maintenance treatment. *Journal of Health and Social Behaviour,* **29,** 214-226.

Bell, J., Hall, W., & Byth, K. (1992). Changes in criminal activity after entering methadone maintenance. *British Journal of Addiction,* **87,** 251–258.

Bell, J., Ward, J., Mattick, R.P., Hay, A., Chan, J., & Hall, W. (1995). *An evaluation of private methadone clinics* (National Drug Strategy Report Series No. 4). Canberrra, Australia: Australian Government Publishing Service.

Bracy, S.A., & Simpson, D.D. (1982-83). Status of opioid addicts 5 years after admission to drug abuse treatment. *American Journal of Drug and Alcohol Abuse,* **9,** 115-127.

Cochrane, A.L. (1972). *Effectiveness and efficiency: Random reflections on health services.* Abingdon, United Kingdom: The Nuffield Provinical Hospitals Trust.

Cohen, J. (1992). A power primer. *Psychological Bulletin,* **112,** 155-159.

Collins, D.J., & Lapsley, H.M. (1991). *Estimating the economic costs of drug abuse in Australia* (National Campaign Against Drug Abuse Monograph Series No. 15) Canberra, Australia: Australian Government Publishing Service.

Cook, T. D., & Campbell, D.T. (1979). *Quasi-experimentation: Design and analysis issues for field settings.* Chicago: Rand McNally

Darke, S., Hall, W., Heather, N., Ward, J., & Wodak, A. (1992). Development and validation of a multi-dimensional instrument for assessing outcome among opiate users: The Opiate Treatment Index. *British Journal of Addiction,* **87,** 773-742.

D'Aunno, T., & Vaughn, T.E. (1992). Variations in methadone treatment practices: Results from a national study. *Journal of the American Medical Association,* **267,** 253-258.

Dole, V.P., & Nyswander, M. (1965). A medical treatment for diacetylmorphine (heroin). addiction. *Journal of the American Medical Association,* **193**, 80-84.

Dole, V.P. & Nyswander, M.E. (1967). Heroin addiction – a metabolic disease. *Archives of Internal Medicine,* **120**, 19-24.

Dole, V.P., Robinson, J.W., Orraca, J., Towns, E., Searcy, P., & Caine, E. (1969). Methadone treatment of randomly selected criminal addicts. *New England Journal of Medicine,* **280**, 1372-1375.

English, D., Holman, C.D.J., Milne, E., Winter, M.G., Hulse, G.K., Codde, J.P., Corti. B., Dawes, V., de Klerk, N., Knuiman, M.W., Kurinczuk, J.J., Lewin, G.F., & Ryan, G.A. (1995). *The quantification of drug caused morbidity and mortality in Australia - 1995 edition.* Canberra, Australia: Commonwealth Department of Human Services and Health.

Fisher, R.A. (1949). *The design of experiments.* Edinburgh: Oliver & Boyd.

Friedmann, P., Des Jarlais, D.C., Peyser, N.P., Nichols, S.E., Drew, E., & Newman, R.G. (1994). Retention of patients who entered methadone maintenance via an interim methadone clinic. *Journal of Psychoactive Drugs,* **26**, 217-221.

Freiman, J.A., Chalmers, T.C., Smith, H., & Kubler, R.R. (1978). The importance of beta, the type II error and sample size in the design and interpretation of the randomized control trial. *New England Journal of Medicine,* **299**, 690-694.

Gardner, M.J., & Altman, D.G. (1989). *Statistics with confidence.* London: British Medical Journal.

Gearing, F.R., & Schweitzer, M.D. (1974). An epidemiologic evaluation of long-term methadone maintenance treatment for heroin addiction. *American Journal of Epidemiology,* **100**, 101-112.

General Accounting Office. (1990). *Methadone maintenance: Some treatment programs are not effective; greater federal oversight needed.* Report to the Chairman, Select Committee on Narcotics Abuse and Control, House of Representatives. Washington DC: General Accounting Office.

Gerstein, D.R., & Harwood, H.J. (1990). *Treating drug problems Volume 1: A study of effectiveness and financing of public and private drug treatment systems.* Washington DC: National Academy Press.

Grönbladh, L., & Gunne, L. (1989). Methadone-assisted rehabilitation of Swedish heroin addicts. *Drug and Alcohol Dependence,* **24**, 31-37.

Gunne, L-M. & Grönbladh, L. (1981). The Swedish methadone maintenance program: A controlled study. *Drug and Alcohol Dependence,* **7**, 249-256.

Hall, W. (1993). Perfectionism in the therapeutic appraisal of methadone maintenance. *Addiction,* **88**, 1181-1182.

Hill, A.B. (1951). The clinical trial I. *British Medical Bulletin,* **7**, 278. Reprinted in: A.B. Hill (1962). *Statistical methods in clinical and preventive medicine.* Edinburgh: E & S Livingstone.

Hill, A.B. (1965). The environment and disease: Association or causation. *Proceedings of the Royal Society of Medicine,* **58,** 295-300.

Hubbard, R.L., Rachal, J.V., Craddock, S.G., & Cavanaugh, E.R. (1984). Treatment Outcome Prospective Study (TOPS): Client characteristics and behaviors before, during and after treatment. In F.M. Timms & J.P. Ludford (Eds.), *Drug abuse treatment evaluation: Strategies, progress and prospects* (NIDA Research Monograph 51, pp. 42-68). Rockville, MD: National Institute on Drug Abuse.

Hubbard, R.L., Marsden, M.E., Rachal, J.V., Harwood, H.J., Cavanaugh, E.R., & Ginzburg, H.M. (1989). *Drug abuse treatment: A national study of effectiveness.* Chapel Hill, NC: University of North Carolina Press.

McGlothlin, W.H., & Anglin, M.D. (1981). Shutting off methadone: Costs and benefits. *Archives of General Psychiatry,* **38,** 1055-1063.

McLelland, A.T., Luborsky, L., Cacciola, J., Griffith, J. Evans. F., Barr, H.L., & O'Brien, C.P. (1985). New data from the Addiction Severity Index: Reliability and validity in three centers. *Journal of Nervous and Mental Disorders,* **173,** 412-423.

McMaster Department of Clinical Epidemiology (1981). How to read clinical journals IV: To determine disease etiology and causation. *Canadian Medical Association Journal,* **124,** 985-990.

Mattick, R.P.M., & Hall, W. (eds). (1993). *A treatment outline for approaches to opioid dependence: Quality assurance project* (National Drug Strategy Monograph No. 21). Canberra, Australia: Australian Government Publishing Service.

Newman, R.G., & Whitehill, W.B. (1979). Double-blind comparison of methadone and placebo maintenance treatments of narcotic addicts in Hong Kong. *Lancet,* September 8, 485-488.

Newman, R.G., & Des Jarlais, D.C. (1991). Criteria for judging methadone maintenance programs. *Journal of Psychoactive Drugs,* **23,** 115-121.

Schuster, C. R. (1989). Methadone maintenance: An adequate dose is vital in checking the spread of AIDS. *NIDA Notes,* **4,** 3 & 33.

Simpson, D.D. (1981). Treatment for drug abuse: Follow-up outcomes and length of time spent. *Archives of General Psychiatry,* **38,** 875-880.

Simpson, D.D., & Sells, S.B. (1982). Effectiveness of treatment for drug abuse: An overview of the DARP research program. *Advances in Alcohol and Substance Abuse,* **2,** 7-29.

Simpson, D.D., Joe, G.W., & Bracy, S.A. (1982). Six-year follow-up of opioid addicts after admission to treatment. *Archives of General Psychiatry,* **39,** 1318-1323.

Strain, E.C., Stitzer, M.L., Liebson, I.A., & Bigelow, G.E. (1993). Dose-response effects of methadone in the treatment of opioid dependence. *Annals of Internal Medicine,* **119,** 23-37.

Vanichseni, S., Wongsuwan, B., the staff of the BMA Narcotics Clinic No. 6., Choopanya, K., & Wogapanich, K. (1991). A controlled trial of methadone maintenance in a population of intravenous drug users in Bangkok: Implications for prevention of HIV. *International Journal of the Addictions,* **26,** 1313-1320.

Ward, J., Mattick, R. & Hall, W. (1992). *Key issues in methadone maintenance treatment.* Sydney, Australia: New South Wales University Press.

Yancovitz, S.R., Des Jarlais, D.C., Peyser, N.P., Drew, E., Friedmann, P., Trigg, H.L., & Robinson, J.W. (1991). A randomized trial of an interim methadone maintenance clinic. *American Journal of Public Health,* **81,** 1185-1191.

3

THE EFFECTIVENESS OF METHADONE MAINTENANCE TREATMENT 2: HIV AND INFECTIOUS HEPATITIS

JEFF WARD, RICHARD P. MATTICK
AND WAYNE HALL

INTRODUCTION

During the 1980s, one of the most significant factors influencing the provision of resources for the treatment of injecting drug users was the discovery of epidemic HIV infection among this group in many countries of the world (Des Jarlais, 1992). HIV infection with injecting drug use as a probable cause has now been reported in 80 countries, although the prevalence varies from country to country and city to city (Des Jarlais *et al.*, 1995). More recently, concern has been expressed about the discovery of even more widespread epidemics of hepatitis B and C among injecting drug users (e.g., Bell *et al.*, 1990a; Crofts *et al.*, 1993; Levine *et al.*, 1995; MacDonald *et al.*, 1996; Patti *et al.*, 1993; Thomas *et al.*, 1995; van Ameijden *et al.*, 1993). In response to these concerns, many governments around the world have expanded and developed methadone maintenance treatment programs (Gossop & Grant, 1991; Uchtenhagen, 1990). Therefore, as well as reducing heroin use, crime and drug-related mortality, an important aspect of any examination of the effectiveness of methadone maintenance treatment is the extent to which it protects against injection-related infections such as HIV and hepatitis B and C.

The review in this chapter focuses on HIV because there is now sufficient research from which to draw inferences about the contribution of methadone maintenance to HIV prevention. By contrast, there have been few comparable studies that have examined the relationship between exposure to methadone maintenance treatment and hepatitis B and C, and the evidence from these studies is contradictory. To the extent that the transmission characteristics of hepatitis B and C are the same as HIV among injecting drug users, it should be possible to draw conclusions about hepatitis from the evidence concerning HIV. However, as will be seen in the section below, there are a number of caveats that have to be taken into account before any simple translation of this sort can be made.

METHADONE MAINTENANCE TREATMENT AND HEPATITIS B AND C

In one of the few published studies that has evaluated the relationship between methadone maintenance treatment and injection-related hepatitis infections, Joseph (1988) reported that the rapid expansion of the methadone program in New York City in the years 1971 to 1973 was associated with a similar rapid reduction in the number of notified cases of hepatitis B for the same years. However, in contradistinction, van Ameijden *et al.* (1993) found exposure to methadone treatment did not prevent new cases of hepatitis B or C in a cohort of injecting drug users in Amsterdam who were followed during the period 1985 to 1989. In the case of the latter study, under-dosing with methadone cannot be ruled out as a possible cause of the program's failure to prevent these new infections.

As in the case of HIV, it is likely that transmission probabilities of hepatitis B and C depend on the prevalence in the local population, the frequencies of risk behaviours, the number of partners these risk behaviours are carried out with, and, where seroprevalence is low, whether these partners are from high-risk sub groups (Friedman *et al.*, 1995). It is when we consider the factors that might influence the transmission probabilities of hepatitis B and C in relation to HIV that the biggest impediment to making simple inferences about the former on the basis of evidence concerning the latter becomes difficult. It would appear that hepatitis B and C are more readily transmitted than HIV (Levine *et al.* 1994) and that there are, in many countries throughout the world, high levels of infection with these two viruses among populations of injecting drug users. Prevalence studies from around the world show high levels of exposure (50-80%) to hepatitis B and C among injecting drug users who have been injecting for some time (Bell, *et al.,* 1990a; Crofts, *et al.,* 1993; Institute of Medicine, 1995; Levine, *et al.,* 1994; Patti, *et al.,* 1993; van Ameijden, *et al.,* 1993). By the time opioid injectors present for methadone maintenance treatment, they have usually been injecting for a number of years and have already been exposed to these blood borne hepatitis infections (Bell *et al.,* 1990b; Institute of Medicine, 1995). Recent studies show that hepatitis B and C infection spreads rapidly among populations of drug injectors within the first few years of their injecting careers (Crofts, *et al.,* 1993; Levine, *et al.,* 1995; Thomas, *et al.,* 1995). Since many individuals are already exposed before entry to treatment, it is too late for methadone maintenance treatment to protect a significant proportion of patients who attend for treatment. In principle, therefore, the evidence that methadone maintenance treatment protects against HIV infection may be applicable in the case of hepatitis, but only for those individuals who have not been exposed to hepatitis B and C.

METHADONE MAINTENANCE TREATMENT AND HIV

The primary evidence for the contribution of methadone maintenance treatment to the prevention of HIV among injecting opioid users consists of studies of methadone maintenance treatment that suggest that this form of treatment is associated with reduced rates of HIV infection and injection-related risk behaviours among treatment populations. These two issues are examined separately in the two sections that follow. After considering these two issues, possible limitations to the effectiveness of methadone maintenance treatment are considered on the basis of the apparent ineffectiveness of a special case – low threshold methadone programs in The Netherlands.

Preventing HIV Infection

The first published reports attesting to the effectiveness of methadone maintenance in preventing HIV infection came from New York City where HIV had spread rapidly among injecting drug users in the period 1978-1981 (Des Jarlais *et al.*, 1989). In one of the first studies to be published, Abdul-Quader *et al.* (1987) reported an association between length of time in methadone maintenance treatment and lower rates of HIV antibody. In a subsequent study, Schoenbaum *et al.* (1989) found an inverse relationship between total time spent in methadone treatment since January 1978 and level of HIV seropositivity. Novick *et al.* (1990) similarly found no evidence of exposure to HIV among a group of long term, stable methadone patients, even though 91% had been exposed to hepatitis B, indicating that nearly all of them had shared needles at some time. Two other studies also from the United States found that patients in methadone treatment were less likely to be HIV positive than those in detoxification programs (Marmor *et al.*, 1987) and those not yet receiving methadone (Chaisson *et al.*, 1989).

These early studies strongly suggested that methadone maintenance might protect injecting opioid users from HIV infection, but absolute conclusions in this regard could not be drawn because the observed associations may have been due to selection factors, such as the more careful opioid users being more likely to enter treatment. Since the publication of the early studies, the evidence for a protective effect of methadone maintenance treatment has been confirmed in a number of studies that have employed more sophisticated study designs. The weight of the evidence now clearly indicates that being in methadone maintenance treatment leads to a reduced chance of HIV infection.

In the first of these studies, Blix and Grönbladh (1988; 1991) capitalised on the unique situation of the methadone program in Sweden to examine the relationship between what amounted to quasi-random access to methadone treatment and HIV infection. Because places in the program were limited, applicants for treatment were accepted during the 1980s in an almost random fashion depending upon whether a place was available at the time of application or not. When rates of HIV seroprevalence among applicants for treatment were compared with those who remained in treatment, there was strong evidence of a protective effect for methadone treatment. Commencing in 1983, when the first evidence of HIV infection became apparent in stored sera, it was found that the prevalence of

HIV infection increased from 3% for patients who entered methadone maintenance before 1983, to 16% for those who entered during the years 1984 to 1986 and to 57% for those who entered during 1987. The seroprevalence rate for applicants increased again to 59% in 1988, thereafter reducing to 48% in 1989 and 41% in 1990, presumably after prevention programs had been given a chance to have an effect in the community. By comparison, there had been no seroconversion of any methadone patients who had tested negative for HIV antibodies on entry since 1984. This study provides stronger evidence than those reviewed above in that it demonstrates that methadone maintenance treatment protects its recipients from HIV infection and that this appears to be independent of selection bias. A number of subsequent cohort and case control studies have confirmed this finding.

There have been two prospective cohort studies, both of which have been conducted in the United States. In the first of these studies 255 opioid injectors sampled from in- and out-of-treatment sources in Philadelphia were followed over a period of 36 months by Metzger and colleagues (Metzger *et al.*, 1993; see also Institute of Medicine, 1995). While the baseline prevalence of HIV seropositivity almost doubled among those out of treatment from 21% to 39% over the three years, among those in treatment at the commencement of the study it only increased from 13% to 18%. Furthermore, this increase of 5% in the treatment group was wholly accounted for by individuals who had left treatment. When asked about needle sharing at the 18-month follow-up interview, study participants recruited from methadone maintenance clinics were less likely to report sharing needles in the six months prior to their 18-month follow-up interview (34%) when compared with those recruited from out-of-treatment sources (70%).

In the second of these cohort studies, Moss *et al.* (1994) found methadone maintenance to be protective against HIV infection in a cohort of 681 heterosexual opioid injectors who were recruited from methadone maintenance and methadone detoxification programs in San Francisco and followed from 1985 to 1990. After adjusting for other major predictors of infection, individuals who had spent less than one year in methadone maintenance were nearly three times more likely to test positive for HIV antibody than those who had spent at least a year in treatment (Hazard Ratio = 2.7).

The finding of a protective effect of methadone treatment in

Sweden and the United States has also been reported from a nested case control study carried out in Verona, Italy on a subset of participants in a longitudinal study of injecting drug users. In this study, Serpelloni and colleagues (1994) found that participation in methadone maintenance treatment was negatively associated with risk for HIV infection. That is, the risk for HIV infection increased with increasing time spent out of treatment in the year prior to data collection and decreased with increasing average daily methadone dose during the same period. The authors estimated that the risk of HIV infection was increased by 70% for every three months spent out of treatment and that it was reduced by 35% for each 10 mg increase in methadone dose. These findings suggest that methadone maintenance is protective against HIV infection, and the dose-response nature of the evidence supports the notion that methadone is the active ingredient contributing to this protective effect. A relationship between increasing dose of methadone and lower rates of HIV infection has also been reported by Brown *et al.* (1989).

Further support for the effectiveness of methadone maintenance treatment is provided by a case control study of HIV infection among injecting drug users conducted in Miami, Florida (Chitwood *et al.,* 1995). In this study, Chitwood and colleagues found that controls were three times more likely than infected cases to have participated in some methadone treatment during the year prior to interview (unadjusted odds ratio = 0.29, 95% CI 0.09, 0.94). After statistical adjustment for other important variables this relationship was no longer statistically significant (adjusted odds ratio = 0.70, 95% CI 0.18, 2.81). However, unlike the participants in the other studies reviewed in this section, it appears from the authors' description of the sample that not all participants in the Miami study were opioid users, and this may account for the loss of statistical significance once other variables were adjusted for (e.g., the major predictor in the statistical model was cocaine use). While this study provides more mixed evidence that methadone maintenance treatment provides protection against HIV infection, when taken along with the other studies it provides support for the proposition.

The studies reviewed in this section suggest that there is reasonable support for the proposition that methadone maintenance protects its recipients from HIV infection. To the extent that other opioid replacement therapies are demonstrated to be as efficacious in reducing injecting drug use and the risk behaviours associated with it, it can be assumed that they will also be protective. The next section examines the evidence for the role of methadone maintenance treatment in reducing these injection-related risk behaviours, thereby showing evidence of direct reduction in behaviours associated with infection.

Sharing of Injecting Equipment

The principal mode of transmission of HIV and hepatitis B and C among injecting drug users is the sharing of injecting equipment that has been contaminated with the blood of an infected person. Although injecting drug users have responded positively to education campaigns informing them how to inject safely (Friedland, 1989), recent studies of the continued spread of hepatitis C in some populations suggest that there is still reason for concern (e.g., Crofts, *et al.,* 1993). In this section we examine the extent to which methadone maintenance treatment is associated with reduced injecting and needle sharing.

Ball and colleagues (Ball *et al.,* 1988; Ball & Ross, 1991), in their Three Cities Study, examined the influence of treatment on frequency of injecting and needle sharing. For both these outcomes they examined the number of subjects who reported these behaviours and the number of days in the month prior to interview that they engaged in them. Methadone treatment had a marked effect both on injecting and on the frequency of injecting for those who did inject. Of the 388 subjects who had remained in methadone maintenance until the end of the study period, 36% had not injected again after the first month of treatment. A further 22% had not injected in the past year, and a further 13% had not injected for a period of between one and 11 months. The remaining 29% had injected in the last month. Overall, this means that 71% had not injected in the month prior to follow-up. Similar results were found for needle sharing; both the number of sharers and the frequency with which they shared were reduced.

Similar findings have been observed in a number of other studies. Selwyn and colleagues (1987) found that being in methadone treatment was associated with a decrease in both injecting and sharing. The subjects in the Abdul-Quader *et al.* (1987) study described above who had been in treatment the longest had the lowest levels of these risk-taking behaviours. Darke *et al.* (1990) found that 20% of a sample of injecting drug users who were in treatment at the time of the interview (the majority in methadone treatment) reported needle sharing compared with 68% of the subjects who were not in treatment. Similar findings have been reported from the United Kingdom by Klee *et al.* (1991), who reported long-term methadone maintenance to be associated with less needle sharing.

In a study which more specifically isolated needle sharing as opposed to injecting, Longshore *et al.* (1993) surveyed a sample of 258 injecting opioid users in California, 41% of whom were attending for methadone treatment when they were interviewed. Those in methadone treatment were less likely to report sharing in the year prior to interview (63% when compared with 79% of those not in treatment; odds ratio = 0.43). When those who shared were examined, those in treatment shared, on average, on less occasions than those out of treatment. These relationships were relatively unaltered when background characteristics were adjusted for in a multivariate regression. Those in treatment injected less often and there was a relationship between less frequent injecting and sharing. Even after adjusting for frequency of injection, methadone treatment was significantly related to reduced sharing.

Williams *et al.* (1992) reported on 108 injecting opioid users who attended, or at one time attended, a methadone program in Connecticut in the USA. Participants were tested for HIV antibody at enrolment in the study and every six months thereafter. Comparisons were made between subjects who were in treatment continuously during the follow-up period and subjects who did not attend or who had interrupted treatment during the follow-up period. Those who received continuous treatment reported less sharing and shared with less partners than those whose treatment was interrupted. Although there was a trend favouring methadone treatment, there were no differences in HIV seroconversion during the follow-up period between the two groups. However, the number of subjects seroconverting was small and the sample size may have been indadequate and the study period too short to detect a difference.

Stark and Müller (1993), in a survey of 472 injecting drug users recruited from a number of different sources in Berlin during 1992, reported that being enrolled in methadone maintenance treatment was associated with less needle sharing (35% versus 51%). Caplehorn and Ross (1995) report similar findings from an analysis of data collected on 1,241 injecting drug users who participated in a survey conducted during 1989 in Sydney, Australia. Caplehorn and Ross (1995) estimated the odds of needle sharing to be almost halved among methadone maintenance patients compared with injecting drug users not in methadone treatment (odds ratio = 0.55, 95% CI = 0.33 to 0.90).

The studies reviewed in this section have consistently shown methadone maintenance to be associated with reductions in the sharing of injecting equipment, the main risk factor for the transmission of blood-borne viruses among injecting drug users. These findings provide further confirmation that methadone maintenance treatment has an important role to play in preventing such infections among injecting opioid users.

A Cautionary Tale: Low Threshold Methadone Programs in The Netherlands

The studies reviewed above strongly indicate that methadone maintenance is protective against HIV infection and is associated with reductions in injection-related risk behaviour. However, a recent series of studies from The Netherlands have failed to find these associations. The possible reasons for this failure are instructive and, when considered in the light of the other evidence reviewed in this book, suggest that methadone maintenance may only be effective in preventing HIV infection when it is delivered at an adequate dose level.

During the 1980s, innovative methadone programs were developed in The Netherlands which, besides traditional treatment in methadone clinics, offered methadone dispensing through a distribution network of buses and small clinics. These programs, which have become known as "low threshold" programs, have relaxed criteria for enrolment and make few therapeutic demands on clients in terms of attendance, counselling and urine testing (Buning *et al*, 1990). The goals of these programs were initially to stabilise drug use and provide for regular contact with opioid users, so that their social and medical needs might be met (Buning, *et al.*, 1990; van Ameijden *et al.*, 1992). Although it was not originally a specific goal of the program, it was hoped that the provision of methadone would also help in reducing and preventing the spread of HIV and other blood-borne infections through a reduction in injecting frequency and an increased exposure to AIDS education materials.

Hartgers *et al.* (1992) evaluated low threshold methadone programs in Amsterdam for the period 1985 to 1989 and found that they did not reduce the risk for, or the spread of, HIV infection. In a further series of studies that continued to follow the same cohort through to 1992, van Ameijden and colleagues found no evidence of a protective effect for daily methadone attendance on incidence of HIV or hepatitis B or C infection, level of injection-related HIV risk behaviour, or the transition from non-injecting to injecting opioid use (van Ameijden *et al.* 1994a; van Ameijden *et al.*, 1994b; van Ameijden, *et al.*, 1992; van Ameijden, *et al.*, 1993). Hartgers *et al.* (1992) and van Ameijden (1994) speculated that the use of less than optimal doses of methadone (<40 mg per day) may be responsible for this apparent lack of effectiveness and that higher doses of methadone may be necessary to achieve better outcomes. This hypothesis is supported by the two findings reported above of a dose-response relationship between methadone dose and HIV infection (Brown *et al.*, 1989; Serpelloni *et al.*, 1994).

CONCLUSION

On the basis of the research conducted to the present, it can be concluded that methadone maintenance reduces injection-related risk behaviour among injecting opioid users and that this reduction in risk behaviour is reflected in the finding by a number of independent researchers on different continents that enrolment in methadone maintenance treatment protects against HIV infection. An important qualification to this conclusion is that this remains true only while patients remain in treatment and while they are receiving adequate doses of methadone. While this evidence is clear with regard to HIV, it is less clear when hepatitis B and C are considered. The latter two viruses appear to be more virulent than HIV and by the time people who inject opioids present for treatment they have usually already been exposed to these viruses. Where populations of injecting drug users have high carriage rates of hepatitis B and C, it is unlikely that methadone maintenance treatment will have the opportunity to exert a protective effect.

SUMMARY

An important aspect of assessing the effectiveness of methadone maintenance treatment is the extent to which it contributes to preventing the spread of blood-borne viruses, such as HIV and hepatitis B and C, among injecting opioid users. There is now reasonably strong evidence that methadone maintenance treatment reduces injection-related HIV risk-taking behaviour and thereby reduces the risk of infection with HIV among its recipients. However, while in principle this should translate into a similar preventive effect for hepatitis B and C transmission, there is, as yet, little published research with which to evaluate this inference. Moreover, because there is a very high carriage rate for these two viruses among populations of injecting opioid users when they enter treatment, there is much less of an opportunity for preventing infection. The conclusion that methadone maintenance treatment reduces the risk of HIV infection among injecting opioid users is only valid for those programs that use adequate doses of methadone (>60 mg per day) and adopt maintenance rather than abstinence as the goal of treatment. Evidence from The Netherlands suggests that methadone programs that dispense less than adequate doses of methadone will not be effective in preventing the spread of HIV among drug users who inject opioids.

REFERENCES

Abdul-Quader, A. S., Friedman, S. R., Des Jarlais, D., Marmor, M. M., Maslansky, R., & Bartelme, S. (1987). Methadone maintenance and behavior by intravenous drug users that can transmit HIV. *Contemporary Drug Problems, 14,* 425-434.

Ball, J. C., Lange, W. R., Myers, C. P., & Friedman, S. R. (1988). Reducing the risk of AIDS through methadone maintenance treatment. *Journal of Health and Social Behavior, 29,* 214-226.

Ball, J. C., & Ross, A. (1991). *The effectiveness of methadone maintenance treatment: Patients, programs, services, and outcome.* New York: Springer-Verlag.

Bell, J., Batey, R. G., Farrell, G. C., Crewe, E. B., Cunningham, A. L., & Byth, K. (1990a). Hepatitis C virus in intravenous drug users. *Medical Journal of Australia, 153,* 274-276.

Bell, J., Fernandes, D., & Batey, R. (1990b). Heroin users seeking methadone treatment. *Medical Journal of Australia, 152,* 361-364.

Blix, O., & Grönbladh, L. (1988). AIDS and IV heroin addicts: The preventive effect of methadone maintenance in Sweden. Paper presented to 4th International Conference on AIDS, Stockholm, 1988.

Blix, O., & Grönbladh, L. (1991). The impact of methadone maintenance treatment on the spread of HIV among IV heroin addicts in Sweden. In N. Loimer, R. Schmid, & A. Springer (Eds.), *Drug addiction and AIDS* (pp. 200-205). Vienna: Springer-Verlag.

Brown, L. S., Chu, A., Nemoto, T., Ajuluchukwu, D., & Primm, B. J. (1989). Human immunodeficiency virus infection in a cohort of intravenous drug users in New York City: Demographic, behavioral, and clinical features. *New York State Journal of Medicine, 89*, 506-510.

Buning, E. C., Van Brussel, G. H. A., & Van Stanten, G. V. (1990). The 'methadone by bus' project in Amsterdam. *British Journal of Addiction, 85*, 1247-1250.

Caplehorn, J. R. M., & Ross, M. (1995). Methadone maintenance and the likelihood of risky needle sharing. *International Journal of the Addictions, 30*, 685-698.

Chaisson, R. E., Bacchetti, P., Osmond, D., Brodie, B., Sande, M. A., & Moss, A. R. (1989). Cocaine use and HIV infection in intravenous drug users in San Francisco. *Journal of the American Medical Association, 261*, 561-565.

Chitwood, D. D., Griffin, D. K., Comerford, M., Page, J. B., Trapido, E. J., Lai, S., & McCoy, C. B. (1995). Risk factors for HIV-1 seroconversion among injection drug users: A case-control study. *American Journal of Public Health, 85*, 1538-1542.

Crofts, N., Hopper, J. L., Bowden, D. S., Breschkin, A. M., Milner, R., & Locarnini, S. A. (1993). Hepatitis C virus infection among a cohort of Victorian injecting drug users. *Medical Journal of Australia, 159*, 237-241.

Darke, S., Hall, W., & Carless, J. (1990). Drug use, injecting practices and sexual behaviour of opioid users in Sydney, Australia. *British Journal of Addiction, 85*, 1603-1609.

Des Jarlais, D. C. (1992). The first and second decades of AIDS among injecting drug users. *British Journal of Addiction, 87*, 347-353.

Des Jarlais, D. C., Friedman, S. R., Novick, D. M., Sotheran, J. L., Thomas, P., Yancovitz, S. R., Mildvan, D., Weber, J., Kreek, M. J., Maslansky, R., Bartelme, S., Spira, T., & Marmor, M. (1989). HIV-1 infection among intravenous drug users in Manhattan, New York City, from 1977 through 1987. *Journal of the American Medical Association, 261*, 1008-1012.

Des Jarlais, D. C., Hagan, H., Friedman, S. R., Friedmann, P., Goldberg, D., Frischer, M., Green, S., Tunving, K., Ljungberg, B., Wodak, A., Ross, M., Purchase, D., Millson, M. E., & Myers, T. (1995). Maintaining low HIV seroprevalence in populations of injecting drug users. *Journal of the American Medical Association, 274*, 1226-1231.

Friedland, G. (1989). Parenteral drug users. In R. A. Kaslow & D. P. Francis (Eds.), *The epidemiology of AIDS: Expression, occurrence, and control of Human Immunodeficiency Virus type 1 infection* (pp. 153-179). New York: Oxford University Press.

Friedman, S. R., Jose, B., Deren, S., Des Jarlais, D. C., & Neaigus, A. (1995). Risk factors for human immunodeficiency virus seroconversion among out-of-treatment drug injectors in high and low seroprevalence cities. *American Journal of Epidemiology,* **142**, 864-874.

Gossop, M., & Grant, M. (1991). A six country survey of the content and structure of heroin treatment programmes using methadone. *British Journal of Addiction,* **86**, 1151-1160.

Hartgers, C., van den Hoek, A., Krijnen, P., & Coutinho, R. A. (1992). HIV prevalence and risk behavior among injecting drug users who participate in "low-threshold" methadone programs in Amsterdam. *American Journal of Public Health,* **82**(4), 547-51.

Institute of Medicine (1995). *Federal regulation of methadone treatment.* Washington: National Academy Press.

Joseph, H. (1988). The criminal justice system and opiate addiction: A historical perspective. In C. G. Leukefeld & F. M. Tims (Eds.), *Compulsory treatment of drug abuse: Research and clinical practice* (NIDA Research Monograph No. 86, pp. 106-125). Rockville, MD: National Institute on Drug Abuse.

Klee, H., Faugier, J., Hayes, C., & Morris, J. (1991). The sharing of injecting equipment among drug users attending prescribing clinics and those using needle-exchanges. *British Journal of Addiction,* **86**, 217-233.

Levine, O. S., Vlahov, D., Koehler, J., Cohn, S., Spronk, A. M., & Nelson, K. E. (1995). Seroepidemiology of hepatitis B virus in a population of injecting drug users. *American Journal of Epidemiology,* **142**, 331-341.

Levine, O. S., Vlahov, D., & Nelson, K. E. (1994). Epidemiology of hepatitis B virus infections amng injecting drug users: Seroprevalence, risk factors, and viral interactions. *Epidemiologic Reviews,* **16**, 418-436.

Longshore, D., Hsieh, S., Danila, B., & Anglin, M. D. (1993). Methadone maintenance and needle/syringe sharing. *International Journal of the Addictions,* **28**, 983-996.

MacDonald, M., Crofts, N., & Kaldor, J. (1996). Transmission of HCV: Rates, routes and cofactors. Unpublished manuscript, National Centre in HIVEpidemiology and Clinical Research, University of New South Wales, Australia.

Marmor, M., Des Jarlais, D. C., Cohen, H., Friedman, S. R., Beatrice, S. T., Dubin, N., El-Sadr, W., Mildvan, D., Yancovitz, S. R., Mathur, U., & Holzman, R. (1987). Risk factors for infection with human immunodeficiency virus among intravenous drug abusers in New York City. *AIDS,* **1**, 39-44.

Metzger, D. S., Woody, G. E., McLellan, A. T., O'Brien, C. P., Druley, P., Navaline, H., DePhilippis, D., Stolley, P., & Abrutyn, E. (1993). Human Immunodeficiency Virus seroconversion among intravenous drug users in- and out-of-treatment: An 18-month prospective follow-up. *Journal of Acquired Immune Deficiency Syndromes,* **6**, 1049-1055.

Moss, A. R., Vranizan, K., Gorter, R., Bacchetti, P., Watters, J., & Osmond, D. (1994). HIV seroconversion in intravenous drug users in San

Francisco 1985-1990. *AIDS, 8*, 223-231.

Novick, D. M., Joseph, H., Croxson, T. S., Salsitz, E. A., Wang, G., Richman, B. L., Poretsky, L., Keefe, J. B., & Whimbey, E. (1990). Absence of antibody to human immunodeficiency virus in long-term, socially rehabilitated methadone maintenance patients. *Archives of Internal Medicine, 150*, 97-99.

Patti, A. M., Santi, A. L., Pompa, M. G., Giustini, C., Vescia, N., Mastroeni, I., & Fara, G. M. (1993). Viral hepatitis and drugs: A continuing problem. *International Journal of Epidemiology, 22*, 135-139.

Schoenbaum, E. E., Hartel, D., Selwyn, P. A., Klein, R. S., Davenny, K., Rogers, M., Feiner, C., & Friedland, G. (1989). Risk factors for human immunodeficiency virus infection in intravenous drug users. *New England Journal of Medicine, 321*, 874-879.

Selwyn, P. A., Feiner, C., Cox, C. P., Lipshutz, C., & Cohen, R. L. (1987). Knowledge about AIDS and high-risk behavior among intravenous drug users in New York City. *AIDS, 1*, 247-254.

Serpelloni, G., Carrieri, M. P., Rezza, G., Morganti, S., Gomma, M., & Binkin, N. (1994). Methadone treatment as a determinant of HIV risk reduction among injecting drug users: A nested case control study. *AIDS Care, 16*, 215-220.

Stark, K., & Müller, R. (1993). HIV prevalence and risk behaviour in injecting drug users in Berlin. *Forensic Science International, 62*, 73-81.

Thomas, D. L., Vlahov, D., Solomon, L., Cohn, S., Taylor, E., Garfein, R., & Nelson, K. E. (1995). Correlates of hepatitis C virus infections among injection drug users. *Medicine, 74*, 212-220.

Uchtenhagen, A. (1990). Policy and practice of methadone maintenance: An analysis of worldwide experience. In A. Arif & J. Westermeyer (Eds.), *Methadone maintenance in the management of opioid dependence: An international review* (pp. 55-74). New York: Praeger.

van Ameijden, E. J. C. (1994) *Evaluation of AIDS-prevention measures among drug users: The Amsterdam experience.* Doctoral dissertation, University of Amsterdam, Amsterdam, The Netherlands.

van Ameijden, E. J. C., van den Hoek, A. A. R., & Coutinho, R. A. (1994a). Injecting risk behavior among drug users in Amsterdam, 1986 to 1992, and its relationship to AIDS prevention programs. *American Journal of Public Health, 84*, 275-281.

van Ameijden, E. J. C., van den Hoek, A. A. R., Hartgers, C., & Coutinho, R. A. (1994b). Risk factors for the transition from noninjection to injection drug use and accompanying AIDS risk behaviour in a cohort of drug users. *American Journal of Epidemiology, 139*, 1153-1163.

van Ameijden, E. J. C., van den Hoek, A. A. R., van Haastrecht, H. J. A., & Coutinho, R. A. (1992). The harm reduction approach and risk factors for Human Immunodeficiency Virus (HIV) seroconversion among injecting drug users, Amsterdam. *American Journal of Epidemiology,* **136,** 236-243.

van Ameijden, E. J. C., van den Hoek, J. A. R., Mientjes, G. H. C., & Coutinho, R. A. (1993). A longitudinal study on the incidence and transmission patterns of HIV, HBV and HCV infection among drug users in Amsterdam. *European Journal of Epidemiology,* **9,** 255-262.

Williams, A. B., McNelly, E. A., Williams, A. E., & D'Quila, R. T. (1992). Methadone maintenance treatment and HIV type 1 seroconversion among injecting drug users. *AIDS Care,* **4,** 35-41.

4

THE EFFECTIVENESS OF METHADONE MAINTENANCE TREATMENT 3: MODERATORS OF TREATMENT OUTCOME

SHANE DARKE

INTRODUCTION

The preceding chapters examined the evidence for the effectiveness of methadone maintenance. The present chapter addresses potential moderators of methadone maintenance treatment outcome, factors that have been associated with riskier behaviours and may indicate a poorer prognosis. The factors chosen for discussion in this chapter are all pertinent to methadone maintenance patients, and have all been shown to relate to riskier behaviours and poorer psychosocial functioning. These factors fall into three main areas: drug use other than heroin, psychopathology and methadone dose diversion.

DRUG USE OTHER THAN HEROIN

The two drug classes that have been associated in recent years with higher risk behaviours and poorer general functioning are the benzodiazepines and cocaine. Both drug classes are widely used by heroin users, and both appear to indicate poorer treatment prognosis.

Benzodiazepines

Studies conducted in Europe, the US and Australia consistently indicate that benzodiazepine use is widespread among both treated and untreated heroin users (Ball & Ross, 1991; Barnas *et al.*, 1992; Darke, 1994; Darke *et al.*, 1992b; Darke *et al.*, 1994c; Donoghoe *et al.*, 1992; DuPont, 1988; Klee *et al.*, 1990; Stitzer *et al.*, 1981). Three quarters of heroin users in the Treatment Outcome Prospective Study reported using benzodiazepines in the preceding year (DuPont, 1988). Ball and Ross (1991) report a third of clients having used benzodiazepines regularly prior to methadone maintenance, and that a third of clients had used benzodiazepines in the first six months after their entry to treatment. Over a third (37%) of Australian methadone maintenance patients reported benzodiazepine use in the month preceding interview (Darke *et al.*, 1994c). Similar figures have been reported among British heroin users (Donoghoe *et al.*, 1992; Klee *et al.*, 1990). It is worthy of note that there is tentative evidence that the subjective effects of methadone are enhanced by the use of benzodiazepines (Preston *et al.*, 1984).

The widespread use of benzodiazepines constitutes a major clinical problem. The use of these drugs has been linked to higher levels of needle sharing, higher levels of poly-drug use, an increased chance of injecting during methadone maintenance, higher levels of psychopathology, higher levels of criminal activities, as well as poorer health and poorer social functioning (Darke *et al*, 1992a; Darke *et al.*, 1994c; Donoghoe *et al.*, 1992; Klee *et al.*, 1990; Metzger *et al.*, 1991). There is also evidence that the use of benzodiazepines is associated with both fatal (Zador *et al.*, 1996) and non-fatal (Klee *et al.*, 1990, Darke *et al.*, 1996b; Gutierrez-Cebollada *et al.*, 1994) heroin overdose. The overall clinical picture of benzodiazepine users is of a more risky, distressed and chaotic lifestyle than other heroin users.

A worrying trend that has arisen in recent years has been the practice of injecting benzodiazepine tablets (Klee *et al.*, 1990; Darke *et al.*, 1995; Strang *et al.*, 1994; Strang *et al*, 1992). The injection of benzodiazepines presents clinical problems in itself, as the practice is associated with vascular morbidity and mortality (Ralston & Taylor, 1993; Ruben & Morrison, 1992).

One research finding that has direct clinical relevance is that heroin users make meaningful distinctions between different types of benzodiazepines. Heroin users in the U.S., Europe, Australia and Asia show distinct preferences for quick-onset benzodiazepines (such as flunitrazepam and diazepam) and for the easily injectable temazepam gel preparations (Barnas *et al.*, 1992; Darke *et al.*, 1995; Iguchi *et al.*, 1990; Navaratnum *et al.*, 1990).

From a treatment perspective, the evidence clearly indicates that benzodiazepine users require particular attention. They are likely to exhibit overall patterns of increased risk and poorer psychosocial functioning than other clients. Given the strong associations with overall dysfunction, extreme caution should be exercised in prescribing these drugs in the context of methadone maintenance. If benzodiazepines are prescribed, it is recommended that those with particularly high abuse potential (e.g., flunitrazepam, diazepam, temazepam) should be avoided.

Cocaine

The second major drug class that has caused concern among clinicians, particularly in the United States, is cocaine. The use of cocaine is widespread among methadone maintenance patients in the United States (Ball & Ross, 1991; Chaisson *et al.*, 1989; Grella *et al.*, 1995; Kang & DeLeon, 1993; Kosten *et al.*, 1987; Meandzija *et al.*, 1994; Metzger *et al.*, 1993; Schoembaum *et al.*, 1989; Strain *et al.*, 1993). One-half of methadone maintenance admissions in the eastern US reported by Ball & Ross (1991) and by Strain *et al.*, (1993) reported cocaine use in the month preceding admission. Three quarters of admissions to a Los Angeles methadone maintenance program had used cocaine in the year prior to admission (Grella *et al.*, 1995), while a similar proportion of New York methadone maintenance patients reported a history of cocaine injecting (Schoembaum *et al.*, 1989). As with the benzodiazepines, the concomitant use of cocaine by heroin users is widespread, at least in the U.S. and in parts of Europe (e.g., The Netherlands, Switzerland).

Cocaine injecting, both independently and in combination with heroin ('speedballs') has been strongly associated with more frequent injections, more frequent needle sharing, increased sexual risk-taking, more frequent use of shooting galleries, and a higher HIV seroprevalence (Chaisson *et al*, 1989; Schoembaum *et al*, 1989). The association between cocaine use and HIV risk-taking has also been reported in Europe (Darke *et al.*, 1992a) and Australia (Torrens *et al.*, 1991). It is important to note that the link between cocaine use and HIV risk is not restricted to the parenteral use of the drug. Crack smoking has been independently linked to higher levels of needle risk in crack users who also inject, to sexual risk-taking and to HIV serostatus (Grella *et al.*, 1995, Chiasson *et al.*, 1991; Chirgwin *et al.*, 1991; DesJalais *et al.*, 1992).

Two mechanisms may underlie the relationship between cocaine use and higher levels of HIV risk-taking. Firstly, the relatively short half-life of cocaine may result in greater frequency of injecting than that typically seen for heroin. Secondly, disinhibition resulting from cocaine use may lead to higher levels of risky sexual activity and needle use, irrespective of whether the cocaine is smoked or injected.

While use of cocaine is related to continued risk, there is evidence that methadone maintenance tretament reduces the prevalence and frequency of cocaine use, as well as of heroin (Ball & Ross, 1991, Meandzija *et al.*, 1994; Metzger *et al.*, 1993; Strain *et al.*, 1993). Meandzija *et al.*, (1994) reported the total monthly cocaine use of methadone maintenance patients as 60-70% less than non-treatment subjects, with less frequent injecting both of cocaine and of speedballs. A similar disparity was reported by Metzger *et al.* (1993). Ball and Ross (1991) reported that 24% of patients who had been in methadone maintenance for more than six months had used cocaine in the preceding month, compared to 47% of patients enrolled for less than six months. Given that there is no known pharmacologic action between methadone and cocaine, it has been hypothesised that the reduction in cocaine use relates to the reduction of heroin use, *i.e.*, reduced heroin use results in fewer speedball injections, and thus less cocaine use (Strain *et al.*, 1993). The general stabilisation of lifestyle associated with methadone maintenance might also explain some of this reduction.

As with the benzodiazepines, cocaine use is a clear marker of increased risk. Retention in methadone maintenance treatment, however, may significantly reduce this risk.

PSYCHOPATHOLOGY

Antisocial Personality Disorder

A diagnosis of antisocial personality disorder (ASPD), along with mood and anxiety disorders, is one of the three most common psychiatric diagnoses made among injecting drug users. The prevalence of diagnoses of ASPD among heroin users has ranged from 35% to 61% (Brooner *et al.*, 1992; Brooner *et al.*, 1993; Darke *et al.*, 1994a; Rounsaville *et al.*, 1991; Strain *et al.*, 1991a; Woody *et al.*, 1985). Given the estimated lifetime prevalence of 4% among the general population (Robins *et al.*, 1991), in all studies conducted to date the prevalence of ASPD among heroin users has exceeded the population prevalence by many orders of magnitude. To date, there is no known treatment for ASPD (Quality Assurance Project, 1991).

Heroin users with a diagnosis of ASPD have been found to have an earlier onset of drug use and injecting, and to be more likely to meet the criteria for diagnoses of substance abuse and dependence for drugs other than heroin (Brooner *et al.*, 1992; Brooner *et al.*, 1993; Darke *et al.*, 1994a; Gill *et al.*, 1992).

The primary clinical significance of the diagnosis of ASPD concerns the reported association between the diagnosis and higher levels of HIV risk-taking. Heroin users with a diagnosis of ASPD have been reported in these studies to share injecting equipment more frequently, have more needle sharing partners and more sexual partners, as well as a higher HIV seroprevalence than other heroin users (Brooner *et al.*, 1992; Brooner *et al.*, 1993; Nolimal & Crowley, 1989).

The evidence for the broader effects of a diagnosis of ASPD on methadone maintenance outcome are currently ambiguous (Darke *et al.*, 1994a; Gill *et al.*, 1992; Rouser *et al.*, 1994; Rutherford *et al.*, 1994; Woody *et al.*, 1985). Woody *et al.*, (1985) reported that ASPD patients in methadone maintenance treatment performed more poorly at seven-month follow-up than other patients over a range of outcome variables. Several subsequent studies, however, have indicated that ASPD clients may respond as well as other patients to pharmacotherapy (Darke *et al.*, 1994a; Gill *et al.*, 1992; Rouser *et al.*, 1994; Rutherford *et al.*, 1994). Gill *et al.*, (1992) reported no differences in retention, methadone dosage or drug use at one-year follow-up between ASPD and other patients. Rouser *et al.* (1994) also reported no differences between ASPD patients and others in retention in methadone maintenance. Darke *et al.,* (1994a) reported no significant differences in retention or drug use between methadone maintenance patients with a current diagnosis of ASPD and other patients, although the social functioning of ASPD patients was significantly poorer than other clients, findings similar to those reported by Rutherford *et al.,* (1994).

When discussing the clinical significance of a diagnosis of ASPD, problems associated with making this diagnosis among injecting drug users should be borne in mind. There is difficulty in distinguishing between the presence of a personality disorder and similar behaviours generated by the fact that the patients dependent on illegal drugs (Gerstley *et al.,* 1990). It should not be assumed that because a patient has a diagnosis of ASPD that they are "psychopathic", i.e. characterised by an inability to experience guilt, remorse or anxiety (Hare *et al.,* 1991). In a great many cases, the diagnosis may simply be a marker for a more risky, chaotic lifestyle.

Clinically, patients with a diagnosis of ASPD may enter treatment with higher overall risk-taking and longer standing drug problems. Indeed, the diagnosis may merely be a marker for a riskier individual, rather than being psychopathic. As such increased attention to HIV education in the methadone maintenance setting may be appropriate. While there is no demonstrated treatment for ASPD *per se,* the balance of evidence to date indicates that ASPD patients can be successfully retained in methadone maintenance, and perform as well in treatment as other patients.

Psychological Distress

Research has repeatedly shown that heroin users experience high levels of psychological distress (Corty *et al.,* 1988; Khantzian & Treece, 1985; Limbeek *et al.,* 1992; Rounsaville *et al.,* 1982b; Steer *et al.,* 1992). Rounsaville *et al.* (1982b) reported that a quarter of a sample of heroin users currently in treatment met DSM-III criteria for a current affective disorder, with 12% qualifying for a diagnosis of an anxiety disorder. Khantzian and Treece (1985) reported three quarters of a sample of treatment and untreated heroin users met the criteria for an Axis I diagnosis. Sixty percent qualified for a diagnosis of an affective disorder and 11% for an anxiety disorder. Among current methadone maintenance patients, Strain *et al.* (1991b) reported 20% having experienced an episode of major depression. Similarly, Corty *et al.* (1988) found the most common current psychiatric symptoms among methadone maintenance patients were anxiety (23%) and depression (17%).

Among Australian samples, studies employing the General Health Questionnaire have also yielded high levels of distress among heroin users. Swift *et al.* (1990) reported a current prevalence of psychiatric morbidity of 61% among opioid users seeking methadone maintenance treatment, while Darke *et al.* (1994b) reported a similarly high proportion (58%) among current methadone maintenance patients.

The relevance of the high prevalence of psychological distress among opioid users concerns the relationship of distress to poorer treatment outcome (Kosten *et al.*, 1986; McLellan *et al.*, 1983a; McLellan *et al.*, 1983b; Metzger *et al.*, 1991; Rounsaville *et al.*, 1985; Woody *et al.*, 1983; Woody *et al.*, 1987), a number of studies having reported such a relationship. Kosten *et al.* (1986) reported that methadone maintenance patients diagnosed with depression at intake were less likely to be abstinent at 2.5-year follow-up than other patients. McLellan *et al.* (1983a) reported treatment outcome for opiate users at six month follow-up was related to psychiatric severity: high severity patients exhibited poor outcome performance regardless of treatment modality, while low severity patients improved regardless of modality. Metzger *et al.* (1991) reported that among current methadone maintenance patients, needle sharing in the six preceding months was significantly related to higher levels of depression, as measured by the BDI, and higher SCL-90 scores. Higher BDI scores were also related to continued injecting among Australian methadone maintenance patients (Darke *et al.*, 1994d). Finally, Rounsaville *et al.* (1985) reported success of opioid detoxification was best predicted by initial general psychiatric symptomatology, determined by the SCL-90. While the majority of studies have linked psychiatric distress to poorer treatment outcome, Ball and Ross (1991) found no relationship among a large sample of methadone maintenance patients.

The research data overall indicate that psychiatric comorbidity is prevalent among heroin users, and that psychiatric distress is generally associated with poorer treatment performance. The data also indicate that methadone maintenance can reduce levels of patient distress. Rounsaville *et al.* (1982a) found significant improvements in BDI scores and in all areas of the SCL-90 six months after treatment commenced. McLellan *et al.* (1982) reported a significant decrease in scores on the ASI psychiatric severity scale six months after treatment commencement. Woody *et al.* (1987) reported significant reductions in psychological distress among methadone maintenance patients at 12 month follow-up. Patients who had adjunctive psychotherapy exhibited greater improvement in psychological distress, and across a wider range of variables than methadone-only patients.

There is evidence that reductions in psychiatric distress may commence early in methadone maintenance treatment. Strain *et al.* (1991b) reported significant improvements in BDI scores within the first week of treatment, whereas Dorus and Senay (1980) found the greatest reductions in BDI scores to occur within the first four months of treatment.

In summary, a high proportion of methadone maintenance patients experience psychological distress, and high levels of distress may impede treatment outcome. The research also indicates that methadone maintenance treatment may itself contribute to an amelioration of patients' symptoms of depression and anxiety.

METHADONE DIVERSION

The issue of methadone dose diversion is relevant to a chapter of potential moderators of treatment outcome for several reasons. First, patients who divert their doses are not receiving their full medication schedule, and may 'top up' with heroin. Second, diverted doses may also be used by non-treatment users. Finally, diverted doses may be injected, both by methadone maintenance patients and other heroin users.

Despite controls on its the distribution of methadone, dose diversion does occur, and has been a concern for some time. Inciardi (1977), reported that 46% of a sample of U.S. heroin users had used illicit methadone during the week prior to interview, 70% having used illicit methadone in the three months prior to interview. Weppner *et al.* (1972), in 1972, reported a lifetime prevalence of illicit methadone use of 43% among patients admitted to Lexington hospital for opiate detoxification. More recently, 34% of methadone patients interviewed in Spunt *et al.* (1986) reported having diverted their methadone dose. Lauzon *et al.* (1994) reported a lifetime prevalence of illicit methadone use of 59% among a sample of Canadian heroin users, 42% of whom reported having used illicit methadone in the preceding six months. Half (52%) of a sample of Australian heroin users had injected methadone, 29% in the preceding six months (Darke *et al.*, 1996a). In the latter study, current methadone patients were more likely to have recently injected methadone than other heroin users.

The harms associated with methadone diversion, whether to patients or to others, have rarely been investigated. Between the years 1987-1991 in Harris County, Texas, there were 91 deaths in which methadone was detected. Only 20% of these decedents were currently enrolled in methadone maintenance at the time of death (Institute of Medicine, 1995). Methadone injectors in the Australian study cited above (Darke *et al.*, 1995b) were in poorer general health, had more injection-related symptoms, were twice as likely to have been diagnosed with a venous thrombosis, were more likely to have recently overdosed, have higher levels of psychological distress, and to have recently committed criminal acts.

The primary source of diverted methadone appears to be take-away doses (Darke *et al.*, 1996a; Lauzon *et al.*, 1994; Institute of Medicine, 1995; Spunt *et al.*, 1986). Given the harms associated with patients' injecting of methadone, and harms caused by diversion to heroin users not in treatment, caution appears warranted in the provision of take-away doses. This is not to say that clinicians should not prescribe take-away doses. Rather they should be aware that diversion of doses does occur, and that substantial harms can result. Careful monitoring and control of take-away doses, together with cautious clinical judgement, appear warranted.

SUMMARY

The variables discussed in this chapter, independently and in conjunction, may have deleterious effects on the course of methadone maintenance treatment. Several points need to be made regarding these variables. First, there is encouraging evidence that many of these factors respond positively to methadone maintenance. Reductions in psychiatric distress are illustrative. While high levels of distress appear to portend poorer treatment outcome, the evidence indicates that methadone maintenance can *reduce* levels of distress, thus improving the treatment prognosis. A similar argument can be made regarding cocaine use during treatment. Second, methadone maintenance substantially reduces the mortality and morbidity associated with injecting drug use (Caplehorn *et al.*, 1994; Grönbladh *et al.*, 1990).

Keeping patients in the treatment system, even those with factors indicating a poor prognosis, would thus appear to be a priority. Third, at least some of the problem factors discussed in this chapter can be ameliorated by careful clinical management. The prescription of benzodiazepines and of take-away methadone doses are cases in point. Prescribers can reduce the harms associated with these factors in the treatment setting by exercising cautious clinical judgement in prescribing.

In summary, the factors described in this chapter may indeed indicate poorer treatment outcome. However, retention of these patients in the treatment setting may produce substantial clinical improvement, and improve their prognosis.

REFERENCES

Ball, J.C., & Ross, A. (1991). *The effectiveness of methadone treatment. Patients, programs, services, and outcome.* New York: Springer-Verlag.

Barnas, C., Rossman, M., Roessler, H., Reimer, Y., & Fleischhacker, W. (1992). Benzodiazepines and other psychotropic drugs abused by patients in a methadone maintenance program. *Journal of Clinical Pharmacology,* **12,** 397-402.

Brooner, R.K., Greenfield, L., Schmidt, C.W., & Bigelow, G.E. (1993). Antisocial personality disorder and HIV infection in drug abusers, *American Journal of Psychiatry,* **150,** 53-58.

Brooner, R.K., Bigelow, G.E., Strain, E., & Schmidt, C.W. (1990). Intravenous drug abusers with anti-social personality disorder: Increased HIV risk behaviour. *Drug and Alcohol Dependence,* **26,** 39-44.

Brooner, R.K., Schmidt, C.W., Felch, L.J., & Bigelow, G.E. (1992). Antisocial behaviour of intravenous drug abusers: Implications for antisocial personality disorder. *American Journal of Psychiatry,* **149,** 482-487.

Caplehorn, J.R.M., Dalton, M.S.Y.M., Cluff, M.C., & Petrenas, A.M. (1994). Retention in methadone maintenance and heroin addicts' risk of death. *Addiction,* **89,** 203-207.

Chaisson, R.E., Bacchetti, P., Osmond, D., Brodie, B., Sande, M.A., & Moss, A.R. (1989). Cocaine use and HIV infection in intravenous drug users in San Francisco. *JAMA,* **261,** 561-565.

Chiasson, M.A., Stoneburner, R.L., Hildebrandt, D.J., Ewing, W.E., Telzak, E.E., Jaffe, H.W. (1991). Heterosexual transmission of HIV-I associated with the use of smokable freebase cocaine (crack). *AIDS,* **5,** 1121-1126.

Chirgwin, K., DeHovitz, J.A., Dillon, S., & McCormack, W.M. (1991). HIV infection, genital ulcer disease and crack cocaine use among patients attending a clinic for sexually transmitted diseases. *American Journal of Public Health*, **81**, 1576-1579.

Corty, E., Ball, J.C., & Myers, C.P. (1988). Psychological symptoms in methadone maintenance patients: Prevalence and change over treatment. *Journal of Consulting and Clinical Psychology*, **56**, 776-777.

Darke, S. (1994). The use of benzodiazepines among injecting drug users. *Drug and Alcohol Review*, **13**, 63-69.

Darke, S., Baker, A., Dixon, J., Wodak, A., & Heather, N. (1992a). Drug use and HIV risk-taking behaviour among clients in methadone maintenance treatment. *Drug and Alcohol Dependence*, **29**, 263-268.

Darke, S., Hall, W., Ross, M.W., & Wodak, A. (1992b). Benzodiazepine use and HIV risk-taking behaviour among injecting drug users. *Drug and Alcohol Dependence*, **31**, 31-36.

Darke, S., Hall, W., & Swift, W. (1994a). Prevalence, symptoms and correlates of anti-social personality disorder among methadone maintenance clients. *Drug and Alcohol Dependence*, **34**, 253-257.

Darke, S., Ross, J., & Hall, W. (1995). Preferences and routes of administration in the use of benzodiazepines among injecting heroin users. *Medical Journal of Australia*, **162**, 645-647.

Darke, S., Ross, J., & Hall, W. (1996a). Prevalence and correlates of the injection of methadone syrup in Sydney, Australia. *Drug and Alcohol Dependence*, **43**, 191-198.

Darke, S., Ross, J., & Hall, W. (1996b). Overdose among heroin users in Sydney, Australia I. Prevalence and correlates of non-fatal overdose. *Addiction*, **91**, 405-411.

Darke, S., Swift, W., & Hall, W. (1994b). Prevalence, severity and correlates of psycho-logical morbidity among methadone maintenance clients. *Addiction*, **89**, 229-235.

Darke, S., Swift, W., Hall, W., & Ross, M. (1994c). Drug use, HIV risk-taking and psychosocial correlates of benzodiazepine use among methadone maintenance clients. *Drug and Alcohol Dependence*, **31**, 31-36.

Darke, S., Swift, W., Hall, W., & Ross, M. (1994d). Predictors of injecting and injecting risk-taking behaviour among methadone maintenance clients. *Addiction*, **89**, 331-336.

Des Jarlais, D.C., Wenston, J., Friedman, S.R., Sotheran, J.L., Maslansky, R., & Marmor, M. (1992). Crack cocaine use in a cohort of methadone maintenance patients. *Journal of Substance Abuse Treatment*, **9**, 319-325.

Donoghoe, M.C., Dolan, K.A., & Stimsom, G.V. (1992). Life-style factors and social circumstances of syringe sharing in injecting drug users. *British Journal of Addiction*, **87**, 993-1003.

Dorus, W., & Senay, E.C. (1980). Depression, demographic dimensions, and drug abuse. *American Journal of Psychiatry*, **137**, 699-704.

DuPont, R.L. (1988). Abuse of benzodiazepines: The problems and the solutions. *American Journal of Drug and Alcohol Abuse,* 14, *(supp. 1),* 1-69.

Gerstley, L.J., Alterman, A.I., McLellan, A.T., & Woody, G.E. (1990). Antisocial personality disorder in patients with substance abuse disorders: A problematic diagnosis? *American Journal of Psychiatry,* 147, 173-178.

Gill, K., Nolimal, D., & Crowley, T.J. (1992). Antisocial personality disorder, HIV risk behaviour and retention in methadone maintenance therapy. *Drug and Alcohol Dependence,* 30, 247-252.

Grella, C.E., Anglin, M.D., & Wugalter, S.E. (1995). Cocaine and crack use and HIV risk behaviours among high-risk methadone maintenance patients. *Drug and Alcohol Dependence,* 37, 15-21.

Grönbladh, L., Ohland, L.S., & Gunne, L.M. (1990). Mortality in heroin addiction: Impact of methadone treatment, *Acta Psychiatrica Scandinavia,* 82, 223-227.

Gutierrez-Cebollada, J., de la Torre, R., Ortuno, J., Garces, J., & Cami, J. (1994). Psychotropic drug consumption and other factors associated with heroin overdose. *Drug and Alcohol Dependence,* 35, 169-174.

Hare, R.D., Hart, S.D., & Harpur, T.J. (1991). Psychopathy and the DSM-IV criteria for antisocial personality disorder. *Journal of Abnormal Psychology,* 100, 391-398.

Iguchi, M.Y., Griffiths, R.R., Bickel, W.K., Handelsman, L., Childress, A.R., & McLellan, A.T. (1990). Relative abuse liability of benzodiazepines in methadone maintained populations in three cities. In L.S. Harris (Ed.), *Problems of Drug Dependence 1989* (NIDA Research Monograph No. 95, pp. 364-365). Rockville, MD: National Institute on Drug Abuse.

Inciardi, J.A. (1977). *Methadone diversion: Experiences and issues.* Rockville, MD: National Institute on Drug Abuse.

Institute of Medicine. (1995). *Federal regulation of methadone treatment.* Washington, DC: National Academy Press.

Kang. S., & DeLeon (1993). Criminal involvement of cocaine users in a methadone program. *Addiction,* 88, 395-404.

Khantzian, E.J., & Treece, C. (1985). Psychiatric diagnosis of narcotic addicts. *Archives of General Psychiatry,* 42, 1067-1071.

Klee, H., Faugier, J., Hayes, C., Boulton, T., & Morris, J. (1990). AIDS-related risk behaviour, polydrug use and temazepam. *British Journal of Addiction,* 85, 1125-1132.

Kosten, T.R., Rounsaville, B.J., & Kleber, H.D. (1986). A 2.5 year follow-up of depression, life crises, and treatment effects on abstinence among opioid addicts. *Archives of General Psychiatry,* 43, 733-738.

Kosten, T.R., Rounsaville, B.J., & Kleber, H.D. (1987). A 2.5 year follow-up of cocaine use among opioid addicts. *Archives of General Psychiatry,* 44, 281-284.

Lauzon, P., Vincelette, J., Bruneau, J., Lamothe, F., Lachance, N., Brabant, M., & Soto, J. (1994). Illicit use of methadone among IV drug users in Montreal. *Journal of Substance Abuse Treatment,* 11, 457-461.

Limbeek, J.V., Wouters, L., Kaplan, C., Geerlings, P.J., & Alem, V.V. (1992). Prevalence of psychopathology in drug addicted Dutch. *Journal of Substance Treatment,* 9, 43-52.

McLellan, A.T., Luborsky, L., O'Brien, C.P., Woody, G.E., & Druley, K.A. (1982). Is treatment for substance abuse effective? *Journal of the American Medical Association,* 247, 1423-1428.

McLellan, A.T., Luborsky,L., Woody, G.E., O'Brien, C.P., & Druley, K.A. (1983a). Predicting response to alcohol and drug treatments. *Archives of General Psychiatry,* 40, 620-625.

McLellan, A.T., Woody, G.E., Luborsky,L., O'Brien, C.P., & Druley, K.A. (1983b). Increased effectiveness of substance abuse treatment. A prospective study of patient-treatment matching. *Journal of Nervous and Mental Disease,* 171, 597-605.

Meandzija, B., O'Connor, P.G., Fitzgerald, B., Rounsaville, B.J., & Kosten, T.R. (1994). HIV infection and cocaine use in methadone maintained and untreated intravenous drug users. *Drug and Alcohol Dependence,* 36, 109-113.

Metzger, D., Woody, G., DePhilipis, D., McLellan, A.T., O'Brien, C.P., & Platt, J.J. (1991). Risk factors for needle sharing among methadone treated patients. *American Journal of Psychiatry,* 48, 636-640.

Metzger, D.S., Woody, G.E., McLellan, A.T., O'Brien, C.P., Druley, P., Navaline, H., DePhilippis, D., Stolley, P., & Abrutyn, E. (1993). Human immunodeficiency virus seroconversion among intravenous drug users in- and out-of-treatment: An 18 month follow-up. *AIDS,* 6, 1049-1056.

Navaratnum, V., & Foong, K. (1990). Opiate dependence - the role of benzodiazepines. *Current Medical Research and Opinion,* 11, 620-630.

Nolimal, D., & Crowley, T.J. (1989). HIV risk behaviour: Antisocial personality disorder, drug use patterns, and sexual behaviour among methadone maintenance admissions. In L.S. Harris, (Ed.), *Problems of drug dependence 1989* (NIDA Research Monograph No. 95, pp. 405-406). Rockville, MD: National Institute on Drug Abuse.

Preston, K.L., Griffiths, R.R., Stitzer, M.L., Bigelow, G.E., & Liebson, I.A. (1984). Diazepam and methadone interactions in methadone maintenance. *Clinical Pharmacology and Therapy,* 36, 534-541.

Quality Assurance Project (1991). Treatment outlines for antisocial personality disorder. *Australian and New Zealand Journal of Psychiatry,* 25, 541-547.

Ralston, G.E., & Taylor J.A. (1993). Temazepam abuse. *Addiction,* 88, 423.

Robins, L.N., Tipp, J., & Pryzbeck, T. (1991). Antisocial personality. In L.N. Robins, & D.A. Regier (Eds.), *Psychiatric disorders in America. The*

Epidemiologic Catchment Area Study (pp. 258-290). New York: The Free Press.

Rounsaville, B.J., Kosten, T., & Kleber, H. (1985). Success and failure at outpatient opioid detoxification. Evaluating the process of clonidine- and methadone- assisted withdrawal. *Journal of Nervous and Mental Disease,* **173**, 103-110.

Rounsaville, B.J., Kosten, T.R., Weissman, M.W., Prusoff, B., Pauls, D., Anton, S.F., & Merikangas, K. (1991). Psychiatric disorders in relatives of probands with opiate addiction, *Archives of General Psychiatry,* **48**, 32-42.

Rounsaville , B.J., Weissman, M.M., Crits-Cristoph, K., Wilber, C., & Kleber, H.D. (1982a). Diagnosis and symptoms of depression in opiate addicts. *Archives of General Psychiatry,* **39**, 151-156.

Rounsaville , B.J., Weissman, M.M., Kleber, H.D., & Wilber, C. (1982b). Heterogeneity of psychiatric diagnosis in treated opiate addicts. *Archives of General Psychiatry,* **39**, 161-166.

Rouser, E., Brooner, R.K., Regier, M.W., & Bigelow, G.E. (1994). Psychiatric distress in antisocial drug abusers: Relation to other personality disorders, *Drug and Alcohol Dependence,* **34**, 149-154.

Ruben, S.M., & Morrison, C.L. (1992). Temazepam misuse in a group of injecting drug users, *British Journal of Addiction,* **87**, 1387-1392.

Rutherford, M.J., Cacciola, J.S., & Alterman, A.I. (1994). Relationships of personality disorders with problem severity in methadone patients. *Drug and Alcohol Dependence,* **35**, 69-76.

Schoenbaum, E.E., Hartel, D., Selwyn, P.A., Klein, R.S., Davenny, K., Rogers, M., Feiner, C., & Friedland, G. (1989). Risk factors for human immunodeficiency virus infection in intravenous drug users. *New England Journal of Medicine,* **321**, 874-879.

Spunt, B., Hunt, D.E., Lipton, D., & Goldsmith, D.D (1986). Methadone diversion: A new look. *Journal of Drug Issues,* **16**, 569-583.

Steer, R.A., Iguchi, M.Y., & Platt, J.J. (1992). Use of the revised Beck Depression Inventory with intravenous drug users not in treatment. *Psychology of Addictive Behaviours,* **6**, 225-232.

Stitzer, M.L., Griffiths, R.R., McLellan, A.T., Grabowski, J., & Hawthorne, J.W. (1981). Diazepam use among methadone maintenance patients: Patterns and dosages. *Drug and Alcohol Dependence,* **8**, 189-199.

Strain, E.C., Brooner, R.K., & Bigelow, G.E. (1991a). Clustering of multiple substance use and psychiatric diagnoses in opiate addicts. *Drug and Alcohol Dependence,* **27**, 127-134.

Strain, E.C., Stitzer, M.L., & Bigelow, G.E. (1991b). Early treatment time course of depressive symptoms in opiate addicts. *Journal of Nervous and Mental Disease,* **179**, 215-221.

Strain, E.C., Stitzer, M.L., Liebson, I.A., & Bigelow, G.E. (1993). Dose-response of metha-done in the treatment of opioid dependence. *Annals of*

Internal Medicine, **119,** 23-27.

Strang, J., Griffiths, P., Abbey, J., & Gossop, M. (1994). Survey of injected benzodiazepines among drug users in Britain. *British Medical Journal,* **308,** 1082.

Strang, J., Seivewright, N., & Farrell, M. (1992). Intravenous and other abuses of benzo-diazepines: The opening of Pandora's box? *British Journal of Addiction,* **87,** 1373-1375.

Swift, W. Williams, G., Neill, O., & Grenyer, B. (1990). The prevalence of minor psycho-pathology in opioid users seeking treatment. *British Journal of Addiction,* **85,** 629-634.

Torrens, M., San, L., Peri, J.M., & Olle, J.M. (1991). Cocaine abuse among heroin addicts in Spain. *Drug and Alcohol Dependence,* **27,** 29-34.

Weppner., R.S., Stephens, R.C., & Conrad, H.T. (1972). Methadone: Some aspects of its legal and illegal use. *American Journal of Psychiatry,* **129,** 451-455.

Woody, G.E., Luborsky,L., McLellan, A.T., O'Brien, C.P., Beck, A.T., Blaine, J., Herman, I., & Hole, A. (1983). Psychotherapy for opiate addicts. Does it help? *Archives of General Psychiatry,* **40,** 639-635.

Woody, G.E., McLellan, A.T., Luborsky, L., & O'Brien, C.P. (1985). Sociopathy and psychotherapy outcome. *Archives of General Psychiatry,* **42,** 1081-1086.

Woody, G.E., McLellan, A.T., Luborsky, L., & O'Brien, C.P. (1987). Twelve-month follow-up of psychotherapy for opiate dependence. *American Journal of Psychiatry,* **144,** 590-596.

Zador, D., Sunjic, S., & Darke, S. (1996). Heroin-related deaths in New South Wales, 1992: Toxicological findings and circumstances. *Medical Journal of Australia,* **164,** 204-207.

5

THE EFFECTIVENESS OF METHADONE MAINTENANCE TREATMENT 4: COST-EFFECTIVENESS

PAT WARD AND MATTHEW SUTTON

INTRODUCTION

An economic approach to the allocation of resources for the provision of methadone maintenance treatment is premised on the understanding that there are more uses to which resources can be put than can be afforded (Drummond & Maynard, 1993). As a result, choices need to be made about how resources are expended on the basis of "opportunity costs". In situations of scarcity, the decision to allocate resources to one intervention, unit or individual will mean that these resources are no longer available for other purposes and, therefore, the potential benefits that may have been gained from their alternate use will have been lost.

The aim of economic analysis, then, is to provide decision-makers with some relevant and systematic information that will be of assistance when they are confronted with the need to make choices between alternative courses of action. Armed with data on the outcomes obtained relative to the cost invested in achieving them, it is possible to make decisions that will maximise the health benefits to be gained from the limited resources available. Unfortunately, however, economic analysis is often misperceived as being motivated solely by concerns about financial accountability, financial planning and/or cost-containment, with many authors asserting the rationale for their research in terms of these needs for economic scrutiny. But there are 'carrots' as well as 'sticks' to encourage a greater commitment to economic analysis. The results of economic evaluations may be useful for lobbying for additional funds. Moreover, cost considerations can play an important role in the search for the optimal mode of delivering services. If the results are interpreted and utilised appropriately, the investigation of the costs as well as the consequences of services such as methadone maintenance treatment is potentially for the mutual benefit of clients, providers, purchasers and the community.

As in other areas of health however, there has been a general reluctance on the part of researchers, policy makers and service providers to consider the costs as well as the outcomes of methadone maintenance treatment. There are consequently relatively few published economic evaluations of methadone maintenance treatment. Yates (1994) suggests that several perceptions have impeded the incorporation of cost considerations into program evaluations. These include the beliefs that cost-outcome relationships are simple, that cost-analysis is straightforward, that economic evaluation ignores the most important outcomes by focusing only on the quantifiable, and that the aim of economic analysis is to rationalise funding cuts. As Yates (1994) demonstrates, these perceptions have proved to be erroneous: cost analysis is not straightforward or a value-free exercise and involves consideration of intangible items. Therefore, since the cost of providing methadone services represents benefits forgone elsewhere, analysis of the cost of providing methadone treatment should concern researchers as much as the analysis of its effectiveness as a treatment modality.

Economic studies focus generally on three questions which, in relation to methadone maintenance are:

- *Is it worthwhile treating opioid-dependent individuals?*
- *Is methadone maintenance treatment the most efficient way to treat those who are opioid dependent?*
- *What is the most efficient way to deliver methadone maintenance treatment?*

In this chapter, we aim to set out in more detail the rationale for the economic analysis of methadone services, to describe the different types of economic analysis that can be employed in the evaluation of methadone maintenance treatment, to provide an overview of the existing literature and to identify some of the methodological and conceptual issues relevant to the interpretation of economic evaluations.

WHY ENGAGE IN ECONOMIC ANALYSIS?

To Improve Accountability and Financial Planning

Since economics is essentially concerned with the optimal use of a set of scarce and finite resources, economic analysis is an important tool in identifying resource use and guiding allocation. This information provides the framework by which variations in the cost of methadone treatment between individual service providers and according to the model of service delivery adopted can be examined (Coyle *et al.*, 1994). Clearly, such an endeavour is of value to service planners charged with the responsibility of determining what funds should be made available to provide an appropriate level of services in the future, based on predicted demand for treatment and on an analysis of how much these services cost to provide. Throughout the 1980s, when much of the policy debate in health was singularly focused on rising expenditure and paid little heed to the effective and efficient utilisation of funds (Drummond & Maynard, 1993), this became the primary rationale for the economic evaluation of treatment services. The shift from throughput to output measures of performance has, however, broadened the scope of the debate about funding. Rather than simply being an exercise in accountability, economic analysis is increasingly being utilised to support the provision of services such as methadone maintenance treatment by demonstrating that the benefits of doing so outweigh the costs and, having done that, by identifying the optimal or most cost-effective manner in which to deliver these services.

To Assist in the Development of Optimal Models of Service Delivery

Economic analysis is of potential interest for those directly involved in the provision of methadone treatment because, although demand continues to increase, access to resources is limited (at least in the short term). Evidence of the limited nature of public resources abounds, such as waiting lists at clinics, an increased reliance in many countries on the private sector to provide services, limited dosing times and appointments of fixed length. Difficult choices are being made every day about how services can best meet demand within a fixed operating budget. These include choosing between increasing the amount of staff time dedicated to existing clients and increasing the number of clients on the program (the choice between the intensive and the extensive margins as described by Zarkin *et al.*, 1994) and choosing between providing continued treatment to an existing client or providing access for a "treatment naive" individual. Comparisons can be made of effectiveness at any of the intervention points: recruitment, treatment or after-care (Zarkin *et al.*, 1994). Research into the resources used in different approaches to service delivery relative to the outcomes obtained from the use of those resources can improve the delivery of care by maximising the benefits achieved by all concerned.

While most of the research to date has been concerned with evaluating treatment services as provided and demonstrating their effectiveness *per se* (summative), there is no reason why a more proactive or formative approach cannot be taken (Yates, 1994). The aim of the latter is to propose alternative models of service delivery and to evaluate these with the view to developing the most cost-effective service possible (Yates, 1994). The benefit of service providers undertaking such evaluations is that they are more responsive to the needs of the total population of potential clients. Also they have a greater interest in ensuring that, where possible, a broader perspective is taken which assesses the cost and benefits that accrue to governments, the community and service consumers, who are also members of the community. Failure to take a societal perspective means that the consequences of any decision made will be assessed only from the point of view of the decision maker. Where the purchaser is the decision-maker it may be that the net effect of minimising their cost is an overall increase in costs to the community. For example, the imposition of treatment charges for clients may in the short term reduce the purchaser's outlays but may, in the long term, result in increased community costs if charges act as a barrier to treatment access or reduce retention in treatment.

There is also a mistaken view that economic analysis requires comparison of monetary inputs with monetary outcomes. This is not the case. An economic evaluation can be performed on any cost and outcome criteria which capture the most important effects of service delivery or on any value scale, as long as the effects can be measured in commensurate units. Service providers, therefore, have an important role to play in suggesting which treatment outcomes should be considered and how they should be weighted so as to ensure that the values of those who utilise methadone services are not overlooked.

To Support the Appropriate Allocation of Resources

In the allocation of scarce resources, purchasers are looking to support services and programs that can be shown to increase social welfare. As a result, service providers are often asked to demonstrate that they provide 'value for money'. It is precisely because of this that many fear that if they produce figures these will be used against them (Yates, 1994). Nevertheless, methadone treatment has been shown to be effective (see Chapters 2 & 3) and economic evaluations can be used to add further support to claims for additional funding. In this regard, given the nature of the methadone program and its sensitivity to public opinion and political values, economic analysis may prove useful in competing with other important social programs for resources (French, 1995). Of course, the benchmark against which to ascertain 'value for money' is critical. In many cases, providers perceive they are being asked to compete with other units for funds and prefer instead to attempt to differentiate their 'product' from their competitors by claiming they have different 'objectives'. However, services which call on the same pool of resources must be comparable as choices about resource allocation are already being made between them (Hall, 1987). The avoidance of systematic evaluation will not benefit clients in the long run (Peele, 1990).

Cost-of-illness studies, which aim to place a monetary value on the harm caused by particular health problems, have in the past been influential in determining government priorities for health care expenditure. Internationally, several of these have been undertaken for substance use (Collins & Lapsley, 1991; 1996; Rice *et al.*, 1990). Collins and Lapsley's (1991, 1996) analyses of the cost to society of alcohol, tobacco and illicit drug use in Australia indicate that illicit drugs cost less than alcohol and tobacco, primarily because of the lower prevalence of use. It is generally thought that the first of these studies was particularly effective in raising awareness in government of the larger burden of licit substances compared to the illicit substances. However, the use of ever-increasing "shock" figures of the economic burden of different illnesses in priority-setting has been the subject of criticism (Hall, 1987). Some argue (Shiell *et al.,* 1987) that the results do not reflect whether interventions are available which can cost-effectively reduce the burden identified. The shift in emphasis indicated by Collins and Lapsley's (1991, 1996) figures, for example, does not reflect the volume of evidence showing opioid-related harm can be substantially reduced through interventions such as methadone maintenance treatment. Nor does it provide information about the relative cost-effectiveness of methadone maintenance treatment and strategies aimed at reducing the prevalence of tobacco and alcohol use. In addition, cost-of-illness studies have been found to be particularly susceptible to inconsistent measurement (Smith & Wright, 1996) and this is particularly likely to be true in the case of illicit activities. For these reasons, it is likely that economic evaluations that look at both the cost and the *consequences* of intervening will prove to be more valuable in persuading those charged with the responsibility of determining the appropriate allocation of resources of the value of methadone maintenance treatment.

TYPES OF ECONOMIC EVALUATION

Traditionally, economic evaluations are characterised by two principal features: two or more alternatives are compared (one of the alternatives may be to 'do nothing') and both the costs and the consequences of the interventions are considered (Drummond *et al.,* 1987). Based on the ways in which the benefits are measured, economic evaluations are generally categorised into one of four types: cost-minimisation analysis, cost-effectiveness analysis, cost-benefit analysis, and cost-utility analysis. An additional study type, however, cost-offset analysis, which is essentially a subset of cost-benefit analysis, has been popular in the investigation of treatments for substance misuse. The different types of economic evaluation are summarised in Table 5.1.

Costing Studies

Three types of investigation have been included under this classification – cost description, cost-analysis, and cost-minimisation studies – although only the latter meets the criteria of an economic evaluation in that it considers the consequences of the intervention. Although a cost-minimisation study does not involve the collection of outcome data *per se,* sufficient evidence is said to exist to justify the assumption that the outcomes of the interventions under consideration are equal and hence the comparison can be made on cost alone. This type of study is rarely feasible because of the lack of good quality effectiveness information and the improbability of finding two or more interventions that produce the same outcomes.

Accurate data about the cost of interventions is of fundamental importance to the broader economic evaluation of the cost and benefits of services, yet the identification of resource use and its attribution to different types of activity is not straightforward (Yates, 1994; Coyle *et al.,* 1994). Whether resource utilisation is viewed from the perspective of the government, the service provider, the client or

Table 5.1
Types of economic evaluation

Study Type	Comparison	Measurement of Benefits
Costing Studies:		
Cost-Description	Intervention with 'do nothing'	Not considered
Cost-Analysis	Two or more alternatives with 'do nothing'	Not considered
Cost-Minimisation:	Two or more alternatives	Assumed equal
Cost-Effectiveness Analysis	Two or more alternatives	Single outcome dimension
Cost-Utility Analysis	Two or more alternatives	Multiple outcome dimensions combined using preference weights
Cost-Benefit studies:		
Cost-Benefit Analysis	One or more intervention(s) with 'do nothing'	Multiple outcome dimensions combined using monetary values
Cost-Offset Analysis	One or more intervention(s) with 'do nothing'	Reductions in public service expenditure only

society will have a significant impact on the costs derived. So will the types of costs included in the analysis (direct, indirect and intangible) and the way in which the identified costs are measured and valued. Recognition of the importance of accurate costing data, and concern about the lack of consistency in the costing methodology used, have seen an increase in the emphasis placed on cost analysis (Bradley *et al.,* 1994; French *et al.,* 1994; Ward *et al.,* forthcoming) and cost-description studies (Coyle *et al.,* 1994) in the area of addictions generally, and methadone maintenance treatment in particular.

Cost-Effectiveness Analysis

In cost-effectiveness studies, programs are compared on the basis of the costs incurred and the results achieved on a *single* outcome measure. The benefits are measured in natural units, such as years of life saved or heroin-free days, and a cost per unit of effectiveness is derived by relating the outcome to the cost. As the analysis is limited to one treatment outcome, the outcome measure must be identical for all the interventions and it should also be similarly valued by the services under consideration. For example, one of the objectives of methadone treatment is "to facilitate an improvement in social functioning" (National Methadone Working Party, 1993: p.5), which would conceivably include increased employment among clients. However, it would be of doubtful value and validity to make a comparative assessment of the effectiveness of methadone maintenance treatment and a job training program on the basis of their ability to reduce unemployment among their clientele alone given the different priority placed on achieving this outcome by the two programs. It is for this reason that cost-effectiveness studies are often more useful for making choices between alternative interventions within therapeutic categories rather than across broader program categories.

Cost-Utility Analysis

This type of economic evaluation is similar to a cost-effectiveness analysis except that it is not limited to a comparison between interventions on the basis of one outcome measure. Although a single measure is employed, it is one that combines several aspects of the treatment outcome. For example, for interventions which affect health only, quality adjusted life years (QALYs) are often used which consider both the increase in life expectancy and morbidity avoided due to treatment. It, therefore, allows for a comparison of the relative efficiency of interventions for a broad range of health conditions with a variety of different objectives (Drummond & Maynard, 1993). While QALYs have to date been concerned only with evaluating the health outcomes of various treatment and prevention interventions, the method of combining effects with preference weights may have a far broader application. In particular, it may prove extremely useful in evaluating programs such as methadone maintenance treatment which have wider social objectives (Simpson & Sutton, 1996).

Cost-Benefit Analysis

In cost-benefit analysis an attempt is made to measure the benefits of an intervention in terms of monetary value. Therefore, as with a cost-utility analysis, despite the dissimilarity of objectives and outcomes achieved it is possible to compare the relative value of any program with another – for example, methadone maintenance treatment and a job training scheme. The primary advantage of this approach is that as the costs and consequences are measured on the same scale it is theoretically possible to ascertain whether the intervention is worthwhile on balance. However, the utility of finding that a program has net benefits may be of limited value given that resource constraints mean it is rarely feasible to implement all programs with 'benefits greater than costs'. The acceptability of the findings will also depend on who the beneficiaries of the intervention are and who pays for it.

There are inevitably considerable problems in the monetary valuation of some elements of both costs and benefits. Therefore many 'cost-benefit studies' focus on the impact of programs on public expenditure only. This type of analysis is called a cost-offset study since the primary question is whether the intervention brings about "offsets", that is, reductions in public expenditure that are larger than its implementation costs (Godfrey, 1994). Does the intervention, in simple terms, result in cost savings to the government? Given the broad social objectives of methadone treatment and the impact it may have on the work of other government agencies (e.g., reducing calls on welfare services, cutting down the workload of the criminal justice system, or facilitating access to primary health care interventions), this has often been the focus of the economic evaluations undertaken in this area. The main risk of cost-offset studies is that the benefits of treatment are undervalued (Simpson & Sutton, 1996) and are inconsistent with the broader social perspective taken by policy makers (French *et al.*, 1991).

THE EVIDENCE SO FAR

The extensive literature on the effectiveness of methadone treatment presents a stark contrast to the dearth of information available with regard to its costs. As a substitution therapy, methadone maintenance treatment has generated an enormous level of moral and political debate. As such, the question facing governments and health authorities in the 1970s and early 1980s was simply whether to provide the service at all, rather than how to provide it in the most efficient and cost-effective manner. However, the continued demand for treatment in the face of fiscal constraint, as well as the emergence of alternative substitution therapies for the treatment of opioid dependence, has led to the development of alternative models of methadone service delivery, choices between which demand that program evaluations include economic analysis. While the majority of the studies to date have been conducted in the United States, there is a growing literature from the United Kingdom and Australia.

In reviewing the literature, the first section is concerned with presenting the findings from three economic evaluations undertaken to date that have compared methadone maintenance treatment with other alternative interventions for opioid dependence. These studies have sought to provide a response to the first two questions posed in the introduction: namely, is it worthwhile treating opioid-dependent individuals and is methadone treatment the most efficient way to treat those who are opioid dependent? Of these three studies, Goldschmidt (1976), in analysing the marginal cost of retaining clients in treatment for additional six-monthly periods, began to seek answers to the third question. Specifically, he was concerned with investigating how the benefits of treatment varied over different lengths of time spent in and out of treatment. The second section therefore, is concerned with the issue of retention. Given that resources are limited and that pressure is being placed on methadone treatment services because of continuing demand and increased retention rates, this is a logical starting point for service providers, policy makers and researchers interested in maximising total benefits for the treatment-seeking population. Finally, the third section describes the methodological problems encountered that limit the interpretation of the results, and identifies the need to develop a consistent and standardised approach to the measurement of both treatment costs and outcomes.

Findings From the Economic Evaluation of Methadone Maintenance Treatment

Goldschmidt, 1976

The first economic evaluation of methadone treatment was conducted in the early 1970s by Goldschmidt (1976) following a tenfold increase in federal funding for drug abuse programs. It was a cost-effectiveness study that compared therapeutic communities and methadone programs on two measures of effectiveness. The first of these simply measured whether the client had been heroin-free in the two months prior to interview. The second, however, was a composite measure, the "normabider" criterion, which was developed by Goldschmidt (1976) to represent the multiple and varying goals of the two programs. It purported to assess the client's "ability to live by the norms of society" and, as such, involved the derivation of a single composite score which related to the subject's drug use (excluding cannabis), criminal behaviour and employment activity during the same period.

The study involved the evaluation of the effect of treatment on these two criteria for 1,241 individuals admitted to one of ten treatment programs across the United States during a 30-month period from July 1, 1970 to January 31, 1973. Goldschmidt (1976) found that the two treatments were equally effective on both measures. However, the overall measures disguised substantial differences between the effects of the programs. As would be expected, given the restrictive environment, clients in therapeutic communities initially scored better on the heroin-free criterion but worse on the normabider criterion where gainful employment was a consideration. Since the durability of the treatment effect (i.e., the extent to which the outcomes achieved were maintained following the cessation of treatment) for those retained in either program for less than six months was found to be poor, retention became a crucial factor in determining the overall effectiveness of the two treatment modalities. Consequently, despite residential programs achieving greater behaviour change initially (because methadone clients were retained in treatment for longer) both treatment modalities were found to be equally effective over the entire study period. Furthermore, in spite of the higher costs associated with increased treatment duration, methadone treatment was still found to be twice as cost-effective. This was because the cost of providing it per period was one-quarter of that for therapeutic communities.

Much could be said in criticism of the effectiveness criteria selected, especially their insensitivity to small changes in behaviour. The current emphasis in many countries on "harm reduction" as an approach to drug abuse, recognises that although programs may not achieve abstinence, they may reduce the harm associated with opioid dependence. Goldschmidt's measure (1976) did not attribute any utility to the incremental changes in behaviour that may have occurred as a result of treatment. As such, it is likely to have underestimated the effectiveness of the two treatment modalities. In addition, others would argue that the criteria did not measure outcomes but instead related to intermediate behaviour changes (alcohol and illicit drug use) or process (incarceration and enrolment in other treatment programs). The latter is particularly problematic since it relates to the availability of services, the very question the study sought to address. In this regard, it is also of concern that there were no direct measures of improvement in health or social functioning, although death rates were considered but found not to differ significantly between the two types of programs.

Overall, the value of the study is largely theoretical. Goldschmidt (1976) recognised that programs have multiple objectives and that individual agencies are likely to be differentially effective in achieving them. Given this, perhaps the greatest disappointment is that the normabider criterion was binary, so that a positive score on any of the six measures negated a successful outcome on the others. As such, its value as a composite measure that could be used to assess the overall effectiveness of the different services was undermined. Nevertheless, Goldschmidt's (1976) attempt to generate a composite measure challenged the unidimensional nature of cost-effectiveness studies which are of little use when programs, such as methadone maintenance treatment, have multiple objectives across several domains.

Cost-benefit and cost-offset analysis can be used to evaluate the relative effectiveness of programs with multiple and different objectives and to answer questions of allocative efficiency (i.e., how to distribute funds across and within programs to achieve maximum outcomes). Given the controversy that has surrounded the methadone program in the United States and the consequent need to demonstrate that methadone services should be provided at all, it is not surprising that most of the economic evaluations that have been conducted in the States have been of this type.

Harwood, Hubbard, Collins and Rachal, 1988

One of the first cost-benefit studies was undertaken by Harwood and his colleagues (1988) using data from the Treatment Outcome Prospective Study (TOPS) (Hubbard, *et al.*, 1989). Their analysis recognised that crime constituted a significant proportion of the estimated cost to society of drug abuse and that its reduction was a major rationale for the provision of drug treatment. Accordingly, Harwood *et al.* (1988) investigated the cost of providing three types of treatment – residential, outpatient drug-free, and methadone maintenance – by comparing the savings associated with each in terms of reduced crime in the year during and after treatment. Overall they found that the reductions in crime costs from the year before to the year after treatment were 20% for the law-abiding citizen and 8% for society. The principal difference between these two perspectives, as outlined/described by the authors, was that the value of the stolen property was included in estimates of the cost to law-abiding citizens since it directly impacted on the victim, a law-abiding citizen. It was however excluded in calculating the cost to society since theft was not seen to represent an overall net loss to society but rather a transfer of wealth. Likewise, the lost earning potential of drug users was regarded as an overall loss to society's net wealth and was included in estimates of the cost of drug use from a societal perspective but excluded from similar calculations for law-abiding citizens since the effects of unemployment were felt by the drug user and his/her family, not the law-abiding citizen.

As with other studies (Goldschmidt, 1976; Gerstein, *et al.*, 1994), Harwood *et al.* (1988) found that the magnitude of change was greater in the residential group than the outpatient and methadone maintenance treatment groups. However, the lower treatment costs and higher retention rates for the methadone maintenance treatment group meant that from the perspective of the law-abiding citizen it was this modality that yielded the highest benefit to cost ratios in the year following treatment (4.4:1, 3.8:1 and 1.3:1 for the methadone, residential and outpatient groups respectively). With the exception of the outpatient group, the benefits of treatment from a societal perspective were considerably less (0.9:1, 2.1:1 and 4.3:1 for the methadone, residential and outpatient groups respectively). This was largely due to the failure of clients in both residential and methadone programs to obtain employment and the seemingly quicker return to pre-treatment crime rates by those receiving methadone after they left the program. Harwood *et al.* (1988) suggest that the latter could be an experimental artefact given the high non-response rate from the methadone group in the pre-treatment period and the fact that a higher proportion of methadone clients were in more restrictive environments (e.g. prisons) in the year prior to entry to the TOPS program. Overall, however, Harwood *et al.* (1988) concluded that the benefits of treatment were at least of the same magnitude as the cost of providing it and that increased time in treatment resulted in greater cost reductions.

CALDATA Study, 1994

The most recent and comprehensive cost-benefit/offset study to date is that conducted by Gerstein and colleagues in 1994 in California – the California Drug and Alcohol Treatment Assessment (CALDATA) study. The sample consisted of 1,859 individuals who had been discharged in the 12 months through October 1, 1991 to 30 September, 1992 from four treatment modalities: residential programs, residential "social model" programs, outpatient programs and methadone maintenance treatment. The latter group was divided into those who were still in treatment and those who had been on a detoxification program or had remained in treatment for less than 4 months. Gerstein *et al.* (1994) investigated the effect of treatment on alcohol and drug use, criminal activity, health and health care utilisation, and source of income. They also examined the cost of treatment and the economic value of treatment both to taxpayers (the law-abiding citizen in Harwood *et al.*, 1988) and society.

With the exception of employment status, the CALDATA study found improvements on all outcome scales regardless of the treatment modality under consideration. Again, however, there were differences in the patterns of improvement for the different modalities. In particular, reductions in drug and alcohol use were greater for those in residential programs while those continuing in methadone treatment showed the greatest reductions in criminal activity. Those who were discharged from the methadone program produced the poorest outcomes overall.

The differential effects of treatment on criminal activity and employment status had an impact on the results of the economic evaluation. While Gerstein *et al.* (1994) found that overall the benefits of drug treatment were greater than the costs incurred, from a societal perspective this was only of the order of 2:1 compared to 7:1 for the taxpayer. The substantial difference in treatment costs also had a significant impact. Methadone treatment was found, on average, to be one-tenth of the cost of residential treatment which resulted in a superior benefit to cost ratio in the "during" treatment phase. For the continuing methadone group this cost to benefit ratio was almost 5:1 no matter which perspective was taken, while for the discharged methadone group the ratio was of the order of 3:1 and 2:1 for the taxpayer and society, respectively. In contrast, the benefits to taxpayers of residential programs were only slightly higher than the costs (1.1:1), and for society, given the clients' loss of earning potential, the costs exceeded the benefits (0.4:1) in the "during" treatment phase.

Gerstein *et al.* (1994) also found that the benefits following treatment were substantial with the benefit to cost ratio for those in residential treatments being 3.9:1 and 2:1 for the taxpayer and society, respectively. For the methadone discharge group, however, because of increased unemployment, the costs to society exceeded the benefits in the year following treatment. The taxpayer on the other hand, maintained substantial benefits in the order of 10:1 which were attributable to the low cost of treatment.

The conclusions to be drawn from these three studies are that treatment interventions for opioid dependence have been found not only to be effective in achieving their outcomes, but that the value of the benefits obtained have been greater than the cost identified for providing the services. More specifically, methadone treatment has compared favourably with alternative programs for the treatment of opioid dependence. The studies have demonstrated that methadone has produced superior benefit to cost ratios, particularly in the during treatment phase, but also in the year following treatment (if the taxpayer's perspective is taken) largely because of the lower cost of treatment. Both Gerstein *et al.* (1994) and Harwood *et al.* (1988), however, found that the costs exceeded benefits in the year following treatment cessation from a societal perspective. Although promising, the findings, particularly in relation to the magnitude of the effects observed, need to be treated as preliminary and interpreted with caution. The limited application of economic evaluations to the drug and alcohol field mean that there are numerous methodological and conceptual problems that need to be resolved.

Treatment Careers and the Cost of Retention

A major confounder in the evaluation of drug and alcohol interventions is the issue of readmission to, or retention in, treatment. French (1995) points out that studies usually focus on a single episode of treatment and base treatment costs on the mean cost per client day multiplied by the number of days in treatment. This ignores the chronic, relapsing nature of opioid dependence and the extensive treatment careers of those seeking access to services (Zarkin *et al.*, 1994). The attribution of benefits to the particular episode of treatment under consideration, therefore, is problematic because previous treatment experiences may work to either exaggerate or understate the cost-effectiveness of the episode in question. Gerstein *et al.* (1994) recognised this in their study, suggesting that the ratios reported may be "modest overestimates of the net benefits" (p. 87) because there were 35% of clients who re-entered treatment. Treatment expenses should, therefore, have been higher, and the benefits correspondingly adjusted because they cannot be solely attributed to the treatment episode under consideration. Of importance, too, is the need, should treatment effects occur between episodes, to incorporate these future benefits or disbenefits in the estimation of the overall cost-effectiveness of the current intervention.

Similarly, even when estimating the cost of a single episode of treatment (where the average cost of treatment is usually determined by dividing the total cost of providing the service by some measure of the caseload), the failure to recognise varying retention rates can have a significant impact on the treatment costs derived (French *et al.*, 1994). This was borne out in Swensen's (1989) cost-description study of the publicly-run methadone program in Western Australia. Swensen (1989) found that using the number of distinct individuals enrolled in the program for the study year, therefore assuming a full 12 months participation in the program, resulted in a mean cost per client per annum that was 40% less than if the mean cost was calculated on the basis of the average number of clients treated in any given month.

Far more problematic, however, than the methodological issues surrounding multiple admissions or length of time in treatment in the calculation of average treatment costs and the evaluation of the cost-effectiveness of a single episode of treatment is the question of the marginal cost-effectiveness of increased retention. A positive relationship has consistently been found between treatment duration and outcome (see Chapter 12), which has led service providers in many countries to adopt retention as a treatment goal. But in economic terms, retention represents a cost and is therefore not regarded necessarily as an outcome to be valued. Rather than just asking whether additional time in treatment is of benefit to the client or worthwhile, economics poses an additional question. Namely, is keeping a client in treatment for an extra period of time the best way to utilise the limited resources available for the entire treatment population, both those currently in treatment and those seeking admittance to methadone programs.

Indeed, while Gerstein *et al.* (1994) found that longer stays generally led to greater benefits, the anomalies they observed raise important questions about the issue of retention and highlights the need to distinguish between the clinical and economic implications of longer stays in treatment. In particular, Gerstein *et al.* (1994) found that for those in the methadone discharge group who stayed longer than the detoxification period there was an increase in cost to both taxpayers and society. Furthermore, they noted that for the residential treatment group, extensions beyond four months diminished the effect of the shorter stay. The continuing methadone group was by virtue of the pre-post test design excluded from the analysis and the data were not collected in a manner that would allow for an analysis of the marginal cost benefit of providing an additional period of treatment.

Goldschmidt (1976) did, however, attempt to ascertain the marginal cost-effectiveness of an additional six months in treatment, and reported that the longer a client remained in treatment, be it a residential or methadone maintenance program, the more it cost to generate each "effectiveness measure unit" (EMU). While such a finding does not necessarily imply that retaining clients in treatment is not beneficial, it does suggest that in situations of scarcity it may not be as cost-beneficial to provide additional treatment to an existing client as it is to treat a client waiting to commence treatment. The problems already identified surrounding Goldschmidt's selection of outcome criterion and the lack of an appropriate control or "do nothing" group in his study make it difficult to draw any definitive conclusions at this stage about the implications of his findings in relation to optimal treatment length.

Although not directly addressing the issue of the marginal cost-effectiveness of extended periods of treatment, McGlothlin and Anglin (1981) and Anglin and colleagues (1989), following the forced closure of several methadone clinics in California, undertook a cost-benefit/offset analysis that examined the impact of policies that mandatorily limited the duration of treatment on drug use, criminal activity, and general well-being. In both studies it was found that those discharged from treatment reported more crime, higher rates of illicit drug use, and more contact with the criminal justice system. However, despite this, both McGlothlin and Anglin (1981) and Anglin *et al.* (1989), reported overall net social gains as a result of the closure of the clinics.

McGlothlin and Anglin (1981) suggested that the law enforcement strategies in the local area at the time the clinics were closed, and the associated increased cost and reduced purity of heroin, may have minimised the impact of the clinic closures by discouraging clients from returning to pre-treatment levels of use. More recent studies of the impact of law enforcement activities on the drug market (Weatherburn & Lind, 1995; Wagstaff & Maynard, 1988), however, would suggest that this is unlikely to have been the case. On closer examination, the result could be an artefact of the higher initial social cost observed in the continuous treatment group. That is, while the absolute social cost for the continuing group was higher in the post-closure period, the proportional reduction in social cost between discharge and the time of interview was lower at 15% for the discharged group than the 32% reduction found for the continuing treatment group.

More importantly, as Anglin *et al.* (1989) noted, other community agencies were eager to provide alternative treatment to those who were discharged. This may explain the seeming "durability" of the treatment effect, while at the same time it would have underestimated the social cost of closing the clinic because alternative treatment costs were not included in the analysis. In their study, Anglin *et al.* (1989) attributed the increased social cost of closing the clinic to the fact that 67% of the discharged group either transferred or re-entered treatment, with the result that at the time of interview more clients in the discharge group were currently in treatment than those in the continuing treatment group. An additional confounding variable was the fact the one of the clinics in the comparison group had poorer treatment outcomes because of more stringent unit policies such as low methadone doses.

In recognition of the effect of subsequent treatment episodes, an important component of the Anglin *et al.* (1989) study was the comparison of the outcomes of those clients who transferred to a private clinic with those who did not. They found that those who did not choose to transfer had substantially poorer outcomes. Moreover, when they compared the social costs for these two groups for both men and women, discharging clients cost society 2.5 times as much as it did to provide continuing treatment. Interestingly, despite a decrease in the availability of ancillary services in the private methadone clinics, Anglin *et al.* (1989) observed continued improvement in those clients who transferred from public to private programs. While they provided several explanations for this, including maturation and an accumulative treatment effect, it raises important questions about the cost-benefit of providing the resource-intensive ancillary services that are more commonly found in public programs.

Given the overall findings of these two studies, interesting questions still remain as to the extent that treatment may prolong drug using careers, and the subsequent cost of that to both society and the individual. Twenty-seven percent of clients (McGlothlin & Anglin, 1981) believed that they had benefited from the closure in that it had enabled them to remain both methadone – and heroin-free. Furthermore, on only two of nine behaviour scales – heroin use and health – did the majority of clients report that the termination of treatment had a detrimental effect. In relation to other drug use and criminal activity, the majority of clients felt that it had no effect.

In conclusion then, these studies suggest that no definitive conclusion can be drawn as to whether there is an optimal length of methadone maintenance treatment. While methadone maintenance treatment has been shown to be effective (see Chapters 2 & 3) and cost-beneficial (Gerstein *et al.,* 1994, Harwood *et al.,* 1988), it is unclear whether the outcomes achieved are sustained over extended periods as a result of the treatment process alone. It is therefore impossible to ascertain what benefits accrue as a result of an additional period of treatment and whether the benefits come at a greater or lesser cost than the treatment. The results will depend on whether it is appropriate to assume that clients would return to pre-treatment levels of use very quickly and suffer the same degree of social and health problems as previously. If this were the case, given that treatment costs are likely to be reduced over time, it is likely that in situations of scarcity health gains would be maximised by retaining stable clients in treatment rather than admitting new clients with higher intervention costs. However, the studies suggest (despite their many methodological problems) that some clients may not return to pre-treatment drug use and that others who would, may not do so immediately (Gerstein & Harwood, 1990). Where resources are fixed and demand high, there is an argument that resource utility may be optimised by offering treatment to a "naive" or new client rather than an existing one. Far more research, with adequate control groups, needs to be conducted to ascertain the marginal costs and benefits of additional time in treatment so that clients can be more appropriately matched to services and the benefits of treatment maximised. In any such analyses, however, it is important to pay greater heed to the value placed on continued treatment by clients. The accuracy of any marginal cost or benefit figures derived will depend on how inclusive and appropriate the list of costs and benefits identified is and the precision of the measurement techniques employed.

Accurate Assessment of the Costs and Benefits

A consistent and shared understanding of the definition and measurement of the appropriate costs and outcomes associated with the program(s) under consideration is fundamental to the accurate interpretation of any economic evaluation. Unfortunately, to date, it has often been the case that little or insufficient information has been provided about what items have been included in the costing of service provision and the benefits attributed to the program, or how the figures have been derived. Where attention to cost methodology has been provided, as many researchers have indicated (French *et al.*, 1994; Bradley *et al.*, 1994; Apsler & Harding, 1991; French, 1995), the variety of techniques employed make direct comparisons between studies difficult. With the increased recognition of the importance of the costing component of any economic evaluation (Coyle *et al.*, 1994; French *et al.*, 1994), greater emphasis has been placed on the accurate assessment of costs.

Even as early as 1976, Goldschmidt emphasised the importance of obtaining fair cost figures for different treatment programs. He identified three broad cost areas: cost additions, cost reductions and overhead adjustments. Cost additions are made for those items which are received for free by the treatment program but involve a cost to society. These include things such as volunteers' time, donations and rent-free buildings, which are particularly important for services provided by non-government and non-profit organisations. They are added to the financial costs of the program to reflect the *opportunity costs* of those resources on the basis that if they were not expended to provide this service they would have an alternative productive use elsewhere. Cost reductions should be made for those items that appear in the financial budgets but do not actually contribute to service provision. It would, however, be a mistake to exclude administrative or managerial staff without whom the service could not run (Coyle *et al.*, 1994). Overhead adjustments should be made if treatment agencies receive services from parent organisations, such as heating, lighting or accounting services. These are particularly relevant to public services provided within a hospital setting. In comparing three methadone maintenance programs, Bradley *et al.* (1994) found that the hospital-based program was up to 15% cheaper than the free-standing programs which they attributed to the potential benefits it received in capital improvements, shared services and reduced pharmaceutical prices. While some of these cost advantages are "real savings" in costs associated with being sited at a hospital, it may have proved useful to make a comparison of the three programs on the cost categories that could be accurately assessed.

Cost-studies typically derive per-period, average cost figures for the treatment of one client. These figures refer to the allocation of resources to a particular volume of clients receiving a particular level of services. However, with a fixed budget and services operating at near capacity, increased demand may result in a decrease in time spent with existing clients, or reduced quality of care. In this sense, average cost figures are endogenous, that is, they depend on the quality and type of services offered, which in turn are determined by total resources and the number of clients presenting for treatment. It is for this reason that marginal rather than average costs are more useful for predicting the cost implications of treating additional clients. It is also important in estimating the marginal cost of treatment, to consider the extent to which treatment for the additional client has been bought at the expense of other clients or the overall effectiveness of the program.

In a study conducted by Bradley *et al.* (1994) on the cost and financing of methadone programs, they identified that the short-run marginal cost of admitting an additional client to standard treatment amounted to the cost of the direct consumables such as the methadone and medical supplies required. Under this scenario, where there is a core counselling staff, it is assumed that additional counselling and welfare work will be provided through the reallocation of existing counsellor time and resources. Where these sorts of adjustments do occur, and it makes intuitive sense to assume that they occur regularly in response to increased demand, clients will receive on average less staff-time with each additional individual admitted to treatment. The extent to which estimates such as those provided by Bradley *et al.* (1994) are a true reflection of the real marginal cost depends, therefore, on the impact that decreased client-contact time has on other community agencies (do clients seek access to those services previously provided elsewhere?) and on overall treatment outcomes. Given the pressure on service providers to meet continuing treatment demands, greater attention needs to be paid to the real cost of solutions that minimise the tangible short-term service delivery costs but have the potential both to increase the indirect costs of treatment and to reduce the benefits of treatment.

Another solution to the escalating demand for treatment spaces has been the move towards privatising services where the cost of service provision has been increasingly shifted to the client. In assessing the cost-effectiveness of private versus public methadone services it is important to take a societal perspective which would include the often substantial cost borne by the methadone client, since this in fact represents an opportunity cost. Failure to do this introduces a bias. A recent review of methadone services in Australia (Commonwealth Department of Human Services and Health, 1995) illustrates this point well. In adopting a governmental perspective, it was found that in New South Wales services provided privately through general practitioners were approximately one-third of the cost of public methadone clinic services. However, if one assumes that those clients treated by private general practitioners were also dosed privately at clinics, and a societal perspective was taken in which the dosing costs met by clients was included in the estimate of the treatment costs, then the inverse would be true. That is, from a societal perspective the cost of public sector methadone treatment was almost 40% less than that of privately provided methadone services. Likewise, failure to consider client costs can result in an overestimate of the benefits of methadone treatment. Anglin *et al.* (1989) found that it cost 2.5 times as much to discharge clients as it did to provide continued treatment. If, however, they have included the treatment costs passed on to the clients who were compelled to attend private programs the benefits of continued treatment would have been found to be substantially less.

It is also necessary to examine the impact that fees may have on the benefits obtained from treatment since recent studies from the United

States (Britton, 1994; Maddux *et al.*, 1994) suggest that the introduction of charges may have a negative impact on both access to, and retention in, treatment. Britton (1994) found that the mandatory transfer of clients to private programs resulted in a substantial proportion of clients opting to detoxify from methadone treatment. Among those who opted to leave treatment, there was an increase in drug use and high risk HIV practices as compared to those who remained in treatment. Maddux and colleagues (1994) found that those clients required to pay (a modest sum of $2.50 per day compared to that normally incurred) had poorer retention rates after one year than those not charged for treatment. Furthermore, there was evidence that service costs were also higher for the paying group who sought out more counselling sessions with caseworkers because they ran into financial difficulties. While no economic evaluation of the program was conducted, it is likely that this factor alone would have substantially offset the revenue gains generated by charging clients.

Clearly, much needs to be done to develop a standard methodology for ascertaining the cost of methadone service provision and to determine the value of the subsequent benefits obtained. At the very least, there is an onus on researchers to be more rigorous in describing the methodologies employed in their economic evaluations of drug and alcohol interventions. In particular, clear definitions of the perspective adopted and a detailed account of the cost calculations need to be provided if other investigators are to be able to identify those parts of the analysis that are relevant to them and to draw meaningful conclusions. Also, it would be useful if costing results were presented in three stages: (i) the volume of inputs used, measured in natural units (e.g. staff-time); (ii) estimated per-unit costs for each type of input; and (iii) a combination of (i) and (ii) to estimate total costs. This would permit better application of the results to local environments, as the resource-intensity of treatment or input prices may vary considerably between different areas and countries.

Finally, there is a need for researchers to be innovative in their approach to the economic evaluation of methadone programs. In 1976, Goldschmidt challenged the field to consider an appropriate and useful methodology that might assess the effectiveness of programs on multiple dimensions. As yet little has been done in this regard, with researchers pursuing cost-benefit or cost-offset lines of enquiry. Given the difficulty of assigning a monetary value to many of the benefits associated with methadone programs, it may be that a solution lies in the approach recommended by Goldschmidt (1976).

Several reliable and valid multidimensional treatment outcome scales already exist, such as the Opiate Treatment Index (Darke *et al.,* 1992), that measure outcomes in natural units. Using refined scoring technologies, they could provide aggregate scores both within and across the various outcome domains. Simpson and Sutton (1996) have suggested that these instruments may prove to be useful taxonomies in assessing the overall effectiveness of methadone programs, especially if a weight can be attached to each of the outcome measures which reflects the value placed on achieving these goals.

CONCLUSION

Rising demand and limited budgetary increases for treatment for opioid dependence in many countries have heightened the need for good quality evidence on the cost-effectiveness of different interventions and models of service delivery. This evidence may be required for several purposes: to improve financial accountability; to support appropriate allocation of funds to methadone treatment; and to evaluate changes in service provision. Investigations of financial accountability that are motivated by a desire to reduce activities that have no beneficial effect on outcomes (i.e. reducing *technical inefficiencies*) are the least controversial use of economic evaluations. Unfortunately, many economic studies of methadone programs have not attempted to marry cost with outcome information. This raises the risk that cost savings will be sought that reduce the benefits from methadone maintenance treatment substantially.

A more positive role for economic evaluations is to input into discussions about changes in the allocation of funds (i.e. increasing *allocative efficiency*). Previous attempts to influence the funding debate in the addictions arena have been based on cost-of-illness methodology. The results of these studies can be misleading and economic evaluations of methadone maintenance treatment with a comparison intervention that is popular and well-funded may be a more persuasive approach.

Methadone has consistently been found to be an effective intervention for the treatment of opioid dependence and the preliminary research would suggest that it has not been such a leap of faith to assume it is also cost-effective. The few economic evaluations conducted to date suggest that the benefits of treating opioid-dependent individuals are greater than the costs incurred in doing so, and that methadone has generally been found to be more cost-effective than alternative interventions. What remains unclear, however, is what models of methadone service delivery are most cost-beneficial?

It is at this juncture that greater provider involvement in economic evaluations and "bottom-up" development of study designs may be most fruitful. Greater insight may be gained from moving away from program-level evaluations to experimental changes in service provision. As Mooney (1992) has noted, the relevant question is rarely about whether or not to provide a service but rather about "how much" to provide, the answer to which lies in marginal analysis. Economic evaluations are most useful when applied to proposals that result in increased cost and improved effectiveness. The case of client retention is a good example. There is substantial evidence to suggest that the longer an individual remains in treatment the better the outcome, and that for many treatment durations these benefits may be larger than the costs of providing the additional services. However, it is less clear whether offering prolonged treatment for existing clients is as cost-beneficial as admission for a new client.

However, this concern will only be relevant in certain circumstances, and this highlights the importance of pertinent study questions for economic evaluation. As economic analyses are supposed to be motivated by opportunity cost concerns (the next best use of the resources which must be forgone), it is crucial that these opportunity cost comparisons are appropriate. In the case of existing-client retention versus new-client admission, this means that there are potential new clients waiting for services. Similarly, comparisons of different programs should be based on the premise that resources could be reallocated between them to maximise total outcome and comparisons between different interventions based on the belief that they compete for the same client group. The data requirements for such exercises may be best fulfilled by use of routine data sets, exploiting any natural experimental design and using appropriate econometric methods for controlling confounding or extrapolating beyond the study sample.

Enhancing the pertinence of the analysis through increased provider-involvement is not the only challenge that lies ahead for economic evaluations in this area. There are also legitimate concerns about the generalisability of the study results. In particular, authors should give consideration to variability in the costs of different inputs in different areas/countries through sensitivity analysis (Drummond *et al.,* 1987). Moreover, the scale of service delivery over which findings are relevant should be investigated, given substantial cost savings that may accrue from growing larger or that capital expansion may be required for some increases in client numbers.

In addition, the behavioural nature of the condition being treated should be recognised and further attempts made at modelling client costs, effectiveness and treatment careers in a behavioural framework (Hannan, 1975). These models can then take account of the potential impact of environmental variables, such as drug-market conditions. Finally, it should be emphasised that methadone maintenance treatment is in many cases a long-term investment in client outcomes. As such, treatment cost figures may be more illuminating for service planners if they are presented as discounted treatment-career costs, rather than annualised average figures that do not reflect the likely future resource consequences of current changes in service availability.

These challenges to economic study highlight the limitations of existing methods for evaluation and emphasise the need for tentative interpretation of study results. However, initial efforts to measure the effectiveness of treatment can be easily criticised for being too simplistic. Similarly, initial applications of economic techniques will not be sensitive to the intricacies of treatment or particularly proficient at capturing those intangible outcomes that currently defy quantitative measurement. Furthermore, it should be emphasised that economic evaluation is not a value-free exercise and the way in which addiction is conceptualised (as a biological disorder or a disorder with psychological and social antecedents) will influence the perspective taken and the types of costs and benefits included (Buck *et al,* forthcoming; Godfrey & Sutton, 1996).

Various taxonomies of the potential costs and benefits of addictive behaviours and their treatment are beginning to emerge. It is likely that, just as with the assessment of treatment outcomes, various measurement instruments for use in assessing the economic consequences of treatments for opioid dependence will be developed. Differences between these protocols will reflect different values and beliefs and should be subject to tests of validation. In this context, more formative approaches to economic evaluation will prove most useful. Service providers have an important role to play in suggesting what study questions are relevant, what treatment outcomes are pertinent and how they should be valued.

SUMMARY

Economics begins with the premise that "In the beginning, middle and end was, is and will be scarcity of resources" (Mooney, 1992: p. 2). Applied to the area of health, it is concerned with examining the costs involved in, and the benefits obtained from, the provision of various interventions. Through the application of this information to the decision-making process the aim is to maximise the health benefits to be gained by the efficient utilisation of the limited resources available. Unfortunately, many have assumed that the *raison d'être* of health economics is cost containment and financial accountability. We argue, however, that for politically sensitive programs such as methadone maintenance treatment, economics may be a useful ally. Economic evaluations may prove useful in supporting claims for enhanced funding and inject some rationality into the debate about resource allocation. Furthermore, while resources remain limited and demand for treatment high, economic analysis can provide important information about the most cost-efficient way in which to deliver services so as to maximise treatment outcomes. This chapter introduces the reader to the discipline of health economics and reviews the limited literature available on the economic evaluation of methadone treatment.

The research to date suggests that the provision of methadone treatment is cost-beneficial, at least from a taxpayer's perspective, because of the substantial reductions in crime and drug use that occur. Furthermore, methadone compares favourably with alternative interventions for opioid-dependent individuals. As would be expected, the restrictive nature of residential programs results in greater reductions in drug use and criminal activity initially. However, because opioid dependence is a chronic relapsing condition and thus the "durability" of the treatment effect after the cessation of treatment is limited, and because increased time in treatment results in better outcomes, retention is a crucial factor in determining the overall effectiveness of opioid dependence programs. Therefore, because methadone treatment is better able to retain clients, and because it costs less to provide, than other interventions it has been found to be more cost-effective and to yield higher benefit to cost ratios during treatment and up to one year following treatment.

While from a clinical perspective retention is a treatment goal because of its association with improved outcomes, from an economic perspective it represents a cost. Rather than restricting the question to whether increased time in treatment results in greater outcomes, economists ask at what cost. In particular, given that there is a scarcity of resources for methadone service provision and that demand is high, the question is whether keeping someone in treatment for additional time produces greater benefits than an alternative use of the resources, for example, admitting a new client to treatment. To date, only one study has addressed this question directly, the interpretation of which is confounded by methodological problems. It does, however, along with other studies raise important questions about whether there is a point at which retention in treatment results in diminishing returns and, as such, does not represent the most efficient use of program resources.

Before more can be gleaned about the cost-effectiveness of methadone treatment relative to other interventions for opioid dependence or about optimal models of methadone service delivery through the application of marginal analysis, a more consistent and robust methodology needs to be developed. The relevant items to be costed in the delivery of services need to be identified and their measurement standardised. Similarly, there needs to be greater consensus on what the appropriate treatment outcomes are and how they should be valued and measured. In this regard, it is postulated that the application of a methodology that combines treatment effects with preference weights, as was done in the development of QALYs, would be of enormous value in evaluating the effectiveness of programs such as methadone maintenance which produce multiple outcomes across various domains.

Health economics is a relatively new discipline and, consequently, there have been few economic evaluations of methadone maintenance treatment. Since demand for treatment is likely to continue, however, it will be important to pursue lines of economic enquiry to ensure better and more efficient resource utilisation. The answer to this may lie in the transfer of more health resources to the provision of methadone treatment or simply an improved use of those resources already at our disposal.

REFERENCES

Anglin, M.D., Speckart, G.R., Booth, M.W., & Ryan, T.M. (1989). Consequences and costs of shutting off methadone. *Addictive Behaviour,* **14**, 307-326.

Apsler, R., & Harding, W.M. (1991). Cost-effectiveness analysis of drug abuse treatment. In *Background papers on drug abuse financing and services research* (pp.58-81). Rockville, MD: National Institute on Drug Abuse.

Bradley, C.J., French, M.T., & Rachal, J.V. (1994). Financing and cost of standard and enhanced methadone treatment. *Journal of Substance Abuse Treatment,* 11, 433-442.

Britton, B.M. (1994). The privatization of methadone maintenance: Changes in risk behaviour associated with cost related detoxification. *Addiction Research,* 2, 171-181.

Buck, D., Godfrey, C. & Sutton, M. (forthcoming). Economic and other views of addiction: Implications for the evaluation of policy options. *Drug and Alcohol Review.*

Collins, D.J., & Lapsley, H.M. (1991). *Estimating the economic costs of drug abuse in Australia.* National Campaign Against Drug Abuse Monograph Series No. 15. Canberra, Australia: Australian Government Publishing Service.

Collins, D. J., & Lapsley, H.M. (1996). *The social costs of drug abuse in Australia in 1988 and 1992.* National Campaign Against Drug Abuse Monograph Series No. 30. Canberra, Australia: Australian Government Publishing Service.

Commonwealth Department of Human Services and Health. (1995). *Review of methadone treatment in Australia.* Canberra, Australia: Australian Government Publishing Service.

Coyle, D., Godfrey, C., Hardman, G., & Raistrick, D. (1994). *Costing substance misuse services.* YARTIC Occasional Paper 5. York: Centre for Health Economics, University of York.

Darke, S., Hall, W., Wodak, A., Heather, N., & Ward, J. (1992). Development and validation of a multi-dimensional instrument for assessing outcome of treatment among opiate users: The Opiate Treatment Index. *British Journal of Addiction,* 87, 733-742.

Drummond, M.F., & Maynard, A. (1993). *Purchasing and providing cost-effective health care.* London: Churchill Livingstone.

Drummond, M.F, Stoddart, G.L., & Torrance, G.W. (1987). *Methods for the economic evaluation of health care programmes.* Oxford: Oxford University Press.

French, M.T. (1995). Economic evaluation of drug abuse treatment programs: Methodology and findings. *American Journal of Drug and Alcohol Abuse,* 21, 111-135.

French, M.T., Bradley, C.J., Calingaert, B., Dennis, M.L., & Karuntzos, G.T. (1994). Cost analysis of training and employment services in methadone treatment. *Evaluation and Program Planning,* 17, 107-120.

French, M.T., Zarkin, G.A., Hubbard, R.L., & Rachal, J.V. (1991). The impact of time in treatment on the employment and earnings of drug abusers. *American Journal of Public Health,* **81,** 904-907.

Gerstein, D. R., & Harwood, H. J. (Ed.). (1990). *Treating drug problems, Vol. I. A study of the evolution, effectiveness, and financing of public and private drug treatment systems.* Washington: National Academy Press.

Gerstein, D.R., Johnson, R.A., Harwood, H.J, Fountain, D., Suter, N., & Malloy, K., (1994). *Evaluating recovery services: The California drug and alcohol treatment assessment (CALDATA).* Sacramento, CA: California Department of Alcohol and Drug Programs.

Godfrey, C. (1994). Assessing the cost-effectiveness of alcohol services. *Journal of Mental Health, 3,* 3-21.

Godfrey, C. & Sutton, M. (1996). Costs and benefits of treating drug problems. In N. Lunt, & D. Coyle (Eds.), *Welfare and policy: Issues and agenda* (pp. 45-57). London: Taylor and Francis.

Goldschmidt, P.G. (1976). A cost-effectiveness model for evaluating health care programs: Application to drug abuse treatment. *Inquiry, 13 (March),* 29-47.

Hall, W. (1987). Disease costs and the allocation of health resources. *Bioethics, 1,* 211-225.

Hannan, T.H. (1975). *The economics of methadone maintenance.* Lexington, KY: Lexington Books.

Harwood, H.J., Hubbard, R.L., Collins, J.J., & Rachal, J.V. (1988). The costs of crime and the benefits of drug abuse treatment: A cost-benefit analysis using TOPS data. In C.G. Leukefeld, & F.M. Tims (Eds.), *Compulsory treatment of drug abuse: Research and clinical practice* (NIDA Research Monograph, pp. 209-235). Rockville, MD: National Institute on Drug Abuse.

Hubbard, R.L., Marsden, M.E., Rachal, J.V., Harwood, H.J., Cavanaugh, E.R., & Ginzburg, H.M. (1989). *Drug abuse treatment: A national study of effectiveness.* Chapel Hill, NC: University of North Carolina Press.

Maddux, J.F., Prihoda, T.J., & Desmond, D.P. (1994). Treatment fees and retention on methadone maintenance. *The Journal of Drug Issues, 24,* 429-443.

McGlothlin, W.H., & Anglin, D. (1981). Shutting off methadone: Costs and benefits. *Archives of General Psychiatry, 38,* 885-892.

Mooney, G. (1992). *Economics medicine and health care* (2nd ed.). New York: Harvester Wheatsheaf.

National Methadone Working Party, (1993). *National policy on methadone.* Canberra, Australia: Australian Government Publishing Service.

Peele, S. (1990). Research issues in assessing addiction treatment efficacy: How cost effective are Alcoholics Anonymous and private treatment centers? *Drug and Alcohol Dependence, 25,* 179-182.

Rice, D.P., Kelman, S., Miller, L.S, &. Dunmeyer, S. (1990). *The economic costs of alcohol and drug abuse and mental illness: 1985,* Institute of Health and Aging, University of California, San Francisco.

Shiell, A., Gerard, K., & Donaldson, C. (1987). Cost of illness studies: An aid to decision making? *Health Policy,* **8**, 317-323.

Simpson, L., & Sutton, M. (1996). *Putting all the eggs in one basket: A utility based method for evaluating a composite outcome from drug interventions.* Unpublished manuscript, Centre for Health Economics, University of York.

Smith, K, & Wright, K. (1996). Costs of mental illness in Britain. *Health Policy,* **35**, 61-73.

Swensen, G. (1989). The cost of the Western Australian methadone program. *Australian Drug and Alcohol Review,* **8**, 35-37.

Wagstaff, A., & Maynard, A. (1988). *Economic aspects of the illicit drug market and drug enforcement policies in the United Kingdom.* Home Office Research Study 95. London: Home Office.

Ward, P., Sutton, M., & Mattick, R.P. (forthcoming). *A cost-analysis of the public sector methadone program in NSW.* National Drug and Alcohol Research Centre Monograph Series. Sydney, Australia: National Drug and Alcohol Research Centre.

Weatherburn, D., & Lind, B. (1995). *Drug law enforcement policy and its impact on the heroin market.* NSW Bureau of Crime Statistics and Research. Sydney: NSW Government Printing Service.

Yates, B. T. (1994). Towards the incorporation of costs, cost-effectiveness analysis, and cost-benefit analysis into clinical research. *Journal of Consulting and Clinical Psychology,* **62**, 729-736.

Zarkin, G.A., French, M.T., Anderson, D.W., & Bradley, C.J. (1994). A conceptual framework for the economic evaluation of substance abuse interventions. *Evaluation and Program Planning,* **17**, 409-418.

6

THE EFFECTIVENESS OF OTHER OPIOID REPLACEMENT THERAPIES: LAAM, HEROIN, BUPRENORPHINE, NALTREXONE AND INJECTABLE MAINTENANCE

RICHARD P. MATTICK,
DOROTHY OLIPHANT, JEFF WARD
AND WAYNE HALL

INTRODUCTION

The need to consider and develop alternative methods of management of opioid-dependent patients is based on the belief that there is an important element of patient choice that affects the decision to enter and stay in treatment, and hence the benefits achieved. The issue of patient compliance with treatment is well recognised in health care delivery generally. There is no doubt that patient choice in treatment of opioid dependence is an important factor. The experience in one US study was instructive in this regard (Bale *et al.,* 1980). Bale and colleagues (1980) conducted a prospective observational study of treatment outcome among opiate addicted male veterans in which the intention was to randomly assign subjects to either a therapeutic community or to methadone maintenance and to compare their outcome with a detoxification-only control group. This plan had to be abandoned because treatment staff objected to patients being randomly assigned to treatment type. A compromise was reached in which subjects were required to enter the treatment program to which they had been assigned for one month following admission, after which they could change to the program of their choice. Very few of the patients remained in the programs to which they were originally assigned. Specifically, only 18% subjects who were assigned to therapeutic communities entered that modality and only 29% of those assigned to methadone maintenance engaged in that treatment.

We also need to be mindful of the work on heroin maintenance showing that patient choice or preference greatly affects retention (Hartnoll *et al.*, 1980). In that study, at 12 months 74% of patients continued to receive a prescription while only 29% of methadone maintenance patients were still in treatment. Given that retention is associated with other treatment benefits, the better retention of the heroin maintenance group is important; however, it has to be balanced with the issue of treatment response (see later). Even so, it should remain clear that patients have views of the treatments they are offered and these views affect their willingness to enter and stay in treatment. Only the balance of information concerning acceptability of each treatment and the effects achieved will allow a fully informed decision by policy makers and health care workers about the appropriate intervention for management of opioid dependence.

Oral methadone maintenance, like any pharmacotherapy, has some negative characteristics that have led to an interest in alternative pharmacotherapies and methods of treatment delivery (Mattick & Hall, 1993). First, as methadone is a full opioid agonist, it has the potential to produce dependence. Even in those who are suitable for opioid replacement therapy, there have been concerns about maintaining patients on a full agonist for fear of prolonging or worsening their level of dependence on opiates. Second, in overdose, the level of respiratory depression or sedation of methadone can be fatal. Deaths have occurred in patients being stabilised on methadone and in non-tolerant individuals. Third, although methadone is a relatively long-acting opioid, the inconvenience of daily dosing and clinic visits may be unattractive to certain clients, and the restrictions imposed by the daily dosing schedule on clients' opportunities to sustain employment may also limit its suitability. Fourth, the provision of take-away doses has the attendant problem of diversion.

Fifth, "street" myths and the stigma of methadone treatment create a barrier to entering treatment for those who might otherwise benefit from maintenance therapy (Rosenblum *et al.*, 1991), and some argue that the unattractiveness of methadone to many illicit opioid users is a barrier to entering treatment. Finally, there is a desire among some users to be able to inject maintenance medication rather than ingest it orally. Thus, despite its success as a maintenance agent, methadone appears to have some negative characteristics as outlined above, and explored in more detail elsewhere (Mattick & Hall, 1993). These factors may restrict the ability of methadone to attract opioid users into treatment (although the experience is that the demand for treatment with methadone outstrips supply). As a result, interest in the development of alternatives to broaden the range of pharmacotherapies has been the focus of increasing research in recent years.

There are a number of alternatives to methadone as a maintenance agent in the management of opioid dependence. At the basis of methadone maintenance treatment, and all opioid replacement therapy is the observation that, in general, opioid analgesics can be substituted for one another. The cross-tolerance between heroin and other opioids means that a person tolerant to heroin will also be tolerant to a dose-equivalent amount of methadone or other opioids with μ-agonist actions (Jaffe, 1990). Similarly, cross-suppression between heroin and other opioid μ-agonists allows opioid analgesics to prevent or reverse withdrawal symptoms, and thus reduce the need to use illegal heroin.

The most promising of these alternative opioid analgesics for management of opioid dependence in a maintenance regimen involve pharmacotherapies that treat clients with a pharmaceutical grade opioid which has a longer duration of action than methadone. These include the full agonist levo-alpha-acetylmethadol (LAAM), which was approved for use in the United States as a maintenance opioid drug in 1993 (Kreek, 1996a), and the opioid partial agonist buprenorphine. Additionally, diacetylmorphine (heroin) has attracted interest as a possible maintenance agent and is being trialed in Switzerland (Rihs, 1994) and considered for trialing in Australia (Bammer, 1993). Finally, naltrexone, a full opioid receptor antagonist, has been evaluated for the management of opioid dependence. Each of these alternatives to methadone are considered in separate sections below, along with the evidence for the use of injectable medications. Other alternative pharmacotherapies, such as dihydrocodeine (Robertson, 1996) or dextromoramide (Byrne, 1996), are not discussed.

LAAM

LAAM (levo-alpha-acetylmethadol) is a synthetic opioid analgesic (related to methadone) of the morphine type which was extensively investigated in the 1970s as a pharmacological alternative to methadone. Its major advantage compared with methadone is that it has a longer half-life and patients can be dosed every 48 hours, rather than every 24 hours as required with methadone. In some cases three-day dosing has been achieved satisfactorily. Additionally, it is effective when ingested orally, like methadone, meeting a major requirement placed on alternative maintenance pharmacotherapies by some. It was approved for use in treatment of opioid dependence in the U.S.A. in 1993 (Prendergast *et al.*, 1995).

A number of rationales have been put forward to support the use of LAAM in the treatment of opioid dependence. First, its use was to provide better suppression of withdrawal symptoms in patients who reported such symptoms before the end of the usual 24-hour dosing period on methadone. For those patients, and for those who for some reason miss a scheduled dose of methadone, LAAM would reduce the potential need to inject heroin to prevent withdrawal symptoms. Some argue that this benefit is likely to provide somewhat greater protection from transmission of HIV, as the time when patients on LAAM are suffering withdrawal symptoms should be less than for patients maintained on methadone. A second rationale for the use of LAAM rather than methadone was to reduce the need for "take-away" or "take-home" doses of methadone, overcoming problems of diversion and deaths associated with ingestion of the drug by non-tolerant individuals. Ironically, according to some (Kreek, 1996a; Prendergast *et al.*, 1995), the disallowance of take-home privileges for LAAM in the U.S.A. may be counter-productive by reducing patient acceptance of the medication and therefore use of LAAM. A third rationale for the use of LAAM is its potential to offer a more cost-effective intervention than methadone, yielding savings to the health care system through reduced costs of running clinics and to patients through reduced travel costs. A fourth rationale was that the less frequent clinic attendance also brings the additional benefit of reduced congregation at dosing sites because of less frequent clinic visits (Prendergast *et al.*, 1995), potentially providing greater community acceptance of dosing clinics and reduced illicit activity at the clinics.

Pharmacokinetics and Pharmacodynamics

LAAM is a pure μ-type opioid agonist which has a relatively long duration of action due to the fact that its two metabolites are active. Specifically, LAAM metabolises to the active metabolite nor-LAAM, which in turn metabolises to the active metabolite di-nor-LAAM. The half life of LAAM is 2.6 days, of nor-LAAM 2 days, and 4 days for di-nor-LAAM (Kreek, 1996a). While the advantages of the long half-life of LAAM and its metabolites are obvious, Kreek (1996a) has pointed out that these long half-lives can produce potential problems of toxicity, especially if LAAM is rapidly metabolised due to enhanced liver function. In these cases, the potential for toxic levels of LAAM's active metabolites to build up should be noted, especially during the stabilisation phase of maintenance dosing with this medication. Because of these problems, Kreek (1996a) cautions against daily dosing with LAAM, suggesting that 48 hours is the minimum period between doses.

Like methadone, LAAM is well absorbed via the oral route. It is thought that for patients being transferred from methadone to LAAM, the recommended initial dose is 1.2 or 1.3 times the methadone dose in milligrams (Kreek, 1996a). However, there is some evidence that the induction on to LAAM is affected by a delay in opioid activity as LAAM forms the long-acting active metabolites (see earlier), indicating a need for administration of other medications to deal with transient withdrawal symptoms for the initial 96 hours of dosing (Tennant *et al.*, 1986). Once stabilised alternate-day dosing is feasible.

Treatment Effectiveness

Jaffe *et al.* (1972) compared LAAM and methadone with a wait-list control group. Over a 15-week study period, they found no statistical difference in outcome between the methadone and LAAM groups on employment status, drug use, and clinic and therapy group attendance. However, both the LAAM and methadone groups did better in terms of employment than the wait-list group, with the former improving while the employment status of the wait-list group deteriorated.

Others have also found positive results for LAAM. Ling *et al.* (1976) reported on a 40-week double-blind randomised controlled trial to compare the safety and efficacy of LAAM (80 mg thrice weekly with placebo on non-dose days) with that of high-dose (100 mg) and low-dose methadone (50 mg) administered daily. The study was conducted at 12 sites with 430 subjects. Both LAAM and high-dose methadone were found to be more effective treatments than low-dose methadone. The authors concluded that LAAM is as safe and efficacious as high dose methadone. However, a number of caveats have to be taken into account when interpreting the study. First, the study only used fixed doses, whereas in clinical practice it is usual to individualise the dose to suit patient needs. Second, only 42% of the sample completed the full 40 weeks of the trial and most terminations occurred in the early weeks, with more patients leaving the trial in the LAAM group than in the high-dose methadone group. As expected, a greater number of side-effects were reported by the LAAM group than by the low-dose methadone group. It was difficult to compare the extent of side-effects associated with LAAM with that for high-dose methadone because only a few of the LAAM group could be traced to find out why they stopped treatment.

In a second controlled trial from this group, Ling *et al.* (1980) examined the feasibility of maintaining patients on methadone from Monday through to Thursday and then with a single dose of LAAM on Friday until the following Monday. Unfortunately, there was a high drop-out rate in both groups, with 65% of the LAAM subjects and 48% of the methadone subjects leaving the study. The majority of LAAM drop-outs were due to "medication not holding" (48%). The authors concluded that this approach does not have wide general clinical application, but felt it may be useful for particular subjects, because some people found the regimen satisfactory.

Freedman and Czertko (1981) compared the relative clinical efficacy of low-dose daily methadone (mean = 26 mg) with a thrice weekly low-dose LAAM regimen (mean = 24 mg) in a group of employed male heroin addicts. They found that the LAAM subjects used illicit drugs less and had better retention in treatment than the daily methadone subjects. As the LAAM subjects had previously been maintained on methadone, they were asked to complete a drug performance questionnaire to examine their satisfaction with both regimens. Patients preferred LAAM to methadone on nine out of 15 items, which included questions about frequency of dosing, health status and the extent to which each of the drugs reduced craving for heroin. The authors concluded that LAAM was acceptable to patients as a form of opioid maintenance and is particularly indicated for employed patients. It should be stressed that in this study the dose of both methadone and LAAM was kept to the lowest dose possible at which withdrawal symptoms were alleviated and that the low retention rates, especially in the methadone group, are consistent with those observed in other low-dose methadone programs.

Savage and his colleagues (1976) used a double-blind cross-over design to compare the relative safety and effectiveness of LAAM and methadone. A sample of 99 males who had been stabilised on methadone were randomly assigned to one of two groups. One group received methadone for three months and were then switched to LAAM. The other group received LAAM for the first three months and then transferred to methadone. Their results showed that significantly more participants in the LAAM group dropped out of treatment during the first three months, but there was no difference in outcome between the two groups in the second three-month period. Side-effects of the medication were given as the main reason for withdrawing from the study, and this was just as likely for patients on methadone as for patients on LAAM. In addition, there was no association between the type of drug and particular side-effects, and no significant difference between the two drug groups in terms of illicit drug use or absenteeism from the clinic. The authors concluded that for those who remained in treatment, LAAM was at least as effective as methadone and that both were safe treatment procedures.

In a study that examined patient impressions of LAAM, Trueblood and colleagues (1978) canvassed the opinions of subjects who had at least three months experience using both LAAM and methadone. Three groups were surveyed: those currently being maintained on LAAM, those currently on methadone, and a group who were no longer in opioid maintenance, but who had used both LAAM and methadone. LAAM was the preferred maintenance drug, with most subjects believing that it provided better blockade and reduced craving. Subjects claimed that they used less heroin, felt more normal and in better health and were less anxious or nervous while on LAAM. No difference was perceived in sexual performance, sleep problems or appetite. In the setting where this survey was undertaken, LAAM was regarded by staff as an innovative and superior drug and its use was strongly supported.

There has been relatively little study of LAAM since the early

1980s. Clinical experience with the medication has been reported on by Tennant *et al.* (1986). Who provide an overview of clinical experience with LAAM with almost 1,000 patients for periods of up to 36 months. Doses of 20 mg to 140 mg per dosage were used. There was no evidence of long-term toxicological effects. They suggest that the medication is safe, and efficacious for the majority of patients treated.

HEROIN (DIACETYLMORPHINE) MAINTENANCE THERAPY

Heroin (diacetylmorphine) is an opioid analgesic that has not been extensively investigated as a pharmacological alternative for the management of opioid dependence. Its major disadvantage is that it has a shorter half-life than methadone and patients need more frequent dosing. Its use as a therapeutic medication is also affected by its illicit status.

Proponents of heroin maintenance argue that the HIV epidemic requires all approaches to management of illicit drug use to be expanded. Specifically, often arguing for the controlled availability of illicit drugs, they point out that the prohibition of heroin has failed to eradicate the availability of illicit heroin; the unregulated illicit heroin market continues with no control over quality, purity, price, dose, mode of administration or the associated hazards of use; heroin maintenance will attract and retain heroin users who are not interested in entering methadone maintenance treatment; and heroin maintenance is a legitimate intermediate goal in treatment, and can be used in the short term to attract those initially disinterested in methadone to attend treatment settings, thereafter allowing gradual transfer to long-acting opioids for maintenance (Goldstein, 1976).

A number of arguments against heroin maintenance therapy have been made. First, the short duration of action of heroin requires frequent administration at a clinic, which is expensive and inconvenient for all concerned, and which focuses users in a particular geographic area. The alternative to the short half-life problem is to give the patient sufficient supplies to self-administer the drug elsewhere, but this solution risks inappropriate self-administration or significant diversion of the drug to others (Dole & Nyswander, 1965). Moreover, the continued injection practices may result in continued exposure to risk of infection with HIV and other viruses. It has been argued that patients cannot be adequately "stabilised" on short-acting opioids (e.g., morphine, heroin, hydromorphone, codeine, oxycodone, and meperidine) (Fink, 1972), with early attempts at maintenance with short-acting agents reportedly finding that despite frequent injections the patients' condition fluctuated between somnolence and agitation throughout each day, with tolerance increasing over consecutive days to the point where patients were almost continuously agitated even when receiving huge doses of morphine (Dole, 1972; 1988).

Pharmacokinetics and Pharmacodynamics

Heroin is a pure μ-type opioid agonist which has a short duration of action of 4-5 hours, and the plasma half-life of the heroin is reportedly 0.5 hour (Jaffe & Martin, 1990). Relatively little is known about the pharmacodynamics and pharmacokinetics of diacetylmorphine, as its illicit status has not promoted interest in the study of this aspect of the drug. However, it is sufficient to state that heroin has a rapid onset of opioid effects and a short-acting pharmacokinetic profile.

Treatment Effectiveness

The literature on the effects of maintenance prescribing of heroin is markedly different from that available on methadone, buprenorphine and LAAM, being largely dominated by personal views and opinions for and against the approach – views that appear to have more to do with ideological stance, and unfortunately little to do with empirical data. However, some information is available.

On the claim that drug misusers cannot be adequately stabilised on heroin, there appeared to be only limited evidence to support the view (Volavka *et al.*, 1970), in the references cited by those who made the claim (Dole, 1972; 1988; Fink, 1972) or in other literature. There is no doubt that there is a more marked psychotrophic effect from heroin due to the shorter half-life compared to long-acting opioids, such as methadone. However, double-blind randomised research has shown that patients can be adequately stabilised on heroin (Ghodse *et al.*, 1990).

There is only one randomised controlled clinical trial of maintenance on injectable heroin compared against oral methadone maintenance treatment (Hartnoll *et al.*, 1980), conducted in the

United Kingdom. Hartnoll and colleagues studied 96 heroin-dependent subjects who were offered one or other treatment and who were followed for one year, and it was found that the majority of those prescribed injectable heroin continued to inject heroin regularly (daily) and to supplement their maintenance prescription from other sources. Those who received oral methadone were more likely to be abstinent. Those in methadone maintenance treatment who continued to inject were (not surprisingly) more reliant on illegal sources of drugs. The significant differences tended to favour oral methadone maintenance, in that methadone maintenance patients had a significantly lower daily opioid consumption level, injected less frequently, and spent less of their time with other users. However, the drop-out rates differed markedly, with a 26% drop-out rate in the heroin maintenance group and a 71% drop-out rate in the methadone maintenance group. Thus, it appeared that oral methadone forced patients to either become abstinent or to continue illicit involvement. Heroin maintenance patients maintained the status quo. There were no differences in terms of physical health, or employment between the two groups. Crime was not different between the groups once pre-treatment criminal involvement was taken into account.

Hartnoll and colleagues (1980) note that the mixed results "do not indicate a clear overall superiority of either approach. Both treatments have advantages in some areas, but at the expense of disadvantages in other areas. The approach favoured depends on the priorities assigned to the various outcomes" (p. 882). They make the point that the approach taken must reflect the relative "clinical, ethical and political judgements". In an HIV-aware world, the reduced frequency of injecting might be the prime goal, or having more heroin-dependent patients in treatment may be preferred so that risk reduction procedures can be put in place.

Others (Marks, 1991) are more optimistic concerning the value of heroin prescribing. Marks presents results from the Widnes Clinic suggestive of lowered criminal activity, injecting, needle sharing and HIV rates associated with the prescribing of heroin. He provides data comparing Merseyside to the rest of England and Scotland. The results are interesting, but do not equate to a controlled trial, and there are numerous rival hypotheses which could explain the difference in apparent rates.

Most recently, the Swiss have been investigating the value of heroin prescribing in a multi-site trial. Originally, the trial was to assess the effects of injectable heroin and injectable morphine at one site in a randomised controlled trial, and at other sites quasi-experimental studies were to compare those injectable opioids against usual oral methadone treatment. The research is yet to be completed and it will be at that time that the relative benefits and disadvantages of heroin maintenance will be more clearly documented. However, preliminary information (Hall, 1996) suggests that the cost of the delivery of heroin in a clinic-based system is at least double that of the cost of methadone maintenance in Switzerland. The trial has some preliminary data suggesting relatively good retention in the heroin maintenance arm of the study, but the final analysis will be required for firm conclusions.

Not surprisingly, given the lack of empirical data, there appears to be more energy put into debating the issues surrounding heroin maintenance therapy (Bammer, 1992; 1993; Bammer *et al.*, 1994; Fink, 1972; Marks, 1991; Marks, 1990; Parry, 1992; Stimmel, 1975; Stimson & Oppenheimer, 1982; Strang *et al.*, 1994) than into further careful evaluation of the relative efficacy of heroin maintenance, who it is suitable for, whether it can function to attract and retain users who would not otherwise enter treatment, whether it would serve as a bridge to oral long-acting opioid replacement therapy, and whether it can be administered in a fashion that is economic and cost-beneficial to the users and community. Strang and colleagues (1994) concluded a recent consideration of the area by noting the lack of research and stating that "no reliable conclusions can be reached about such prescribing, and the issue is open to hijack by those who wish to reinforce their pre-selected position" within the debate (p. 203). The research currently being carried out in Europe may, however, shed further light on the value of heroin maintenance (Karel, 1993; Rihs, 1994).

BUPRENORPHINE

Buprenorphine is a mixed agonist-antagonist with high affinity at both μ and opioid receptors. It has been used extensively in many countries for the management of acute pain, and is as effective an analgesic as morphine with a longer duration of action and greater safety in overdose (Lewis, 1985). Pharmacologically, buprenorphine invokes morphine-like subjective effects and produces cross-tolerance to other opioids. The mixed opioid-action/blocking-action appears to make buprenorphine safer in overdose and possibly less likely to be diverted than pure opioids. It may also provide a potentially easier withdrawal phase and the unusual receptor kinetics which cause a long duration of action allows for alternate-day dosing. Buprenorphine has been the subject of much recent research, and applications for approval for use of the drug in the U.S.A. (Swan, 1993) and in European countries are in train. It is registered for the treatment of opioid dependence in France.

It was during the initial development of buprenorphine as an analgesic in the 1970s that its potential utility as a substitution agent in the treatment of opioid dependence was recognised. Early work by Jasinski *et al.* (1978), using buprenorphine administered by the subcutaneous route, characterised it as an opioid with low physical dependence liability. This property suggested that at doses somewhat greater than those used for analgesia, it could be used in the treatment of opioid dependence.

A major consideration in the development of a viable treatment product for opioid dependence has been the perceived need to avoid injectable formulations. Since buprenorphine has poor oral bio-availability due to intestinal metabolism, most of the subsequent clinical pharmacology and clinical studies have administered buprenorphine beneath the tongue, via the sublingual route in an ethanol solution. For a time, this offered the most convenient formulation for the range of doses used in the various studies. The successful development of the sublingual analgesic tablet has also proved it to be an acceptable route of administration, albeit with lower bioavailability than the ethanol formulation (Mendelson *et al.*, 1995).

Pharmacokinetics and Pharmacodynamics

Buprenorphine is classified as a mixed agonist-antagonist or as a partial μ-type opioid agonist (Lewis, 1985). The opioid effects of this drug appear to plateau as the dose increases, and this effect may be due in part to the antagonist effect coming into play at higher dose and plasma concentration levels. There is a suggestion that increasing doses beyond the plateau can produce *decreasing* opioid effects as the antagonist action of buprenorphine occurs, and this has been described as a classical bell-shaped or inverted U-type dose response curve (Kreek, 1996b). It appears to be very safe relative to other opioids, such that overdose has not occurred in doses many times the therapeutic dose (Banks, 1979).

It is a potent analgesic considered to be 25-50 times more potent than morphine for pain relief and 30 times more potent than morphine in its ability to produce effects in opioid-dependent subjects (Jasinski & Preston, 1996). Taken orally it is a relatively ineffective drug due to the efficient "first-pass" metabolism by the liver. However, the drug is quite well absorbed sublingually and has been shown to be effective when administed via this route. It is also potent when injected and has the potential for abuse, as the tablet is easily crushed and injected. This property has led to the development of research to evaluate the ability of a combined buprenorphine-naloxone sublingual preparation to prevent injection (Robinson *et al.*, 1993). Various ratios of buprenorphine to naloxone are being trialed (1:1, 4:1, 6:1) to determine the best ratio.

The half-life of buprenorphine in humans by the intravenous route is relatively short, at 3 to 5 hours. However, the drug appears to have the property of binding very tightly to receptor sites causing a very slow release from opioid receptors, and this property produces the kinetics that are important in bringing about the long duration of action (Lewis, 1985). This strong binding has been shown in studies of the effects of pure opioid antagonists which indicate that it is quite difficult to antagonise the effects of buprenorphine once it has bound to opioid receptors (Kreek, 1996b; Lehmann *et al.*, 1988). In a study by Lehmann and colleagues (1988), naloxone did not completely reverse the respiratory depression and other effects induced by buprenorphine in all the cases studied. However, the respiratory depression associated with buprenorphine is quite mild, relative to other pure opioid agonists. This property suggests that it has the potential to markedly reduce the incidence of opioid death in patients and others. Walsh and colleagues (1994) gave 32mg of buprenorphine to non-dependent subjects and estimate this dose to be equivalent to approximately 500mg of intramuscular morphine and to 1000mg of oral methadone. "Those doses (of morphine and methadone) would be in the lethal range; in contrast, buprenorphine produced no serious adverse effects at any dose tested and had only marginal effects on respiratory function" (p. 578).

The tightness of binding of buprenorphine onto opioid receptor sites has been one explanation put forward for the very low level of withdrawal symptoms associated with the abrupt cessation of chronic dosing with buprenorphine compared with other opioids such as morphine (Lewis, 1985). Others have suggested that the mixed agonist-antagonist effects of buprenorphine may reduce the extent of significant physical dependence and this may be the mechanism whereby the less severe withdrawal symptoms occur (Jasinski *et al.*, 1978).

Buprenorphine is well absorbed via the sublingual route (Lewis, 1985), whereas the bioavailability of buprenorphine is decreased if the medication is swallowed, as oral absorption is 15% of sublingual absorption. This poor oral absorption also provides greater safety in the case of overdose, compared to other pure agonists which are well absorbed orally.

As well, there are differences between the ethanol solution and the tablet in terms of bioavailability. Specifically, U.S. researchers (Mendelson *et al.*, 1995) studying a small number of patients have reported that the bioavailability of buprenorphine in the ethanol solution used in most of the pivotal clinical efficacy studies was higher than that of the tablet, which is the commercially available formulation. The tablet produced approximately 50% the bioavailability of the ethanol solution, on average, and had marginally slower absorption. However, there was marked inter-individual variability such that bioavailability for some subjects was essentially equivalent for the two preparations (tablet bioavailability was 85% of ethanol base), but markedly lower for one patient (12%) in the series of six cases reported in the study (Mendelson *et al.*, 1995). The importance of full dissolution of the tablet in patients is highlighted by these findings, as is the need to consider the development of alternative rapid dissolution formulations to maximise absorption.

A series of clinical pharmacology studies have been conducted using volunteer subjects, who were either dependent or non-dependent opioid users, and could recognise and quantify the effects of opioid drugs. In an initial study, Jasinski and colleagues (1989) showed that sublingual buprenorphine in ethanol solution had opioid agonist effects and that its pharmacodynamic activity, based on a number of parameters, was about 70% of that of subcutaneous buprenorphine. In two further studies, a range of buprenorphine doses (up to 32 mg) were compared to methadone using a Latin-square (Walsh *et al.*, 1993) or parallel group (Walsh *et al.*, 1994) design. In both studies, there was a ceiling on the effects of buprenorphine which varied according to the parameter assessed, but in general occurred in the dose range 8-32 mg. The effects of these doses were similar to those produced by 60 mg methadone but the onset of action of buprenorphine was more rapid. In the first study, buprenorphine (8-32 mg) and methadone (60 mg) produced blockade of the effects of an opioid agonist (hydromorphone) 24 hours after drug administration. In the parallel group study, the higher doses of buprenorphine (8-32 mg) had a long duration of effect, which was evident for up to 48 hours after drug administration.

Two further studies have assessed the effects of buprenorphine administration to subjects maintained on methadone or morphine. In a study on methadone-maintained subjects (June *et al.*, 1993), buprenorphine produced dose-related antagonist effects in subjects maintained on 60 mg/day of methadone, but this effect was less evident in subjects maintained on 30 mg/day of methadone. This result suggests that abrupt transition from methadone to buprenorphine may produce unacceptable discomfort and that the transition should be accomplished gradually.

The clinical pharmacology studies have clearly identified the potential utility of buprenorphine as a substitution agent in the treatment of opioid dependence, as shown by its opioid agonist effects and its ability to produce prolonged blockade of subsequently administered opioid agonists.

Treatment Effectiveness

As with methadone, the number of randomised controlled trials that compare buprenorphine with a relevant comparison treatment are few. Fortunately, the recent interest (both scientific and financial) provoked by government and community recognition of the necessity for alternative pharmacological interventions for opioid dependence has proved a boon for such research, as evidenced by the number of recent randomised controlled clinical trials that have been published.

The majority of clinical studies have been conducted in the USA, and have used opioid dependent subjects, many of whom were unemployed and were using a range of drugs in addition to opioids, especially cocaine, but also benzodiazepines, amphetamines, etc. Based on the clinical pharmacology and initial clinical studies, a sublingual buprenorphine dose of 8 mg/day in an ethanol solution was identified as potentially offering the best maintenance dose and was used in most of the comparative studies. In nearly all of these studies, which range in duration from 3 weeks to one year, methadone was used as the reference therapy.

Bickel, Stitzer, Bigelow, Liebson, Jasinski and Johnson (1988)

Bickel and colleagues (1988) were the first to conduct a randomised, double-blind trial that compared buprenorphine with methadone. Forty-five opioid-dependent male subjects were randomised to receive either 2mg/day of buprenorphine or 30 mg/day of methadone for the first three weeks of the study. Following this stabilisation, doses were reduced over a 4-week period, after which placebo was administered for the final 6 weeks. No differences were observed between buprenorphine and methadone with respect to retention in treatment, symptom report or reduction of illicit opioid use. However, the study demonstrated that 2 mg of sublingual buprenorphine in ethanol solution was less effective than 30 mg of oral methadone in its ability to attenuate the physiological and subjective effects of a 6 mg hydromorphone challenge.

Johnson, Jaffe and Fudala (1992)

In a longer randomised double-blind trial, Johnson and colleagues recruited 162 volunteers seeking treatment for their opioid dependence (Johnson *et al.*, 1992). All subjects received both an oral (methadone or placebo) and a sublingual (buprenorphine or placebo) dose on each day of treatment ("double-dummy"). Three treatment groups were used: 8 mg per day sublingual buprenorphine in ethanol solution (n=53), 20 mg/day oral methadone (n=55) and 60 mg/day oral methadone (n=54). The study was conducted over 180 days, which included 120 days of induction and maintenance, and 60 days of dose reduction and placebo dosing.

The primary outcome measures were retention in treatment and illicit opioid use. The percentage of subjects retained in treatment for the 25 weeks of the study were 30%, 20% and 6% for buprenorphine, methadone 60 mg and methadone 20 mg respectively, with the methadone 20 mg group showing significantly poorer retention than either the buprenorphine or methadone 60 mg groups. There was no difference between the buprenorphine or the methadone 60 mg groups on the retention measure. For the second outcome measure, the analysis showed that buprenorphine-maintained subjects produced an average of 53% of urine samples negative for opioids, methadone 60 mg an average of 44% and methadone 20 mg an average of 29%. Both buprenorphine and methadone 60 mg were significantly better than methadone 20 mg on this measure. When the data were analysed for the patients who completed the maintenance phase only, buprenorphine was associated with significantly more urines negative for opioids than either methadone 20 mg or 60 mg.

The authors concluded that buprenorphine 8 mg/day was at least as effective as methadone 60 mg/day and both were superior to methadone 20 mg/day in reducing illicit opioid use and maintaining patients in treatment. The results were indicative of buprenorphine being as effective as methadone at the fixed doses given.

Kosten, Schottenfeld, Ziedonis and Falcioni (1993)

Kosten and his colleagues compared sublingual buprenorphine (2 mg or 6 mg/day) with methadone maintenance (35 mg or 65 mg/day) in a 24-week double-blind, double-dummy, randomised clinical trial (Kosten *et al.*, 1993). The 125 subjects received fixed doses of both an oral syrup and sublingual ethanol solution (active and placebo). Comparison of the two buprenorphine groups revealed that there was less illicit opioid abuse in the 6 mg group than in the 2 mg group, as demonstrated by fewer opioid-positive urines and self-reported illicit opioid use. Continued opioid withdrawal symptoms were also associated with the 2 mg group. Treatment retention was better in the methadone groups (20 weeks) compared to the buprenorphine groups (16 weeks), and opioid-free urines were higher for methadone than for buprenorphine (51% vs. 27%), as was abstinence for at least 3 weeks (65% vs. 27%). The authors concluded that both buprenorphine doses were clearly less effective than methadone, and that comparison studies of buprenorphine and methadone need to utilise higher doses of buprenorphine. Again, the suggestion of a dose response is clear, and others have been critical of the low doses used (Newman, 1994). It is unfortunate that most researchers have used fixed-dose rather than flexible-dose regimens, as there is a lack of information about the relative dose equivalence of buprenorphine and methadone.

Strain, Stitzer, Liebson and Bigelow (1994)

The assessment of possible dose-equivalence was undertaken in a 26-

week study in which the dose received by 164 subjects was varied to obtain optimum response after initial stabilisation at doses of 8 mg/day sublingual buprenorphine or 50 mg/day methadone (Strain *et al.*, 1994). Participants were randomly assigned to one of two treatment groups: sublingual buprenorphine in ethanol solution or oral methadone. The first four days comprised the induction phase of treatment, subjects received daily doses of 2, 4, 6, and 8 mg buprenorphine or 20, 30, 40, or 50 mg methadone, in a double-blind and double-dummy dosing regimen, until stabilised. From weeks 3 to 16, subjects could receive double-blind dose increases and decreases (in increments of either 10 mg methadone or 2 mg buprenorphine) to a maximum of 4 increases (90 mg methadone or 16 mg buprenorphine) spaced at least one week apart. During the last 10 weeks doses were tapered by 10% per week to placebo. Outcome measures included retention in treatment, attendance and opioid positive urines.

The mean doses during the stable dosing period were 8.9 mg/day buprenorphine and 54 mg/day methadone. There were no group differences in the number of subjects requesting or receiving dose increases. Fifty-six percent of subjects in each group completed the 16-week induction/maintenance phase. No differences were observed between the two groups with respect to retention time in treatment or to urine samples found to be positive for opioids. Buprenorphine and methadone were also equally effective in sustaining compliance with medication and counselling. These data suggest that a dose of 8 mg buprenorphine is equivalent to a moderate dose of methadone.

Johnson, Eissenberg, Stitzer, Strain, Liebson and Bigelow (1995a)

These investigators were the first to use a placebo-controlled design in their buprenorphine research, in which buprenorphine treatment is compared with a placebo control condition, rather than with methadone (as in previous studies) (Johnson *et al.*, 1995a). This was a 2-week (14 day) double-blind study, which was part of a 20-week study. Participants were randomly assigned to one of 3 treatment conditions in a 2:2:1 ratio: placebo (n=60), sublingual buprenorphine 2 mg (n=60), or buprenorphine 8 mg (n=30). On days 6 to 13 patients could request to change to another dose condition, which would be randomly chosen from the two to which they had not been originally assigned. Outcome measures included the percentage of patients on initial dose, percentage of opioid-positive urines, and dose adequacy, as measured by patients' responses to a visual analogue scale incorporating such questions as "How well has this dose of medicine been holding you?".

Analyses showed that subjects given buprenorphine showed greater time on initial dose, requested fewer dose changes, used less illicit opioids, and rated dose adequacy higher than those on placebo, but that the two active medication groups did not differ from each other. This result is somewhat surprising given other results suggestive of a dose response for buprenorphine, but the failure to detect differences between the two buprenorphine dose levels may have been due to the short duration of the study period.

Ling, Wesson, Charuvastra, and Klett (1996)

These investigators (Ling *et al.,* 1996) recently reported on a trial comparing 30 mg methadone, 80 mg methadone and 8 mg buprenorphine in ethanol solution with 225 opioid dependent individuals. The trial was of one-year duration with data collected at study midpoint and at one year. Patients were randomly allocated to groups and the blind was adequately maintained.

The results showed that 80 mg methadone was superior to both 30 mg methadone and to 8 mg buprenorphine in retaining patients in treatment, reducing illicit opioid use, and decreasing craving for opioids. The 30 mg methadone and 8 mg buprenorphine were largely equivalent to each other in their effects on these variables. Ling and colleagues noted the 8 mg of buprenorphine in ethanol solution was not an optimal dosage, and that higher doses would probably provide a better outcome. They also noted the discrepancy between their results and those of earlier research (Johnson *et al.,* 1992), and pointed out the need for research to address the dose levels of buprenorphine that are effective, rather than predetermine doses. Such research is in train in the USA and Australia.

Dosage and Alternate-Day Dosing

Dose induction has been studied (Johnson *et al.,* 1989) with 19 subjects given sublingual buprenorphine in ascending daily doses of 2 mg, 4 mg, and 8 mg, then maintained on 8 mg for 15 days. Results from the first 4 days showed subjects reported significantly elevated ratings of "good effects" and "overall well-being" and decreased ratings of "overall sickness", and correctly identified buprenorphine as an opioid (not an opioid antagonist). It was concluded that buprenorphine was acceptable to heroin-dependent users, and that rapid dose induction causes minimal withdrawal symptoms.

Doses of buprenorphine between 2 mg and 16 mg have been assessed, and 32 mg doses have been evaluated in some trials. Currently, the maximum safe dose that has been tested for buprenorphine appears to be 32 mg per day. There may be a ceiling on the effects of buprenorphine at doses beyond 32 mg per day in terms of its ability to produce further opioid effects. Because of this ceiling effect, the benefit of higher doses may not be increased efficacy through increasing agonist effects, but rather increased duration of action. Given the potential for longer duration of dosing, alternate-day dosing with buprenorphine has been examined and found acceptable to many patients. The feasibility of dosing on alternate days has been investigated in a number of studies.

In the first study (Fudala *et al.*, 1990), 19 male volunteers were randomly assigned to one of two groups. All received sublingual buprenorphine in ascending daily doses of 2 mg, 4 mg and 8 mg and were maintained on 8 mg/day through to study day 18. On study days 19 to 36, group one continued on daily dosing, whereas group two received buprenorphine or placebo on alternate days. From days 37 to 52 all subjects received placebo. Alternate-day recipients reported significantly greater urge for an opioid, increased dysphoria scores and pupillary dilation on placebo days. Daily dosing provided greater control of subtle opioid withdrawal symptoms, but subjects could tolerate a between-dose interval of 48 hours.

In a second study (Amass *et al.*, 1994), following stabilisation on sublingual buprenorphine (4 mg/70 kg or 8 mg/70 kg), 13 opioid-dependent subjects were treated with their stabilisation dose daily or double their stabilisation dose every other day for 21 days each. There were no observable differences between the two treatment regimes for the great majority of parameters assessed, suggesting that sublingual buprenorphine can be administered every 48 hours at double the subjects' normal daily maintenance dose. Specifically, 16 out of 17 measures of opioid agonist and withdrawal effects did not differ between the two schedules. However, the subject-rated agonist effects did differ, being lower for alternate-day dosing.

Resnick and his colleagues (Resnick *et al.*, 1994), studied alternate-day dosing in a single-blind study of 31 abstinent subjects who had been stabilised on buprenorphine (4-16 mg/day) for 1 to 12 months. The 31 patients were switched to double their daily dose on alternate days. All subjects continued in treatment and remained abstinent. Of the 31 subjects, 28 had no abstinence symptoms for 48 hours after receiving their double dose. Reports on this measure were dose related. Patients expressed appreciation for the decreased number of clinic visits.

Most recently, Johnson and colleagues (Johnson *et al.*, 1995b) examined alternate-day dosing in 99 subjects who were stabilised on 8 mg daily sublingual buprenorphine in an 11-week randomised, double-blind, parallel group study. Subjects either received daily 8 mg buprenorphine or alternate-day 8 mg buprenorphine and placebo. Outcome measures included retention in treatment, opioid positive urines, percentage of cocaine positive urines, clinic attendance, dose adequacy and opioid withdrawal symptoms. There was a non-significant trend for the superiority of the daily dosing schedule. However, the authors concluded that the results were generally consistent with prior research that alternate-day dosing can be effective in and acceptable to a substantial number of opioid-dependent patients.

Buprenorphine misuse

Buprenorphine has abuse potential, as do all other psychotrophic medications available to injecting drug users. Early research showed that the medication had the potential to produce opioid-like effects. Both acute and chronic administration of subcutaneous buprenorphine produces euphoria and ratings of "drug liking" (Jasinski *et al.*, 1978). Similar results were also obtained by others (Pickworth *et al.*, 1993). Abuse has been reported in Western Australia, Scotland and New Zealand (Robinson *et al.*, 1993). This has led to some experimentation with the combination preparation of buprenorphine with naloxone in New Zealand (Robinson *et al.*, 1993) and the research is currently being pursued further in the U.S.A. The concerns about injection of the mono-therapy buprenorphine may lead to the combination buprenorphine-naloxone preparation being the preferred formulation.

Conclusion

It is apparent from the research to date that buprenorphine is at least
as effective as methadone as a maintenance agent. Specifically, open
trials (Johnson *et al.*, 1989) and randomised research have
demonstrated that buprenorphine is as effective as methadone as a
maintenance medication in reducing illicit opioid use, in retaining ·
patients in treatment (Johnson *et al.*, 1992; Kosten *et al.*, 1993), and
as a detoxification agent (Bickel *et al.*, 1988). Double-blind research
has also demonstrated that maintenance buprenorphine is effective in
reducing heroin craving and use (Resnick *et al.*, 1992). Further large-
scale double-blind randomised controlled clinical trials have recently
been completed in the U.S.A. and have produced positive results for
buprenorphine as a maintenance medication.

Buprenorphine also appears to possess markedly greater safety in
overdose than methadone since it produces relatively limited
respiratory depression, and is extremely well tolerated by non-
dependent humans (Walsh *et al.*, 1994). The safety margin means that
it also has the potential for alternate-day dosing (i.e. double dosing on
alternate days). Utilisation of this capability would provide a
significant advantage over methadone as a maintenance medication in
terms of patient convenience, risk of diversion of take-home doses,
and the economic costs of treatment delivery.

Finally, there is evidence that the mixed agonist-antagonist action of
buprenorphine makes withdrawal from this medication less severe
than withdrawal from pure agonists, such as methadone or heroin.
This has led some to suggest that withdrawal from maintenance
therapy would be easier, and to speculate that because of the mixed
action "the endogenous opioid system may indeed be set closer to
normal baseline functioning when chronically exposed to the partial
antagonist buprenorphine rather than to the pure agonist methadone"
(Kosten *et al.*, 1992).

The issue of patient acceptance must be studied, as much of the
research has occurred in the U.S.A., where the poor availability of
access to opioid replacement therapy arguably makes patients more
compliant. It may prove that patients in other countries will find
buprenorphine's antagonist properties unattractive. Alternatively, it
may be that the large pool of patients who feel unable to withdraw
from methadone, and who wish to cease opioid replacement therapy,
will find buprenorphine a boon.

Of course, the research literature generally raises some important issues for considering the dose equivalence of buprenorphine and methadone. First, dose equivalence has not yet been adequately determined, and the issue is complicated by the partial agonist nature of buprenorphine which makes plateau effects likely with buprenorphine and reduces the extent to which a linear dose-response relationship is present. Ideally, dose equivalence would be determined using a within-subject research design wherein subjects are stabilised on methadone or buprenorphine and then crossed over to the other drug in a randomised double-blind fashion. Alternatively, patients randomised to either drug in a flexible dosage study could be split into deciles and doses compared.

Second, the research cited earlier has used fixed and sometimes low doses of methadone, and this has important implications for understanding the possible efficacy of buprenorphine. If patients in methadone treatment were maintained on a sub-optimal dose, it is possible that they were in a low-grade withdrawal. To the extent that this occurred, it is possible that buprenorphine (as a partial agonist) also leaves patients in a low-grade withdrawal. Increasing doses of methadone to maximise patient comfort will, we believe, reduce withdrawal symptoms and craving, but it is possible that increasing buprenorphine doses will not yield the same result. As such, buprenorphine may never have the ability to suppress withdrawal symptoms and craving that a full agonist possesses.

NARCOTIC ANTAGONISTS

Rationale

Opioid antagonists such as naloxone and naltrexone have been considered as maintenance drugs for treatment of opioid dependence. These opioid antagonists are typically used to reverse the effects of opioid agonists in cases of overdose. They competitively displace opioids from μ-opioid receptor sites. The rationale for their use as a maintenance treatment was that an individual being maintained on an opiate antagonist will not experience any opioid agonist effects after use of heroin. It was proposed that this lack of effect from injecting opioids in the presence of pre-treatment with an antagonist might result in a decline in injecting drug use.

Naloxone

Naloxone was thought suitable as an opiate replacement therapy as it does not produce dependence and does not have serious side-effects (Kurland *et al.*, 1975). However, it has the disadvantages that oral doses as high as 2-3 gm were necessary to provide 24-hour blockade, making it costly to use. The alternative of parenteral route of administration by injection was not thought appropriate for obvious reasons.

Trials of naloxone maintenance were carried out by Kurland and his colleagues (Kurland & Hanlon, 1974; Kurland *et al.*, 1975) with a group of parolees who were required to attend a clinic, to provide daily urines, and to receive weekly psychotherapy sessions after they had been discharged from U.S. correctional institutions. Pilot studies established that an oral regimen of naloxone was feasible and that there were no serious side-effects or toxicity associated with long-term administration. Subsequent controlled trials were carried out to assess the effectiveness or otherwise of naloxone maintenance.

In the first controlled trial, 119 parolees were randomly assigned to one of three groups: a no-treatment control condition in which no medication was prescribed; a group that received naloxone; and a group that received a placebo in place of naloxone (Kurland & Hanlon, 1974). All participants had to provide regular urine samples and attend a weekly psychotherapy group. Outcome was measured by opioid use and retention in treatment over the nine months of the study. The results failed to show any difference between the placebo and naloxone on retention in treatment or opioid use.

Subsequently these investigators examined the effects on treatment retention and opiate use of administering increasing doses of naloxone when either opiate use was detected or suspected (Kurland *et al.*, 1975). This contingent administration of naloxone was proposed as a way of reducing the high cost of providing large quantities of naloxone on a daily basis. These trials found no advantage to the use of contingent naloxone administration. The authors identified lack of compliance with naloxone ingestion as being a major impediment to success with naloxone. While naloxone adequately blocked the effects of opioids, lack of motivation to ingest the medication was the main reason identified for high rates of relapse to heroin use.

Naltrexone

Naltrexone is a long-acting (up to 72 hours, depending on the dose) opioid antagonist with many advantages as a maintenance drug. It can be administered orally, it blocks both the analgesic and euphoric effects of opioids, and it has only minor side-effects. Despite these advantages, many of the programs using naltrexone report substantial drop-out rates early in the program, in some cases, even before the first dose of naltrexone is given.

There have been a number of controlled trials comparing naltrexone with methadone or placebo. Compared with methadone maintenance, naltrexone treatment retained fewer patients over a 12-week study period, although there were no differences between the two regimens in terms of extent of illicit drug use (Osborn *et al.*, 1986). When compared with a placebo, there was a trend towards naltrexone patients having less illicit drug use and better retention; however, the data remained equivocal because of a high drop-out rate in both groups (National-Research-Committee-on-Clinical-Evaluation-of-Narcotic-Antagonists, 1978).

In another study, 117 patients who had completed a trial of LAAM were given the opportunity to transfer to naltrexone (Judson & Goldstein, 1984). Forty patients entered treatment and 77 did not. At the follow-up, more patients who had received naltrexone were opioid-free compared with those who did not receive naltrexone. The authors make the point that the two groups were not comparable in motivation at the outset.

More recently, Israeli researchers (Shufman *et al.*, 1994) have reported on a double-blind trial that demonstrated that naltrexone had a superior impact on heroin use compared with placebo. However, possibly because of the small sample size the differences between naltrexone and placebo were non-significant. Spanish research had also failed to detect significant differences in favour of naltrexone above placebo (San *et al.*, 1991).

Although retention in naltrexone maintenance has proved difficult for even short periods of time with illicit drug using populations, it has been found to be quite successful with highly motivated individuals who wish to cease opioid use. Thomas and her colleagues first described success with naltrexone maintenance in a small sample of opiate-dependent medical professionals (Thomas *et al.*, 1976). In a subsequent study, 114 opiate-dependent businessmen and 15 opiate-dependent physicians were treated with naltrexone as part of a structured aftercare program following clonidine detoxification (Washton *et al.*, 1984). More than 80% of the patients completed at least six months of treatment and remained drug-free 12 to 18 months later.

It is clear that naltrexone has a potential role as a maintenance medication with these selected and highly motivated patients, but the target population is small. It may prove with time that it also has a role in gradually transferring patients from full opioid agonist therapy to partial agonist treatment and eventually to full antagonist treatment as a method of withdrawing those who wish to cease all maintenance therapy.

ROUTE OF ADMINISTRATION: ORAL OR INJECTABLE?

Rationale for Alternative Routes of Administration

The dominant form of opioid maintenance therapy involves oral administration. Some have argued that the availability of injectable maintenance medications is warranted, because *some* patients find oral maintenance "unhelpful" (Brewer, 1991) and unattractive. The United Kingdom Advisory Council on the Misuse of Drugs has reportedly recommended that prescribing of injectable drugs may occur in the "exceptional cases" for very short time periods of up to three months with an aim of weaning patients on to oral replacement therapy. (Battersby *et al.*, 1992) Intractable cases where injecting continues unabated, and where risk of death or serious infectious disease is present, appear to be the target group. However, according to others the risks associated with injectable drugs makes it preferable to provide all drugs orally (Ghodse *et al.*, 1990).

Effects on Drug Use

There is a dearth of research on the impact of injectable drugs in a maintenance orientation. Hartnoll and colleagues (1980) in their controlled trial of injectable heroin against oral methadone (reviewed earlier) found that while those given injectable heroin were retained in treatment longer than methadone maintenance patients, there was no differential improvement in health, employment, or crime (once pre-treatment criminal activity was accounted for) compared with those patients who were not given a prescription for injectable drugs. As Mitcheson (1994) recently pointed out, these "are all areas where proponents for legal prescribing, then and now, believe there should be a harm reduction effect" (p. 182). Patients in the oral methadone group injected less frequently, consumed less opioid drugs daily, spent less time with other drug users and were more likely to be abstinent or stable than patients in the injecting group, although they were less likely to stay in treatment than those provided with injectable heroin.

In a second study of the value of injectable opioids, Battersby and colleagues (1992) conducted an audit of 40 opioid-dependent patients prescribed injectable methadone or heroin. The patients generally requested long-term injectable prescriptions (more than one year). They were characterised by chronic injecting opioid use and a refusal to comply with oral-only prescribing, and would appear to be just the target group that the proponents of the prescribing of injectable opioids suggest would be likely to benefit from injectables. The aim of the program was to attract these entrenched injectors into treatment and to promote a move to oral maintenance and reduce HIV risk. They stayed a mean of 45 weeks in treatment, but at the point of last contact, 80% remained injecting illicit drugs. Life-threatening illness, continued dangerous injecting practices, and deteriorating stability of patients while receiving prescribed injectable drugs, led the authors to highlight "the high risk nature of this prescribing practice, where short-term benefit and consumer satisfaction may need to be balanced against the possibility of adverse consequences in the longer term" (p. 40). They did note some beneficial outcomes among some patients including dose reductions, inpatient attendance, and positive life changes.

Battersby and colleagues (1992) make the obvious point that it is impossible to provide conclusive evidence of either benefit or harm as a consequence of the prescribing of injectable opioids. They note that had injectable drugs not been offered, many patients may have accepted oral maintenance. In conclusion, the authors point out that more "careful consideration needs to be given to the role of injectable prescribing in the case of the entrenched drug addict if the drug worker is to avoid complicity with continued high-risk behaviours behind a presumption of health promotion and harm minimisation" (p. 41).

Finally, Reynolds (1994) has reported on the use of intravenous methadone in Australia for 17 patients who appeared unresponsive to other forms of treatment. The program admitted patients from 1970 until 1976, and four patients still receive injectable methadone. Six transferred to oral methadone, three left the programme, and four died (two of drug overdose). Reynolds concluded that the programme had been successful, although it must be acknowledged that the evaluation can provide no information on the relative value of injectable methadone compared with oral methadone.

It is likely that a small group of treatment-resistant patients may benefit from access to prescribed injectable opioids (Strang *et al.*, 1994). Identifying these patients, monitoring their progress, and being aware of the warning of Battersby (Battersby *et al.*, 1992) to avoid complicity with continued high-risk behaviours behind a presumption of health promotion and harm minimization, remain the challenges. Taking up these challenges would be made easier if there were some reasonable research on the topic.

SUMMARY

LAAM has been shown to be an effective maintenance agent in a number of randomised clinical trials. It has advantages over methadone as a maintenance drug: its longer half-life allows alternate- or three-day dosing; it provides greater flexibility for the patient; and there is less opportunity for illicit diversion. It should be considered as a contender in a range of pharmacological approaches to opioid dependence. The evidence to date suggests that the necessary research and application procedures for the registration of LAAM for clinical use in Australia would provide a useful additional alternative to methadone.

Proponents of heroin maintenance argue that the HIV epidemic, the failure of prohibition, the lack of control over heroin quality and the potential of heroin maintenance to attract and retain heroin users in treatment, make heroin maintenance a legitimate approach. Arguments against heroin maintenance include: the short half-life of heroin requires frequent administration being costly and/or risking diversion, and the difficulty of stabilising patients adequately. Heroin maintenance treatment is not well researched. There is little evidence that patients cannot be adequately stabilised on heroin, and some research that shows that they can. The one randomised controlled clinical trial completed to date provided mixed advantages and disadvantages for heroin maintenance compared to methadone maintenance. Methadone was associated with poorer retention in treatment, but also produced lower levels of daily opioid use, less injecting and less time spent with other drug users. However, this single trial is an insufficient basis for drawing confident conclusions about the relative impact of heroin maintenance.

Generally, studies have shown buprenorphine to be as effective as methadone in reducing illicit opioid use, retaining clients in treatment, and in reducing withdrawal symptoms. Studies have also shown that buprenorphine is acceptable to heroin addicts; has few side-effects; binds well to opioid receptors; appears to induce a low level of physical dependence; diminishes self-administration of heroin; has subjective effects that are opioid-agonist-like; blocks or greatly attenuates the self-reported drug effects of concurrently administered opioids; induces a relatively mild withdrawal syndrome; is safe, because agonist effects such as respiratory depression reach a ceiling at sub-toxic but clinically useful doses; and has a long duration of action that may allow for less than daily dosing.

There are a number of limitations associated with buprenorphine: the sublingual route of administration may prove cumbersome and inconvenient; the medication is water soluble and highly concentrated so can be absorbed sublingually, and because of this it is relatively easy to inject; and a ceiling effect may limit its applicability to certain individuals, especially the more severely dependent. Nevertheless, it is likely to find a place as an alternative pharmacotherapy in the treatment of opioid dependence.

Naloxone is a doubtful alternative to methadone as a replacement therapy in view of its high cost and the lack of evidence of its effectiveness. Naltrexone treatment has more potential as a useful treatment option as has been demonstrated with selected patients. It has mild side-effects and can be used on flexible dosage regimens ranging from daily to thrice weekly, depending on patients' needs. Medical practitioners, business executives, parolees and other groups who are highly motivated to remain drug-free in environments where their drug of choice is freely available have responded well to naltrexone maintenance.

The dominant form of drug substitution maintenance therapy involves oral administration, but some have argued that the availability of injectable maintenance medications is warranted as *some* patients find oral maintenance unhelpful, unattractive, and have suggested that prescribing of injectable drugs may occur in the "most exceptional cases" for very short time periods. Others point out that risks associated with injectable drugs make it preferable to provide all drugs orally. There was no research found that could be used to convincingly argue that prescribing injectable opioids in a maintenance fashion is able to promote healthy behaviour or reduce risk of infectious disease beyond oral maintenance. Randomised research and program evaluation research suggests that there may be significant risks and some possible benefits associated with such practices.

REFERENCES

Amass, L., Bickel, W. K., Higgins, S. T., & Badger, G. J. (1994). Alternate-day dosing during buprenorphine treatment of opioid dependence. *Life Sciences,* **54,** 1215-1228.

Bale, R. N., Stone, W. W., Kuldau, J. M., Engelsing, T. M. J., Elashoff, R. M., & Zarcone, V. P. (1980). Therapeutic communities versus methadone maintenance - A prospective controlled study of narcotic addiction treatment: Design and one-year follow-up. *Archives of General Psychiatry,* **37,** 179-193.

Bammer, G. (1992). A trial of controlled availability for heroin for the ACT? In J. White (Ed.), *Drug problems in society: Dimensions and perspectives* (pp. 57-62). Adelaide: S.A. Drug and Alcohol Services Council.

Bammer, G. (1993). Should the controlled provision of heroin be a treatment option? Australian feasibility considerations. *Addiction,* **88,** 467-475.

Bammer, G., McDonald, D. N., Jarrett, R. G., Solomon, P. J., & Sibthorpe, B. M. (1994). *Issues for designing and evaluating a 'heroin trial': Three discussion papers.* (Vol. 8). Canberra: National Institute of Epidemiology and Population Health, Australian Institute of Criminology.

Banks, C. D. (1979). Overdose of buprenorphine: Case report. *New Zealand Medical Journal,* **89,** 255-256.

Battersby, M., Farrell, M., Gossop, M., Robson, P., & Strang, J. (1992). 'Horse trading': Prescribing injectable opiates to opiate addicts. A descriptive study. *Drug and Alcohol Review,* **11,** 35-42.

Bickel, W. K., Stitzer, M. L., Bigelow, G. E., Liebson, I. A., Jasinski, D. R., & Johnson, R. E. (1988). A clinical trial of buprenorphine: Comparison with methadone in the detoxification of heroin addicts. *Clinical Pharmacology and Therapeutics,* **43,** 72-78.

Brewer, C. (1991). Intravenous methadone maintenance: A British response to persistent opiate injectors. In N. Loimer, R. Schmid, & A. Springer (Eds.), *Drug addiction and AIDS* (pp. 187-199). Vienna: Springer-Verlag.

Byrne, A. (1996). Use of dextromoramide to stabilize a heroin addict. *Drug and Alcohol Review,* 15, 200.

Dole, V. P. (1972). Comments on "Heroin maintenance". *Journal of the American Medical Association (JAMA),* 220(11), 1493.

Dole, V. P. (1988). Implications of methadone maintenance for theories of narcotic addiction. *Journal of the American Medical Association (JAMA),* 260, 3025-3029.

Dole, V. P., & Nyswander, M. (1965). A medical treatment for diacetylmorphine (heroin) addiction: A clinical trial with methadone hydrochloride. *Journal of the American Medical Association,* 193, 80-84.

Fink, M. (1972). Heroin maintenance. *Journal of the American Medical Association (JAMA),* 221(6), 602.

Freedman, R. R., & Czertko, G. (1981). A comparison of thrice weekly LAAM and daily methadone in employed heroin addicts. *Drug and Alcohol Dependence,* 8, 215-222.

Fudala, P. J., Jaffe, J. H., Dax, E. M., & Johnson, R. E. (1990). Use of buprenorphine in the treatment of opioid addiction. II. Physiologic and behavioral effects of daily and alternate-day administration and abrupt withdrawal. *Clinical Pharmacology and Therapeutics,* 47, 525-534.

Ghodse, A. H., Creighton, F. J., & Bhat, A. V. (1990). Comparison of oral preparations of heroin and methadone to stabilise opiate misusers as inpatients. *Lancet,* 300, 719-720.

Goldstein, A. (1976). Heroin addiction: Sequential treatment employing pharmacologic supports. *Archives of General Psychiatry,* 33, 353-358.

Hall, W. (1996). The Swiss scientific studies of medically prescribed narcotics: A personal view. National Drug and Alcohol Research Centre, University of New South Wales, Sydney.

Hartnoll, R. L., Mitcheson, M. C., Battersby, A., Brown, G., Ellis, M., Fleming, P., & Hedley, N. (1980). Evaluation of heroin maintenance in controlled trial. *Archives of General Psychiatry,* 37, 877-884.

Jaffe, J. H. (1990). Drug addiction and drug abuse. In A. G. Gilman, T. W. Rall, A. S. Nies, & P. Taylor (Eds.), *The pharmacological basis of therapeutics* (8th ed., pp. 522-573). New York: Pergamon Press.

Jaffe, J. H., & Martin, W. R. (1990). Opioid analgesics and antagonists. In A. G. Gilman, T. W. Rall, A. S. Nies, & P. Taylor (Eds.), *The pharmacological basis of therapeutics* (8th ed., pp. 485-521). New York: Pergamon Press.

Jaffe, J. H., Senay, E. C., Schuster, C. R., Renault, P. R., Smith, B., & DiMenza, S. (1972). Methadyl acetate vs methadone. *Journal of the American Medical Association,* 222, 437-442.

Jasinski, D. R., Fudala, P. J., & Johnson, R. E. (1989). Sublingual versus subcutaneous buprenorphine in opiate abusers. *Clinical Pharmacology and Therapeutics,* 45(5), 513-519.

Jasinski, D. R., Pevnick, J. S., & Griffith, J. D. (1978). Human pharmacology and abuse potential of the analgesic buprenorphine. *Archives of General Psychiatry, 35,* 501-516.

Jasinski, D. R., & Preston, K. L. (1996). Laboratory studies of buprenorphine in opioid abusers. In A. Cowan & J. W. Lewis (Eds.), *Buprenorphine: Combatting drug abuse with a unique opioid* (pp. 189-211). New York: Wiley-Liss.

Johnson, R. E., Cone, E. J., Henningfield, J. E., & Fudala, P. J. (1989). Use of buprenorphine in the treatment of opiate addiction. I. Physiologic and behavioral effects during a rapid dose induction. *Clinical Pharmacology and Therapeutics, 46,* 335-343.

Johnson, R. E., Eissenberg, T., Stitzer, M. L., Strain, E. C., Leibson, I. A., & Bigelow, G. E. (1995a). A placebo controlled clinical trial of buprenorphine as a treatment for opioid dependence. *Drug and Alcohol Dependence, 40,* 17-25.

Johnson, R. E., Eissenberg, T., Stitzer, M. L., Strain, E. C., Liebson, I. A., & Bigelow, G. E. (1995b). Buprenorphine treatment of opioid dependence: Clinical trial of daily versus alternate-day dosing. *Drug and Alcohol Dependence, 40,* 27-35.

Johnson, R. E., Jaffe, J. H., & Fudala, P. J. (1992). A controlled trial of buprenorphine treatment for opioid dependence. *Journal of the American Medical Association (JAMA), 267*(20), 2750-2755.

Judson, B. A., & Goldstein, A. (1984). Naltrexone treatment of heroin addiction: One-year follow-up. *Drug and Alcohol Dependence, 13,* 357-365.

June, H. L., Preston, K. L., Bigelow, G. E., & Stitzer, M. L. (1993). Buprenorphine effects in methadone-maintained subjects. In L. Harris (Ed.), *NIDA Research Monograph 132 - Problems of drug dependence: Proceedings of the 54th annual scientific meeting the College on Problems of Drug Dependence, Inc.* (pp. 334). Rockville, MD.: U.S. Department of Health and Human Services.

Karel, R. (1993). New Swiss program will distribute hard drugs to addicts. *Drug Policy Letter, 21,* 10-11.

Kosten, T. R., Morgan, C., & Kleber, H. D. (1992). Phase II clinical trials of buprenorphine: Detoxification and induction onto naltrexone. In J. D. Blaine (Ed.), *NIDA Research Monograph: Buprenorphine An alternative treatment for opioid dependence* (pp. 101-119). Rockville, MD: U.S. Department of Health and Human Services.

Kosten, T. R., Schottenfeld, R., Ziedonis, D., & Falcioni, J. (1993). Buprenorphine versus methadone maintenance for opioid dependence. *Journal of Nervous and Mental Disease, 181*(6), 358-364.

Kreek, M. J. (1996a). Long-term pharmacotherapy for opiate (primarily heroin) addiction: Opioid agonists. In C. R. Schuster & M. J. Kuhar (Eds.), *Pharmacological aspects of drug dependence: Toward an integrated neurobehavioral approach* (Vol. 118, pp. 487-562). Berlin: Springer.

Kreek, M. J. (1996b). Long-term pharmacotherapy for opiate (primarily heroin) addiction: Opioid antagonists and partial agonists. In C. R. Schuster & M. J. Kuhar (Eds.), *Pharmacological aspects of drug dependence: Toward an integrated neurobehavioural approach* (Vol. 118, pp. 563-598). Berlin: Springer.

Kurland, A. A., & Hanlon, T. E. (1974). Naloxone and the narcotic abuser: A controlled study of partial blockade. *International Journal of the Addictions, 9,* 663-672.

Kurland, A. A., McCabe, L., & Hanlon, T. E. (1975). Contingent naloxone (N-allylnoroxymorphone) treatment of the paroled narcotic addict. *International Pharmacopsychiatry, 10,* 157-168.

Lehmann, K. A., U., R., & Wirtz, R. (1988). Influence of naloxone on the post-operative analgesic and respiratory effects of buprenorphine. *European Journal of Clinical Pharmacology, 34,* 343-352.

Lewis, J. W. (1985). Buprenorphine. *Drug and Alcohol Dependence, 14,* 363-372.

Ling, W., Charuvastra, C., Kaim, S. C., & Klett, C. J. (1976). Methadyl acetate and methadone as maintenance treatments for heroin addicts. *Archives of General Psychiatry, 33,* 709-720.

Ling, W., Klett, J. C., & Gillis, R. C. (1980). A cooperative clinical study of methadyl acetate: II. Friday-only-regimen. *Archives of General Psychiatry, 37,* 908-911.

Ling, W., Wesson, D. R., Charuvastra, C., & Klett, C. J. (1996). A controlled trial comparing buprenorphine and methadone maintanence in opioid dependence. *Archives of General Psychiatry, 53,* 401-407.

Marks, J. (1991). The practice of controlled availability of illicit drugs. In N. Heather, W. R. Miller, & J. Greeley (Eds.), *Self-control and the addictive behaviours* (pp. 304-316). Melbourne: Maxwell MacMillan.

Marks, J. A. (1990). The prescribing debate (continued). *British Journal of Psychiatry, 157,* 460.

Mattick, R. P., & Hall, W. (Eds.). (1993). *A treatment outline for approaches to opioid dependence: The quality assurance in the treatment of drug dependence project.* (Vol. 21). Canberra: Australian Government Publishing Service.

Mendelson, J., Upton, R., Jones, R. T., & Jacob, P. (1995). *Buprenorphine pharmacokinetics: Bioequivalence of an 8mg sublingual tablet formulation.* Paper presented at the Problems of drug dependence, 1995: Proceedings of the 55th annual scientific meeting of the College on problems of drug dependence, Inc, Phoenix, AZ.

Mitcheson, M. (1994). Drug clinics in the 1970s. In J. Strang & M. Gossop (Eds.), *Heroin addiction and drug policy: The British system* (pp. 178-191). Oxford: Oxford University Press.

National-Research-Committee-on-Clinical-Evaluation-of-Narcotic-Antagonists. (1978). Clinical evaluation of naltrexone treatment of opiate-dependent individuals. *Archives of General Psychiatry,* **35,** 335-340.

Newman, R. G. (1994). Comparing buprenorphine and methadone maintenance. *Journal of Nervous and Mental Disease,* **182,** 245-246.

Osborn, E., Grey, C., & Reznikoff, M. (1986). Psychosocial adjustment, modality choice, and outcome in naltrexone versus methadone treatment. *American Journal of Drug and Alcohol Abuse,* **12,** 383-388.

Parry, A. (1992). Taking heroin maintenance seriously: The politics of tolerance. *Lancet, 8 February,* 350-351.

Pickworth, W. R., Johnson, R. E., Holicky, B. A., & Cone, E. J. (1993). Subjective and physiologic effects of intravenous buprenorphine in humans. *Clinical Pharmacology and Therapeutics,* **53,** 570-576.

Prendergast, M. L., Grella, C., Perry, S. M., & Anglin, M. D. (1995). Levo-alpha-acetylmethadol (LAAM): Clinical, research, and policy issues of a new pharmacotherapy for opioid addiction. *Journal of Psychoactive Drugs,* **27,** 239-247.

Resnick, R. B., Galanter, M., Pycha, C., Cohen, A., Grandison, P., & Flood, N. (1992). Buprenorphine: An alternative to methadone for heroin dependence treatment. *Psychopharmacology Bulletin,* **28**(1), 109-113.

Resnick, R. B., Pycha, C., & Galanter, M. (1994). Buprenorphine maintenance: Reduced dosing frequency. *Psychopharmacology Bulletin,* **30,** 123.

Reynolds, A. (1994). A clinical review of the use of intravenous methadone in the treatment of opiate drug dependence in Queensland. Queensland Health Department.

Rihs, M. (1994). *The prescription of narcotics under medical supervision and research relating to drugs at the Federal Office of Public Health.* Bern: Swiss Federal Office of Public Health.

Robertson, J. R. (1996). Dihydrocodeine-a second strand treatment for drug misusers. *Drug and Alcohol Review,* **15,** 200-201.

Robinson, G. M., Dukes, P. D., Robinson, B. J., Cooke, R. R., & Mahoney, G. N. (1993). The misuse of buprenorphine and buprenorphine-naloxone combination in Wellington, New Zealand. *Drug and Alcohol Dependence,* **33,** 81-86.

Rosenblum, A., Magura, S., & Joseph, H. (1991). Ambivalence towards methadone treatment among intravenous drug users. *Journal of Psychoactive Drugs,* **23,** 21-27.

San, L., Pomarol, G., Peri, J. M., Olle, J. M., & Cami, J. (1991). Follow-up after a six-month maintenance period on naltrexone versus placebo in heroin addicts. *British Journal of Addiction,* **86,** 983-990.

Savage, C., Karp, E. G., Curran, S. F., Hanlon, T. E., & McCabe, O. L. (1976). Methadone/LAAM maintenance: A comparison study.

Comprehensive Psychiatry, 17, 415-424.

Shufman, E. N., Porat, S., Witztum, E., Gandacu, D., Bar-Hamburger, R., & Ginath, Y. (1994). The efficacy of naltrexone in preventing reabuse of heroin after detoxification. *Biological Psychiatry,* 35, 935-945.

Stimmel, B. (1975). Heroin maintenance. In B. Stimmel (Ed.), *Heroin dependency: Medical, economic and social aspects* (pp. 219-231). New York: Stratton Intercontinental Medical Book Corporation.

Stimson, G. V., & Oppenheimer, E. (1982). *Heroin addiction: Treatment and control in Britain.* London: Tavistock.

Strain, E. C., Stitzer, M. L., Liebson, I. A., & Bigelow, G. E. (1994). Comparison of buprenorphine and methadone in the treatment of opioid dependence. *American Journal of Psychiatry,* 151(7), 1025-1030.

Strang, J., Ruben, S., Farrell, M., & Gossop, M. (1994). Prescribing heroin and other injectable drugs. In J. Strang & M. Gossop (Eds.), *Heroin addiction and drug policy: The British system* (pp. 192-206). Oxford: Oxford University Press.

Swan, N. (1993). Two NIDA-tested heroin treatment medications move toward FDA approval. *NIDA Notes,* 8(1), 4-5.

Tennant, F. S., Rawson, R. A., Pumphrey, E., & Seecof, R. (1986). Clinical experiences with 959 opioid-dependent patients treated with levo-alpha-acetylmethadol (LAAM). *Journal of Substance Abuse Treatment,* 3, 195-202.

Thomas, M., Kauders, F., Harris, M., Cooperstein, J., Hough, G., & Resnick, R. (1976). Clinical experiences with naltrexonein 370 detoxified addicts. In D. Julius & P. Renault (Eds.), *Narcotic antagonists: Naltrexone* (Vol. 9, pp. 88-92). Rockvile, MD.: National Institute on Drug Abuse.

Trueblood, B., Judson, B. A., & Goldstein, A. (1978). Acceptability of methadyl acetate (LAAM) as compared with methadone in a treatment program for heroin addicts. *Drug and Alcohol Dependence,* 3, 125-132.

Volavka, J., Zaks, A., Roubicek, J., & Fink, M. (1970). Electrographic effects of diacetylmorphine (heroin) and naloxone in man. *Neuropharmacology,* 9, 587-593.

Walsh, S. L., Preston, K. L., Stitzer, M. L., Cone, E. J., & Bigelow, G. E. (1994). Clinical pharmacology of buprenorphine: Ceiling effects at high doses. *Clinical Pharmacology and Therapeutics,* 55, 569-580.

Walsh, S. L., Preston, K. L., Stitzer, M. L., Liebson, I. A., & Bigelow, G. E. (Eds.). (1993). *Comparison of the acute effects of buprenorphine and methadone in non-dependent humans.* (Vol. 132). Rockville, MD: National Institute on Drug Abuse.

Washton, A. M., Pottash, A. C., & Gold, M. S. (1984). Naltrexone in addicted business executives and physicians. *Journal of Clinical Psychiatry,* 45, 4-6.

II PROCESS

7

DELIVERING EFFECTIVE METHADONE TREATMENT

JAMES BELL

INTRODUCTION

The aim of this chapter is to discuss the practical task of delivering methadone maintenance treatment. Despite an extensive research literature, there is no broad consensus on the role of methadone maintenance treatment, or on how treatment should be delivered. Even where there is firm empirical evidence, such as the importance of adequate methadone dose, treatment practices are often out of line with research evidence (D'Aunno & Vaughn, 1992). The disparity between research findings and clinical practice is not unique to methadone treatment, but has been a feature of treatments for drug and alcohol dependence (Miller & Hester, 1986). It is partly explained by the fact that much clinical practice ignores research findings, and partly by the fact that much research is only marginally relevant to clinical realities. However, the major factor in the disparity between research and practice is that there is profound disagreement over such basic issues as the nature of the problem being treated and the goals of treatment (Newman, 1987). Both research and treatment require a frame of reference within which observations can be made, hypotheses generated and clinical practices evaluated. The absence of such a frame of reference explains why, despite extensive research validation, methadone maintenance continues to be referred to as "controversial" (Dole, 1989).

Given the lack of consensus around this modality of treatment, the emphasis in this chapter is not on trying to define how treatment should be delivered, but on making sense of the clinician's role in methadone treatment. It is an attempt to integrate research findings with clinical experience. The starting point for this account is an analysis of the rationale for treatment, the core components of treatment and the importance of how these are integrated and applied. Finally, data from an observational study of methadone clinics are presented suggesting some specific ways in which treatment can be more or less effective.

METHADONE MAINTENANCE AS TREATMENT

Methadone maintenance as a treatment of dependency

Vincent Dole has claimed that in early experiments in which heroin users were regularly administered a variety of opioid drugs, those maintained on morphine appeared apathetic, preoccupied with when their next dose of morphine was due, and constantly requested increasing doses (quoted in Courtwright *et al.,* 1989). He has hypothesised that the use of short-acting opioids as maintenance therapy leads to the persistent pursuit of intoxication through seeking for more drug, rather than to stabilisation (Dole, 1980). In contrast, those maintained on methadone ceased being focused on when their next dose was due, or on how much drug they would receive, and became interested in other, everyday activities. He explained these observations as being due to methadone's slow absorption and slowly declining blood levels between doses, which avoided the cycle of intoxication and withdrawal experienced by addicts using short-acting drugs (Dole, 1980).

What Dole was describing was a lessening in the severity of dependence in patients by abolishing the cycle of intoxication and withdrawal through the administration of a daily dose of methadone. The change from the behavioural features of dependency – being preoccupied with drug seeking and drug use – to being able again to focus on "normal" pursuits is the primary means by which methadone contributes to the rehabilitation of heroin addicts. Effective treatment can restore a greater degree of autonomy and flexibility in their lives primarily by reducing the severity of their dependence.

Methadone Maintenance as a Treatment of Individuals

In recent years it has become customary to present methadone maintenance treatment as a public health measure, rather than a treatment to assist individuals. Such public health or community benefits as reduced risk of HIV spread, and reduced involvement in acquisitive crime, flow directly from the reduction in heroin injection by people entering methadone treatment. The demonstrated benefits of methadone maintenance are for the individuals in treatment and any community benefits are secondary.

This chapter focuses on the clinicians involved in treatment, rather than on the larger policy and administrative issues about how treatment should be structured. There are important policy issues over whether methadone treatment is based on prescribing or dispensing, or whether it is delivered in primary care settings or in large specialist clinics. However, in this paper the focus is on the core elements of treatment, clinical issues that in some degree are independent of context. In seeking to present an approach to delivering methadone treatment, treatment is somewhat arbitrarily divided into four components – symptom relief, structure, information, and affirmation and validation.

Relief of Symptoms

The effectiveness of methadone maintenance depends on the patient's perception of the advantages of entering and remaining in treatment. As pointed out in a recent authoritative report from the Institute of Medicine in the USA, the major reason why drug users are reluctant to enter treatment is that treatment is not perceived to offer them any advantage over their drug-using state (Gerstein & Harwood, 1990).

Heroin addiction involves many stresses. The cycle of withdrawal symptoms, crime and drug seeking makes for a demanding and uncertain way of life, and the commonest reason given by heroin addicts for entering treatment is that they are "sick of the lifestyle". The fact that methadone programs provide a stable, predictable supply of a drug removes the pressures of maintaining a heroin habit.

Treatment offers time out, a respite from the risks and rigours of addiction. This is the simplest and most obvious level at which methadone treatment offers symptomatic relief, and is the major reason why people seek and remain in treatment.

The fact that treatment represents a refuge from the difficulties of addiction does not sit comfortably with most people. Our governing image of addiction is as a form of deviance, and from that moral perspective it does not seem appropriate to protect people from the adverse consequences of deviant behaviour. Thus, providing relief from distress resulting from the addicted lifestyle is seen not only as unnecessary, but as counterproductive. As will be discussed in a later section, this attitude constitutes one of the major obstacles to delivering effective methadone treatment.

It is helpful to look beyond the narrow framework of addiction as deviance in order to understand the role of methadone in providing symptomatic relief. What is remarkable is not that addicts should seek respite by entering treatment, but that despite family and community disapproval, legal sanctions, and a difficult, often degraded lifestyle, people continue to use heroin. Even after quite prolonged periods of abstinence, relapse to dependent heroin use is the rule for most opioid addicts who have sought treatment. Once stabilised on methadone, and even with successful social reintegration, people continue to attend for a daily dose of methadone for many years. It is apparent that just as heroin users value heroin, most patients in treatment value methadone. Given that discontinuing drug use provides relief from the stresses of the addicted lifestyle, it is apparent that the benefits of methadone treatment extend beyond simply providing relief from the travails of addiction.

"Disease" theories of addiction, like disease theories of alcoholism, emphasise that the primary problem for the addict is addiction, and that other problems of psychosocial dysfunction are the result of drug addiction. However useful this conventional approach may be in treatment, it sits uncomfortably with the observation that many addicts exhibit problems of adjustment independent of their use of drugs (McClellan *et al.,* 1981). There have been a variety of hypotheses put forward to account for drug dependence. One plausible hypothesis is that for some people with significant adjustment difficulties, and a pervasive mood of frustration, the use of opioids is one of the few mechanisms available to achieve a sense of well-being. Viewed in this light, heroin use serves an adaptive purpose, a way of dealing with alienation and frustration (Martin *et al.*, 1973; Khantzian, 1985).

In the last decade, it has become apparent that most people seeking treatment for drug dependence use multiple drugs, rather than being dependent on a single drug. This observation provides further evidence that drug dependence is difficult to explain simply in terms of exposure to a drug leading to neurochemical changes that are experienced as craving. Rather, drug dependence appears to be a reliance on external sources of control over moods and feelings (Dodes, 1990). Individuals with an entrenched sense of helplessness and lack of control over their moods are particularly vulnerable to becoming drug dependent. The experience of helplessness and loss of control is central to the phenomenology of addiction.

Thus in treating drug-dependent people the task is to aid them in their adjustment and temperament difficulties – difficulties for which dependent individuals have found drug use helpful. The basis of the effectiveness of methadone treatment is the pharmacological effect of methadone in stabilising and attenuating dysphoria. The disadvantage of such drug effects may be a degree of emotional blunting, but people seem to value this (for example, many patients report reduced libido, but few complain that this is a problem to them). Those patients who value the effect of methadone remain in treatment for prolonged periods, bearing the stigma associated with being in treatment (Murphy & Irwin, 1992) but still attending and valuing the effect of the drug. The clinical importance of the pharmacological action of methadone is that higher doses contribute to this effect, and this explains the observation that doses higher than are needed to block withdrawal for 24 hours convey greater efficacy.

Methadone is not a panacea for all distressing symptoms. Patients with specific disorders, such as anxiety and depression, require additional specific treatment – either using pharmacotherapy or psychotherapy.

Structure

"Structure" refers to the behavioural component of treatment – the way treatment is organised. There is little specific empirical evidence on the role of structure in treatment efficacy. The only research has focused on one particular approach to treatment structure, the use of rewards and/or punishments in contingency management approaches designed to improve treatment outcomes. Although there have been some claims for effectiveness of positive reinforcers, by and large the results of contingency management have been surprisingly disappointing (Hall, 1983). Possible reasons for this will be discussed below.

Although it has been little investigated, the organization of treatment is almost certainly an important component of effectiveness. Indeed, it is only when confronted with the chaos and confusion of a poorly organised methadone clinic that the importance of structured treatment becomes apparent (Bell *et al.,* 1995b).

The goal of delivering structured treatment is to ensure that the treatment space is safe. Safety for patients and staff includes freedom from harassment (by staff and other patients), fairness, and the sense that the treatment constitutes a reliable, consistent experience. While punitive responses from staff towards acting out behaviour need to be avoided, maintaining safe limits needs to be enforced – a difficult balancing act for which clear rules and expectations need to be spelt out and consistently applied.

Daily attendance to receive a dose of methadone is one aspect of the structure of treatment. Although not all methadone treatment is initiated in this way (for example, in the United Kingdom), daily attendance for supervised dosing is probably valuable during the early phases of treatment. At the very least, it provides an alternative structure to the daily routine of income-generating crime and drug seeking. It is also the basis for a relationship between the patient and the person dispensing methadone. Most importantly, for people with little sense of control over their lives, externally imposed controls such as daily attendance for dosing can be a valuable component of treatment. By minimising the risk of diversion, injection, and taking erratic quantities of methadone, it makes treatment safer. Although some patients find daily attendance irksome, others acknowledge that safety from the temptation to sell or inject doses is appreciated.

However, treatment needs to be individualised to the circumstances of individual patients. While daily attendance for dosing is probably desirable early in treatment, and for chaotic patients, it becomes irksome for people who are stable and functional. For these patients, daily attendance for dosing can become an obstacle to social reintegration.

Provision of Information

Information is the cognitive component of treatment, and the current vogue for cognitive-behavioural approaches has highlighted the importance of providing patients with information. There is a wealth of simple information relevant to the needs of opioid addicts at different stages of treatment, and a useful approach to structuring treatment is to provide information over time.

Early in treatment, often the relevant information concerns methadone and its side-effects, and access to welfare support. Information about high-risk behaviours and health issues such as dental care and hepatitis C, is usually better received once a patient is stabilised on treatment.

Early in treatment, and in periodic reviews, it is helpful to establish realistic goals of treatment. Often, patients have quite unrealistic expectations of what methadone will do, and what they can achieve, and it is important not to set them up to fail. Throughout treatment, it is important to address patients' ambivalence about being on methadone, and their anxieties about taking high doses.

Providing information is an acquired clinical skill. To be most effective, it should be personalised to the circumstances of the individual patient. The clinical interview is a sophisticated, personalised way of providing patients with information about themselves. As a patient recounts their drug use and psychosocial functioning, it provides the clinician with information, but more importantly should reflect back to the patient in an organised way aspects of their life. This is an important process in the addictions, where many individuals are chaotic and avoidant, and seem unwilling or unable to see what is happening to them and their lives. By taking a detailed psychosocial and drug use history, it is possible to reflect back to the individual what has been happening to them over a period of months or years. Such information about drug use and the effect it is having on a person's life is probably a far more powerful therapeutic tool than insight into why they are using drugs.

In its most sophisticated form, information presents not merely facts, but offers the patient a different perspective or understanding. One of the most common therapeutic activities in treatment of dependence is helping people to "reframe" how they see themselves – a process neatly captured in the title of an article written by Marie Nyswander "From drug addict to patient".

Affirmation and Validation

The therapeutic relationship established between the patient and his/her caseworker or prescriber is a critical component of treatment. Providing the patient with the experience of acceptance and validation is central to establishing a therapeutic relationship. Most heroin users have long histories of experiencing invalidation, rejection, and punishment. This experience entrenches their alienation and sense of antagonism. Treatment is an opportunity to provide them with a different experience – of safety and containment instead of confrontation and rejection. Without such experience, it is difficult to establish a sense of safety and trust in the clinical interaction.

In passing, it is worth noting that the act of providing a daily dose of methadone in itself is an important validation. Instead of challenging and negating drug use, methadone treatment affirms the validity of the addict's need for drugs. This is a liberating experience for people who have found that drugs work for them, but have been told repeatedly that they are expected to do without them.

In their study of methadone clinics in North America, Ball and Ross identified the importance of a good relationship with a staff member as one of the important determinants of outcome. Most interestingly, in their examination of the work carried out by clinic staff, Ball and Ross concluded that most of the work of methadone clinic staff can more properly be described as casework rather than counselling (Ball & Ross, 1991). They deal with day-to-day issues, mostly of a practical nature. How these interactions are conducted, and particularly the attitude of staff members, is probably the next most important determinant of treatment effectiveness after an adequate dose of methadone.

The Whole is Greater Than the Sum of the Parts

The components of treatment need to be provided in a coherent way. It is contradictory to provide patients with acceptance and validation while at the same time adopting punitive and controlling policies designed to enforce compliance with the therapist's expectations. Treatment of dependence problems is permissive, allowing change to occur rather than predictably causing individuals to change. People on methadone are given the opportunity to change, by being freed from their dependency on illicit opioids and the uncertain rigours of the addicted lifestyle, but are not always able to take full advantage of the respite offered by treatment to make changes in their lives. In part, this is a volitional problem, and it is always important to recognise that drug users may want something different for themselves from what we want for them. In part, it also reflects the social disadvantage and personal disabilities of many addicted patients.

Insofar as treatment policies seek to control patients' behaviour and impose the therapist's goals on patients, they negate the sense of acceptance and validation which is one of the fundamentals on which effective treatment is based. This is probably the reason for the limited effectiveness of contingency management policies that reward compliance and/or punish continued drug use. Prima facie, such schemes seem like a potent tool to improve treatment outcomes. However, they are not congruent with one of the basic components of effective treatment – validation and acceptance of the patient. The result is that while a few patients may benefit from a system of rewards and punishments, most do not, and overall results tend to be poor (e.g., Saxon *et al.*, 1993).

In seeking to find what makes treatment effective, most research, driven by the dictates of methodology, has focused on specific interventions or techniques – such as dose levels, the role of counselling or contingency management schemes. This emphasis on specific interventions or techniques may well have overlooked what it is in staff-patient interactions that is of most therapeutic importance, leading to some anomalous research findings. Some of the difficulties with research into specific aspects of treatment may be illustrated by considering two recent randomised trials. The first study (McLellan *et al.*, 1993) investigated what constitutes adequate level of services in methadone maintenance clinics. This is a crucially important research question, since around the world ways of improving access to treatment within limited resources is a problem. The results appear to demonstrate conclusively that the greater the level of services provided, the better the treatment outcomes. Patients randomised to basic methadone did very poorly, with "unremitting use of opiates or cocaine, or medical/psychiatric emergencies" occurring in more than two-thirds of subjects in that group.

This appalling result does not fit with most clinicians' experience, which is that about 50% of patients want and need very little except reliable, predictable safe provision of an adequate dose of methadone. Furthermore, these findings do not fit with another apparently methodologically sound study – an investigation of interim methadone maintenance. In that randomised trial (Yancovitz *et al.*, 1991), patients were allocated to essentially the same, fairly minimalist treatment as in the basic methadone group in McLellan's study. The control group consisted of patients placed on a waiting list. However, far from doing terribly, the interim treatment group did quite well.

Clearly, it is impossible to be certain that the "basic methadone" and "interim methadone" groups in the two different studies did receive similar levels of intervention. However, it seems likely that what these two contrasting studies demonstrate is that non-blinded studies can produce anomalous results. Patients receiving interim methadone treatment were aware that the alternative was a waiting list, and staff were keen to demonstrate the benefits of interim methadone (Newman & Peyser, 1991). Under such positive circumstances, it is not surprising that they did well. In contrast, the group receiving methadone only in the McLellan (1993) study were aware that they were receiving what staff members believed was less than optimal care; and indeed, this proved to be the case. A more appropriate and unsurprising conclusion to both studies would appear to be that if staff believe in the treatment they deliver, it works better.

BARRIERS TO EFFECTIVE TREATMENT

There are many obstacles to delivering good treatment. One major obstacle is that people do not see symptom relief as valid or necessary for treatment of dependency. Treatment services all too often start with the assumption that clients want to be drug-free, to "recover", rather than start with the assumption that they want to feel better. Such people tend to adopt models of treatment based on short-term, curative approaches; symptomatic relief is seen as not only not useful, but positively unhelpful in fostering change. The result is barriers to treatment to test motivation (Bell *et al.*, 1994), low doses of methadone, time-limited treatment, and an orientation to abstinence – all notions that would be quite acceptable if there was not evidence that they are associated with worse treatment outcomes, even judged on the very outcomes they seek to achieve (Bell *et al.*, 1995a).

A second major obstacle is that the regulations and policies governing treatment are frequently designed not for therapeutic benefit, but as a regulatory exercise based on a perceived need to maintain control. Regulations are sometimes externally imposed, reflecting community negativity towards drug addicts and methadone maintenance as a treatment modality. However, many clinicians are also reluctant to affirm and validate people in treatment. Instead, they tend to adopt controlling policies that lead to an adversarial relationship between staff and patients.

Finally, given that positive staff attitudes towards treatment are important, one of the major obstacles to optimising the benefits of treatment is low morale. Methadone clinics are a stressful environment in which to work. Often, there is conflict and inconsistency over the goals of treatment, suggesting little cohesion in the team delivering treatment. To exacerbate these difficulties, clinics are often poorly funded and poorly maintained, thus further diminishing morale.

RITUAL AND STYLE IN METHADONE TREATMENT

A recent study of methadone clinics in Sydney (Bell *et al.,* 1995b) provided some useful insights into how treatment effectiveness might be improved. In the Sydney study, one clinic was strikingly less effective than the others. This provided some valuable insights into factors that detracted from the effectiveness of treatment.

The first clinic was highly organised, and could best be characterised as businesslike (right down to the fact that the administrator regularly undertook time and motion studies to ensure that dispensing of methadone was being carried out efficiently). Patients in this clinic received higher doses of methadone (mean daily dose 76 mg), and this clinic had least heroin use, a result probably attributable to the higher doses of methadone being prescribed. The clinic functioned as a highly efficient methadone dispensary, with little attention to "treatment". Clinical records were poorly kept.

The second clinic was less highly organised, but more individualised. Instead of a businesslike approach, the ethos in this clinic was "medical", with well-maintained clinical records, and attention paid to individual problems. Lower doses of methadone were prescribed (mean 53 mg). Heroin use in this clinic was higher than in the first clinic, but fell progressively over the 12 months of the study. Non-opioid drug use and crime were lowest among patients attending this clinic, and it was rated highest of the three clinics by the patients themselves.

In the third clinic, the atmosphere was chaotic. Staff worked in an atmosphere of perpetual crisis, but made little or no attempt to alter this reactive mode of operating. On one occasion when researchers were in the clinic, an arbitrary and abrupt change in policy regarding take-home medication led to a wave of anxiety and resentment among the patients. There was a pervasive sense of disorganisation and frustration within the clinic. Clinical records were very poorly maintained. Methadone doses were moderate (mean 55 mg), but the outcomes of treatment were poor. Adjusting for subject variables, this clinic had significantly worse outcomes in terms of retention in treatment, heroin use, non-opioid drug use, and crime. Perhaps most tellingly, patients asked to rate their treatment also rated this clinic lowest of the three.

Despite the different ethos in the three clinics, in many key respects treatment delivered was remarkably similar. The clinics had similar admission policies. Patients were almost never involuntarily withdrawn from treatment in any of the clinics. The clientele in the three clinics was similar. Levels of services, staff training, and treatment philosophy were similar. However, where the clinics differed was in the "style" of treatment, and these differences in style were associated with significant differences in outcomes.

Equally striking as the differences between the clinics was the observation that in all three of them, for most staff and patients, methadone maintenance treatment was something of a ritual, with little clear rationale for what was occurring. The absence of a frame of reference for approaching methadone treatment was apparent, not just in the differences between the clinics, but in the interaction between staff and patients within each clinic. These observations lead to three suggestions as to how treatment could be improved.

1. Treatment ethos

Many clinicians and researchers see methadone maintenance treatment as a "program", a preventive or public health measure rather than a treatment of individuals. While this perspective undoubtedly has validity, it can contribute to significant problems in the delivery of effective care. "Treatment" brings with it assumptions of attention to individuals and good clinical practice, assumptions more rigorous than any regulations stipulating minimum standards of care. These assumptions include the necessity for good clinical records. More importantly, a "treatment" ethos provides a framework in which all interactions with patients are understood as part of the care of the individual. Thus issues of anger, conflict and acting out become part of the material being worked with, rather than an irritation or obstacle to the smooth running of the clinic.

In large methadone clinics, it is probably more difficult to maintain an ethos of individualised treatment. This is a strong argument for locating methadone treatment in primary care settings. This has obvious advantages in making treatment more anonymous, less stigmatised, and more accessible. It avoids the problems of loitering associated with large methadone clinics. It also locates methadone maintenance in a setting where the "treatment" framework is assumed, and where the governing assumption is the care of individuals rather than providing a social service.

2. Dose setting

Research has been reasonably consistent in demonstrating that an adequate dose of methadone is an important determinant of treatment efficacy (Hargreaves, 1983). Many patients are ambivalent about being on methadone, and fear that higher doses will have adverse effects. However, in the studies of methadone clinics in North America (Ball & Ross,1991), and in Sydney (Bell *et al.*, 1995b), it is apparent that clinic policies influence dose levels. Thus, sub-optimal doses cannot be primarily attributed to patients' reluctance to be placed on higher doses. It is the clinician's responsibility to address ambivalence and encourage patients to take adequate doses.

3. Organisation

Working with heroin users is stressful for a variety of reasons, not the least being negative community attitudes towards treatment. Staff are at risk of burn-out, disillusionment and cynicism. Such consequences are an unacceptable cost for health professionals, and are probably also potent factors reducing the effectiveness of treatment. Structured and well-organised treatment, with clear rationale and objectives, is one way of minimising these problems.

Staff should have job descriptions, with clear delineation of roles and responsibilities. Lines of communication need to be clear and observed. (This applies as much in a clinic as in a primary care setting between physician and dispensing pharmacist.) Regular team meetings to discuss problems and review policies allow staff to clarify their responses to the pressures of working in methadone treatment.

A structured approach to treatment is helpful, as long as the structure does not constitute a barrier to entering treatment or is an intrusive burden on patients. For example, intake into treatment should be prompt, based on an interview focused on establishing the patient's suitability for treatment, rather than following exhaustive assessment. At the initial visit, treatment policies, and what staff expect of patients should be clarified. Such issues as frequency of attendance for review or counselling sessions, dosing times and rules regarding payment, need to be clearly spelt out. During subsequent weeks of treatment a more detailed assessment, and formulation of a treatment plan can be undertaken. Clinical records should clearly document the important issues in each individual's treatment.

REFERENCES

Ball, J.C., & Ross, A. (1991). *The effectiveness of methadone maintenance treatment: Patients, programs, services and outcome.* New York: Springer-Verlag.

Bell, J., Caplehorn, J., & McNeil, D. (1994). The effect of intake procedures on performance in methadone maintenance. *Addiction, 89,* 463-472.

Bell, J., Chan, J., & Kuk, A. (1995a). Investigating the effect of treatment philosophy on outcome of methadone maintenance. *Addiction,* 90, 823-830.

Bell, J., Ward, J., Mattick R.P., Hay, A., Chan, J., & Hall, W. (1995b). *An evaluation of private methadone clinics* (National Drug Strategy Research Report No 4). Canberra, Australia: Australian Government Publishing Service.

Courtwright, D., Joseph, H., & Des Jarlais, D. (1989) *Addicts who survived: An oral history of narcotic use in America, 1923-1965.* Knoxville, TN, University of Tennessee Press.

D'Aunno, T., & Vaughan, T.E. (1992). Variations in methadone treatment practices: Results from a national study. *Journal of the American Medical Association, 267,* 253-258.

Dodes, L.M. (1990). Addiction, helplessness and narcissistic rage. *Psychoanalytic Quarterly, 59,* 398-419

Dole, V.P. (1980). Addictive behaviour. *Scientific American, 243,* 136-143.

Dole, V.P. (1989). Methadone treatment and the acquired immunodeficiency syndrome epidemic. *Journal of the American Medical Association, 262,* 1681-1682.

Gerstein, D.R., & Harwood, H.J. (1990). *Treating drug problems Volume 1: A study of effectiveness and financing of public and private drug treatment systems.* Washington DC: National Academy Press.

Hall, S.M. (1983). Methadone maintenance; an overview of research findings. In J. R. Cooper, F. Altman, B. S. Brown, & D. Czechowicz (Eds.), *Research on the treatment of narcotic addiction: State of the art* (pp. 575-632). Rockville, MD: National Institute on Drug Abuse

Hargreaves, W. A. (1983). Methadone dosage and duration for maintenance treatment. In J. R. Cooper, F. Altman, B. S. Brown, & D. Czechowicz (Eds.), *Research on the treatment of narcotic addiction: State of the art* (pp. 19-79). Rockville, MD: National Institute on Drug Abuse.

Khantzian, E.J. (1985). The self medication hypothesis of addictive disorders: Focus on heroin and cocaine dependence. *American Journal of Psychiatry,* 142, 1259-1264.

McLellan, A.T., Arndt, I.O., Metzger, D.S., Woody, G.E., & O'Brien C.P. (1993). The effects of psychosocial services in substance abuse treatment. *Journal of the American Medical Association,* 269, 1953-9.

McClellan, A.T., Luborsky, L., Woody, G.E., O'Brien , C.P., & Kron, R. (1981). Are the "addiction-related" problems of substance abusers really related? *Journal of Nervous and Mental Diseases,* 169, 232-239.

Martin, W.R., Jasinski, D.R., Haertzen, C.A., Kay, D.C., Jones, B.E., Mansky, P.A., & Carpenter, R.W.(1973). Methadone: A re-evaluation. *Archives of General Psychiatry,* 28, 286-295.

Miller, W.R., & Hester, R.K. (1986). The effectiveness of alcoholism treatment: What research reveals. In W.R. Miller and N. Heather (Eds.), *Treating addictive behaviours: Processes of change* (pp. 121-174). New York: Plenum Press.

Murphy, S., & Irwin, J. (1992). "Living with the dirty secret:" Problems of disclosure for methadone maintenance clients. *Journal of Psychoactive Drugs,* 24, 257-264

Newman, R.G. (1987). Methadone treatment: Defining and evaluating success. *New England Journal of Medicine,* 317, 447-450.

Newman, R.G., & Peyser, N. (1991). Methadone treatment: experiment and experience. *Journal of Psychoactive Drugs,* 23, 115-121.

Saxon, A.J., Calsyn, D.A., Kivlahan, D.R., & Roszell, D.K. (1993). Outcome of contingency contracting for illicit drug use in a methadone maintenance program. *Drug and Alcohol Dependence,* 31, 205-14.

Yancovitz, S.R., Des Jarlais, D.C., Peyser, N.P., Drew, E., Friedman, P., Trigg, H.L., & Robinson, J.W. (1991). A randomised trial of an interim methadone maintenance clinic. *American Journal of Public Health,* 81, 1185-1191.

8

ASSESSMENT FOR OPIOID REPLACEMENT THERAPY

JEFF WARD, RICHARD P. MATTICK AND WAYNE HALL

INTRODUCTION

Assessing people for opioid replacement therapy involves two tasks: to determine whether therapy is appropriate for a given individual and, once suitability is established, to identify areas other than opioid dependence where medical care or some other form of therapy or assistance might be provided. Drug maintenance regimens, such as those using opioids, involve exposing patients to risks that have to be weighed against the benefits to be gained. Diagnosis is very important in deciding who should receive treatment in such cases, so that individuals who do not have the target condition are not exposed to unnecessary risks. The key risk in the case of opioid replacement therapy is an iatrogenic opioid dependence that may result from the daily administration of an opioid. Accordingly, a major concern is ensuring that non-dependent individuals do not become dependent as a result of treatment. In this chapter, we examine the criteria for deciding who should receive opioid replacement therapy. Put simply, opioid replacement therapy is only suitable for individuals who are either opioid dependent, or for whom the risks associated with continued illicit opioid use outweigh those associated with being maintained on a licit opioid such as methadone. We also examine issues related to how an assessment of the need for opioid replacement therapy should be conducted, and at the role the assessment plays in the initiation of a therapeutic relationship.

A BRIEF HISTORY OF ADMISSION CRITERIA FOR OPIOID REPLACEMENT THERAPY

Dole and Nyswander (1965) established stringent criteria for entry when they established the first methadone maintenance program in New York some 30 years ago. To be considered suitable for this program, applicants had to be at least 21 years of age, had to have been dependent on opioids for at least four years, had to have no serious psychopathology, alcohol or other non-opioid drug problems, and had to have failed repeatedly in other forms of treatment for their opioid dependence. These criteria reflected medical and societal concerns about maintaining individuals in a drug-dependent state. The consequence was that methadone treatment was restricted to applicants who were considered to be untreatable by other methods. They also ensured that patients admitted to the program would be recidivist opioid addicts whose primary problem was their opioid dependence.

In the three decades since the introduction of methadone maintenance, assessment criteria have been liberalised in most parts of the world by reducing both the patient's age and the length of dependence necessary for entry (Gossop & Grant, 1991; Uchtenhagen, 1990). Changing patterns of illicit drug use have also meant that it has become impractical to exclude individuals who use drugs other than opioids. Twenty to 30 years ago, it was common for applicants for methadone maintenance treatment to present with a clearly defined opioid dependence that was not complicated by the frequent use of other illicit drugs. Now the applicant for opioid replacement therapy is more likely to use a variety of illicit drugs (e.g., Bell *et al.,* 1990). Accepting poly-drug users into treatment is problematic because it is only illicit opioids for which substitution is provided and the continued use of other drugs (e.g., benzodiazepines) may be unsafe in combination with opioids such as methadone or LAAM. However, given the virtual disappearance of the opioid-only drug user, it would be impractical to continue to exclude individuals on the basis of multiple drug use.

Another factor that has influenced assessment policy is the advent of the HIV epidemic among injecting drug users in many countries. For example, in The Netherlands, admission criteria have been reduced to a minimum in some programs as a specific measure to try to reduce the spread of HIV among the injecting drug using population (Gossop & Grant, 1991; van Ameijden *et al.,* 1992). Such programs have become known as 'low threshold' programs.

OPIOID DEPENDENCE

The basis for opioid replacement therapy as an intervention is the phenomenon of cross-dependence. This refers to the capacity of one drug of a class to replace another drug of the same class upon which an individual is dependent, without inducing a withdrawal syndrome (Jaffe, 1990). For example, a person who is dependent on heroin can successfully substitute methadone for heroin and not experience any discomfort; they will, however, be dependent on methadone thereafter. Given this pharmacological rationale for the use of methadone, there has always been an understandable concern about iatrogenic dependence – that is, that providing methadone will induce an opioid dependence in individuals who are not opioid dependent. Concern about iatrogenic dependence has often given rise to the requirement that an individual be *physically* dependent on opioids in order to be eligible for treatment.

Physical Dependence

According to Jaffe (1990), the term 'physical dependence' refers to :

> an altered physiological state (neuroadaptation) produced by the repeated administration of a drug, which necessitates the continued administration of the drug to prevent the appearance of the withdrawal or abstinence syndrome that is characteristic for the particular drug (p. 523).

Physical dependence is closely related to the phenomenon of tolerance in which, with repeated administration of a drug, increasing doses are necessary in order to achieve the desired effect. Opioids have their main effects on the body within the brain by acting on specific receptor sites in certain clusters of neurones. The phenomenon of tolerance is thought to be a result of these neurones adapting, via down-regulation, to chronic exposure to "exogenous" (i.e., externally administered) opioids. The term neuroadaptation refers to this adaptive process and is responsible, through a rebound effect, for the withdrawal syndrome when the use of the drug ceases or the dose is sharply reduced. The extent to which neuroadaptation has been established in an individual is assessed by the severity of the withdrawal syndrome that occurs when use of the drug is suddenly stopped (Jaffe, 1990).

Edwards and colleagues (1981) have pointed out that the term 'physical dependence' is imprecise and have suggested that it be replaced by the more correct and specific term 'neuroadaptation'. The word dependence has connotations that suggest that the person concerned finds the drug in question necessary for the conduct of their life. Edwards *et al.* point out that some patients become neuroadapted to opioids when they are used for the purposes of pain management and experience a withdrawal syndrome when they are stopped, but they neither wish to continue taking, nor seek out opioid drugs again. Such patients, while certainly neuroadapted to opioids, would not by any criteria be considered dependent in the sense that the term heroin dependence is used. It is useful, therefore, to conceptually distinguish between the physiological adaptive processes induced by the chronic administration of opioids and the drug-seeking behaviour that characterises dependence.

The Opioid Dependence Syndrome

A major implication of the observation that a person can be neuroadapted to opioids and yet not be dependent on opioids is that neuroadaptation, by itself, cannot account for the typical clinical picture seen in cases of opioid dependence. That is, the fact that a person has had sufficient opioid exposure for neuroadaptation to take place does not explain their inability to cease its use, even though dependent individuals often attribute their inability to stop solely to neuroadaptation (Edwards *et al.*, 1981; Jaffe, 1990). In order to provide a more adequate characterisation of the phenomenon of drug addiction, Edwards *et al.* (1981) developed a model of the drug dependence syndrome which has been extremely influential in the development of definitions of drug dependence by both the World Health Organisation and the American Psychiatric Association (Kosten *et al.*, 1987).

The drug dependence syndrome was defined by Edwards *et al.* (1981) as a cluster of phenomena that include:

- neuroadaptation as evidenced by tolerance or withdrawal;
- a compulsive desire to use the drug, especially when trying to reduce or stop use of the drug;
- being unable to stop use of the drug even though wanting to;
- a well-developed narrow repertoire of behaviours associated with use of the drug;
- using the drug of dependence to prevent or relieve withdrawal;
- drug-seeking behaviour having become more important than other previously more important activities;
- early relapse after withdrawal.

Edwards *et al.* emphasised that neuroadaptation should not be given special importance over and above any of the other criteria. They acknowledged that it would not be possible, given the little that is known about drug taking, to clearly make a distinction between dependent and non-dependent drug use. At the same time, they pointed out that a person need not be dependent to be beset with difficulties as a result of their drug use, nor need they necessarily experience such difficulties if they were dependent. A dependent physician, for example, need not experience any of the drug-related problems that usually beset the street addict (Rounsaville *et al.*, 1987). Rounsaville, Spitzer and Williams (1986) point out that although drug-related problems are often the reason that treatment is sought, it is still important to maintain a clear distinction between a disorder and the social problems that arise from having the disorder. Psychotic individuals, for instance, experience many problems within society but these problems are considered to be a consequence of the presence of these disorders, rather than an aspect of the disease process itself. Problems as a result of drug use were therefore not included in the definition of the drug dependence syndrome proposed by Edwards *et al.* (1981).

The most important implications of this definition of the drug dependence syndrome are that a diagnosis of drug dependence does not require the presence of all of these phenomena and that dependence is a condition that can be more or less severe, rather than simply present or absent. Another implication is that some individuals who do not currently use the drug of dependence, and who are therefore not neuroadapted, could be considered to be dependent if the presence of cues associated with drug taking evokes in them an overbearing desire to take the drug.

ICD-10 and DSM-IV Diagnostic Criteria

There are two internationally accepted diagnostic criteria that cover psychoactive substance use disorders, including drug dependence: the tenth revision of the *International Classification of Diseases* (ICD-10) dealing with mental and behavioural disorders published by the World Health Organisation (WHO, 1992), and the fourth edition of the *Diagnostic and Statistical Manual of Mental Disorders* (DSM-IV) published by the American Psychiatric Association (American Psychiatric Association, 1994). Both of these sets of criteria for diagnosing drug dependence have been based on the conceptual framework developed by Edwards *et al.* (1981). These sets reflect current knowledge based on research and expert clinical opinion (e.g. Feingold & Rounsaville, 1995; Langenbucher *et al.*, 1994; Woody *et al.*, 1993). They have been found to be reasonably reliable in terms of arriving at diagnoses (Rounsaville *et al.*, 1993), and provide a useful guide for diagnosing opioid dependence to determine eligibility for admission to opioid replacement therapy.

The ICD-10 and DSM-IV criteria for the diagnosis of opioid dependence are set out below.

ICD-10: Dependence Syndrome (WHO, 1992, pp. 75-76)

A cluster of physiological, behavioural, and cognitive phenomena in which the use of a substance or a class of substances takes on a much higher priority for a given individual than other behaviours that once had greater value. A central descriptive characteristic of the dependence syndrome is the desire (often strong, sometimes overpowering) to take psychoactive drugs (which may or may not have been medically prescribed), alcohol, or tobacco. There may be evidence that return to substance use after a period of abstinence leads to a more rapid reappearance of other features of the syndrome than occurs with nondependent individuals.

Diagnostic Guidelines

A definite diagnosis of dependence should usually be made only if three or more of the following have been present together at some time during the previous year:

(1) a strong desire or sense of compulsion to take the substance;

(2) difficulties in controlling substance-taking behaviour in terms of its onset, termination, or levels of use;

(3) a physiological withdrawal state when substance use has ceased or been reduced as evidenced by: the characteristic withdrawal syndrome for the substance; or use of the same (or a closely related) substance with the intention of relieving or avoiding withdrawal symptoms;

(4) evidence of tolerance, such that increased doses of the psychoactive substance are required in order to achieve effects originally produced by lower doses (clear examples of this are found in alcohol- and opiate-dependent individuals who may take daily doses sufficient to incapacitate or kill nontolerant users);

(5) progressive neglect of alternative pleasures or interests because of psychoactive substance use, increased amount of time necessary to obtain or take the substance or to recover from its effects;

(6) persisting with substance use despite clear evidence of overtly harmful consequences, such as harm to the liver through excessive drinking, depressive mood states consequent to periods of heavy substance use, or drug-related impairment of cognitive functioning; efforts should be made to determine that the user was actually, or could be expected to be, aware of the nature and extent of the harm.

DSM-IV: Criteria for substance dependence (American Psychiatric Association, 1994, p. 181)

A maladaptive pattern of substance use, leading to clinically significant impairment or distress, as manifested by three (or more) of the following, occurring at any time in the same 12-month period:

(1)　tolerance, as defined by either of the following:

    (a)　a need for markedly increased amounts of the substance to achieve intoxication or desired effect

    (b)　markedly diminished effect with continued use of the same amount of the substance;

(2)　withdrawal, as manifested by either of the following:

    (a)　the characteristic withdrawal syndrome for the substance

    (b)　the same (or a closely related) substance is taken to relieve or avoid withdrawal symptoms;

(3)　the substance is often taken in larger amounts or over a longer period than was intended;

(4)　there is a persistent desire or unsuccessful efforts to cut down or control substance use;

(5)　a great deal of time is spent in activities necessary to obtain the substance (e.g., visiting multiple doctors or driving long distances), use the substance (e.g. chain-smoking), or recover from its effects;

(6)　important social, occupational, or recreational activities are given up or reduced because of substance use;

(7)　the substance use is continued despite knowledge of having a persistent or recurrent physical or psychological problem that is likely to have been caused or exacerbated by the substance (e.g. current cocaine use despite recognition of cocaine-induced depression, or continued drinking despite recognition that an ulcer was made worse by alcohol consumption).

Specify if:

With physiological dependence: evidence of tolerance or withdrawal (i.e., either item 1 or 2 is present)

Without physiological dependence: no evidence of tolerance or withdrawal (i.e. neither item 1 nor 2 is present).

In each of these diagnostic systems the presence of three or more of the criteria are necessary in order to establish a diagnosis of opioid dependence. The two systems differ slightly in that the ICD-10 has a separate item for craving or compulsion to take opioids. Furthermore, the ICD-10 manual emphasises that this item is central to the ICD-10 definition of the substance dependence syndrome (WHO, 1992). Both systems have supplementary criteria that allow for a specification of whether the individual is physically dependent or not, as indicated by the presence of tolerance or withdrawal. Both systems also recommend indicating the current status of the individual. For example, the ICD-10 (WHO, 1992, p. 77) gives the option of noting the following indicators of current status (only those relevant to opioid dependence have been included):

• Currently abstinent
• Currently abstinent but in a protected environment (e.g., in hospital, in a therapeutic community, in prison, etc.)
• Currently on a clinically supervised maintenance or replacement regime [controlled dependence] (e.g., with methadone)
• Currently abstinent but receiving treatment with aversive or

blocking drugs (e.g., naltrexone)
- Currently using the substance [active dependence]

THE ASSESSMENT OF OPIOID DEPENDENCE

This section examines various procedures that have been developed to assess the presence and severity of opioid dependence and evaluates their practicality and desirability as assessment procedures for opioid replacement therapy. The approach that will be recommended here is to take a careful clinical history to assess the current status of the individual using the ICD-10 or DSM-IV criteria.

Naloxone Testing

Opioid substances can be classified according to whether they are agonists or antagonists (Jaffe & Martin, 1990). Opioid agonists (e.g., morphine and methadone) act by occupying and stimulating receptor sites within the brain, thereby producing their well known effects of analgesia, sedation, etc. Opioid antagonists, on the other hand, have an affinity for the same receptor sites but do not produce these effects and when administered after the administration of opioid agonists have the capacity to reverse them. Naloxone is a pure opioid antagonist and is widely used to reverse the effects of opioid agonists in cases of overdose. When it is administered by injection to individuals who are neuroadapted to opioids, it produces a withdrawal syndrome in a matter of minutes which is not unlike the withdrawal that occurs after the abrupt cessation of opioid use. Naloxone-induced withdrawal lasts for about two hours.

The first use of naloxone in combination with a scoring system for assessing physical dependence was reported by Blachly (1973) and there have been a number of other tests developed since (Judson *et al.*, 1980; Peachey & Lei, 1988; Wang *et al.*, 1974; Zilm & Sellers, 1978). The procedure involves scoring for the presence and intensity of signs (and at times symptoms) associated with the opioid withdrawal syndrome. These signs include gooseflesh, sweating, rhinnorrhea (running nose), vomiting, lacrimation (tears in the eyes), restlessness, yawning and increased blood pressure. Some tests weight these items and priority is usually given to the first four listed. Patients are usually assessed prior to and then 20 to 30 minutes after the intramuscular or subcutaneous administration of naloxone. If there is no response to the first injection, it is usual to proceed with a second injection given intravenously followed by another assessment for withdrawal signs.

There is some debate concerning what is an adequate dose of naloxone for use in these tests. Judson and Goldstein, who reviewed the literature on naloxone testing in 1983, argued that the use of 0.18 mg of naloxone should be a sufficient dose for both the first and second injections. They suggested that individuals who required higher doses should not be considered as dependent. Recently, however, Jacobsen and Kosten (1989; see also Kosten *et al.*, 1989) have argued that a dose of 0.8 mg may be necessary, because previous studies had found that when doses lower than 0.8 mg were used, fewer patients were assessed as opioid dependent. Kauffman and Woody (1995) have recently recommended doses in the 0.4-0.8 mg range.

The difficulty evident in establishing an appropriate dose of naloxone for testing for physical dependence raises the difficult issue of what constitutes a significant level of neuroadaptation to opioids. There is a demonstrable quantitative relationship in both animals and humans between the chronic dose of an opioid and the severity of a naloxone-induced withdrawal syndrome (Judson & Goldstein, 1983; O'Brien *et al.*, 1978; Wang, *et al.*, 1974), but this relationship may become unreliable at the lower end of the scale. As Jaffe (1990) notes, an individual who has been administered therapeutic doses of morphine for two to three days will manifest a withdrawal syndrome when administered naloxone, but would not do so if administration of the drug was suddenly stopped.

Resnick (1983), in a commentary on Judson and Goldstein's 1983 review raised what now seems to be the most serious problem with the naloxone test. Using the term 'psychological dependence', he suggested that there may be individuals who use opioids compulsively for their psychotropic effects without becoming neuroadapted. He wondered whether, when refused opioid replacement therapy, these people would not increase their heroin use in order to meet the criteria for admission. Kanof and colleagues (1991) point out that even without escalating their drug use, such individuals will continue to be at risk for the social, legal and health problems associated with habitual illicit opioid use.

An important disadvantage of naloxone testing is the discomfort involved for the patient. Kreek (cited in Cooper *et al.*, 1983), for example, is opposed to naloxone testing because she believes the discomfort involved is unnecessary (along with the cost) when a careful history and physical examination would suffice. A number of other reviewers have emphasised this disadvantage and have recommended against naloxone testing (e.g., Langrod, 1993; Mattick & Hall, 1993).

Sanchez-Ramos and Senay (1987) attempted to obviate the discomfort involved in the procedure by administering naloxone in eye drops unilaterally to methadone maintenance patients and measuring the subsequent change in pupil diameter (the expected response being mydriasis, i.e., dilation of the pupil). However, four out of the five patients in this case study experienced dysphoria as a result of the naloxone administration. They concluded that administering naloxone to the eye in opioid-dependent individuals can induce a typical withdrawal syndrome and therefore is not indicated as a routine assessment procedure. The procedure is still advocated by some practitioners, even though one in five patients receiving methadone maintenance (and therefore dependent on methadone) are not dependent according to the test (e.g., Ghodse *et al.*, 1995). In the light of the discomfort that may be caused and the possibility that dependent individuals may be screened out, we do not recommend the use of this procedure as a routine component in the assessment of suitability for opioid replacement therapy.

Methadone Challenge

Higgins and colleagues (1985) report a procedure for assessing level of neuroadaptation to opioids by measuring the amount of miosis (pupil constriction) in response to a 20 mg dose of methadone. They found a strong relationship between amount of pupil constriction and reported current levels of heroin use and length of time since first opioid use (these two measures together accounted for 60% of the variance in pupillary response). The authors of the study argue that this relationship demonstrates that pupillary response to a challenge dose of methadone is a valid measure of dependence. Given the necessary equipment (Polaroid camera with 3X magnification) and the time involved (a two-hour wait for maximum response to methadone), an alternative interpretation of these results is that the methadone challenge test provides good evidence for the validity of a carefully taken history as a measure of dependence.

Urinalysis

Urine samples are sometimes taken at assessment and tested for the presence of opioids. An opioid-positive urinalysis result establishes recent opioid use but does not reveal any information about the extent of use or dependence. It is apparently common knowledge among drug users that the production of an opiate-positive urine at the assessment interview (if the unit concerned takes a urine sample) for opioid replacement therapy will help in establishing suitability. The use of this criterion may therefore encourage the use of opioids prior to attending for an assessment (Bell, *et al.*, 1990). Judson *et al.* (1980) concluded that since a urine sample only establishes recent use, and not dependence or pattern of use, urinalysis had no place in assessment for opioid replacement therapy. Although of limited use for this purpose, urinalysis during assessment may be useful in determining the range of other drugs currently used by the applicant.

The Severity of Opiate Dependence Questionnaire

The Severity of Opiate Dependence Questionnaire (SODQ) was developed to assess the drug dependence syndrome for opioids as developed by Edwards *et al.* (1981). Accordingly, the SODQ consists of five main sections, each devoted respectively to quantity and pattern of opiate use, physical symptoms of withdrawal, affective symptoms of withdrawal, withdrawal relief drug-taking and the rapidity with which withdrawal symptoms recur on resumption of opioid use after a period of abstinence (Sutherland *et al.*, 1986). The SODQ has been trialled on British, American and Australian samples and found to have good psychometric properties (Burgess *et al*, 1989; Phillips *et al.*, 1987; Sutherland, *et al.*, 1986; Sutherland *et al.*, 1988). Mattick and Hall (1993) recommend its use as a means of structuring the clinical interview.

Clinical Assessment and History Taking

A clinical assessment for opioid dependence involves the taking of a drug use history, an examination for physical signs of injecting drug use (e.g., puncture marks and scars), and noting the presence or absence of signs of opioid intoxication or withdrawal. The main criticism of a clinical assessment is that applicants for opioid replacement therapy may exaggerate the severity of their problems in order to ensure that they are admitted to treatment. This criticism presupposes that neuroadaptation is a necessary condition for entry in to opioid replacement therapy. This will not be discussed any further because, as argued above, it does not take into account the compulsive aspect of opioid use and the harm associated with it, nor does it take into account individuals who have previously been dependent and are at current risk for relapse.

A second presumption is that applicants are likely to exaggerate the extent of their opioid use and dependence. Jaffe (1990) has drawn a useful distinction between purposive and non-purposive behaviour associated with the withdrawal syndrome that can be applied to the assessment process. According to Jaffe, some of the behaviours associated with the withdrawal syndrome are only apparent in specific places (e.g., methadone clinic, doctor's surgery) in the presence of certain other people (person who has power to dispense opioids) and have the sole purpose of obtaining drugs. These behaviours, which include a manipulative communication style and simulated withdrawal symptoms, run the full gamut of behaviours possible in the situation. However, other signs are not dependent on place and the presence of an observer (e.g., puncture marks, gooseflesh, pinpoint pupils). Experienced clinicians are fully aware of this distinction and through their knowledge of the opioid-using lifestyle would usually be able to select out a person with little or no history of opioid use. This kind of clinical assessment by experienced clinicians is, at this time, probably the best method for assessing opioid dependence in opioid replacement therapy programs.

It would, however, be useful for basic assessment criteria to be used by clinicians. Such criteria should be based on well-researched instruments such as the SODQ and well developed criteria such as those outlined in the ICD-10 and the DSM-IV. We have emphasised the importance of clinical experience because of the possible consequences that may result from inexperienced clinicians inadvertently overdosing individuals with little or no tolerance (see Chapter 9 for a full discussion of this issue). A practical solution to this problem is appropriate training for medical practitioners who prescribe opioids for replacement therapy (see Chapter 14).

OTHER AREAS OF ASSESSMENT

Although the drug dependence syndrome is considered to be

independent of the problems associated with drug use, the latter are important in assessing applicants for opioid replacement therapy, because an effective response to these problems is an important predictor of length of stay and response to treatment (see Chapter 12). Opioid dependence may have a range of medical, social, legal and psychological costs associated with it. According to Jaffe (1990):

> The medical complications common among drug users include infections (e.g., septicemia, endocarditis, hepatitis, acquired immune deficiency syndrome, tetanus, tuberculosis, and pulmonary, cerebral, and subcutaneous abscesses) due to shared needles and unhygienic procedures, foreign body emboli, granulomata due to injection of contaminants, and a variety of neurological, musculoskeletal, and other lesions that may be due to hypersensitivity reactions or to toxic impurities in drugs produced in illicit laboratories (p. 533).

People who inject opioids are also at risk of dying through overdose or toxic reactions to contaminated drug supplies (for a full discussion of the health complications of injecting drug use see Levine & Sobel, 1991). Social complications include unemployment, poverty and disruption to personal relationships, while the legal complications include arrest and imprisonment for both drug and drug-related (e.g., breaking and entering) crimes. Psychological difficulties associated with opioid dependence would include a range of reactions to the stress associated with maintaining a drug-dependent lifestyle. A full assessment should include a detailed exploration of the individual's history and current status in each of these areas.

An assessment of the problems and risks associated with the applicant's current lifestyle and state of health is also of relevance in assessing his or her suitability for opioid replacement therapy. Just as an individual does not have to be neuroadapted to opioids to be diagnosed as being dependent, he or she does not have to be neuroadapted to experience serious drug-related problems. There is a growing body of evidence that opioid replacement therapy can be an effective intervention in the lives of many drug users (see Chapters 2 & 3). If there is a concern on the part of the clinician about the possibility of iatrogenic opioid dependence, then the harm associated with not taking the person into treatment has to be weighed against the benefits of reducing the severity of their drug-related problems.

There is no established procedure for assessing the problems associated with opioid dependence, and, as already noted, there is no necessary relationship between the extent of these problems and the level of dependence. For example, a street-dwelling, sporadic (but compulsive) heroin user who injects himself or herself with syringes found on the street may suffer more harm from drug use than a severely dependent heroin dealer who injects with relatively pure heroin five or six times a day but uses a clean needle every time.

A physical examination (which may involve laboratory tests such as liver function tests) and the taking of a history of infections and other drug-related medical problems would establish the extent to which the applicant has suffered physical harm as a result of his or her drug use. Questions concerning the applicant's involvement in prostitution, crime, loss of employment, broken relationships and loss of housing, etc. would indicate the extent to which his or her social life has been disrupted. Past and current involvement in HIV risk-taking behaviours is another important area of potential harm that needs to be assessed. Psychological harm as a result of drug use would involve the extent to which the applicant's drug use and the problems outlined above have led to anxiety and depression. Through this process the consequences of accepting or rejecting the applicant could be evaluated. If the predominant drug of choice is an opioid and there is significant harm, then opioid replacement therapy is indicated.

There is a need perhaps to formalise the assessment of drug-related problems for both research and clinical purposes. Two assessment instruments that have been developed for this purpose are the Addiction Severity Index (McLellan *et al.*, 1980) and the Opiate Treatment Index (Darke *et al.*, 1992). These instruments assess a range of outcomes (health, involvement with crime, psychological and social functioning) as well as estimates of current drug use. The Opiate Treatment Index also assesses extent of recent HIV risk behaviour. The use of such instruments would help to systematise and standardise the assessment process and would provide standardised data that would be useful for program evaluation.

INCLUSION CRITERIA BASED ON PREDICTORS OF SUCCESS

Diagnosing that a condition is of sufficient severity to warrant an intervention is often only one step in deciding whether a particular treatment is indicated or not. Another important issue is whether a particular treatment will help a given patient or not. This issue is especially important in the treatment of opioid dependence because there are often long waiting lists for treatment places. Though an applicant may fulfil the criteria for entry to a treatment program, it may be a waste of time for all concerned if it can be predicted that he or she will not respond positively to the program (Baekeland & Lundwall, 1975). In the case of the opioid dependent, it is well known that there is a minority of patients who continue to use illicit drugs heavily after entering treatment and then leave or are expelled from treatment quickly. If early drop-outs from opioid replacement therapy, and patients who from any viewpoint would be considered failures, could be somehow identified prior to admission, then opioid replacement programs would be freed from their disruptive influence. Applicants who were more likely to benefit from treatment could then be given places, and the overall performance of opioid substitution programs would be improved.

The evidence reviewed in Chapter 12 on predictors of retention during opioid replacement therapy, provides some direction on how to identify applicants who probably would not respond to opioid replacement therapy. Individuals who use opioids more heavily, who have used them for longer and who have more extensive criminal histories tend not to respond to treatment as well as individuals with less severe problems. However, there are two immediate problems associated with such a statement. First, individuals with more severe problems are those most in need of assistance and they are the population that opioid replacement therapy was originally introduced to treat (the recidivist addict). Second, the statement is very general and applies equally well to a proportion of patients who have similar backgrounds but do respond to treatment. Therefore, at this stage, there are no reliable criteria to distinguish these two groups of patients and individuals should not be excluded from treatment because of the extent and severity of their problems.

THE FATE OF UNSUCCESSFUL TREATMENT APPLICANTS

Bell *et al.* (1990) describe the characteristics of 767 individuals who applied for methadone maintenance treatment in Western Sydney between 1986 and 1988. Fifteen per cent either did not complete the assessment process or were unsuccessful in gaining a place. Most of the applicants were either poly-drug users or had used a range of different drugs at different times in their lives. Bell *et al.* suggest that their patterns of drug use suggest a wish to be intoxicated as the central phenomenon in compulsive drug taking, rather than neuroadaptation and its consequences as being the central phenomenon. They also point out that if the drug dependence syndrome as formulated by Edwards *et al.* (1981) had been used as the assessment criteria, then nearly all the applicants would have been assessed as suitable for treatment.

In a follow-up study of 84 applicants who either did not complete the assessment process (n = 26) or who were not accepted (n = 58) for treatment, Bell, Digiusto and Byth (1992) found that the fate of unsuccessful applicants was poor. When the decision process of whether to accept an applicant or not was examined, it was found that daily opioid use, producing an opiate-positive urine, and having an extensive criminal record were the distinguishing criteria for acceptance into the program. This implies that as a group, the unsuccessful applicants had less reported drug use at the time of assessment and less extensive criminal histories.

Just over half of the unsuccessful applicants subsequently entered methadone maintenance at an average of 16 months after being rejected for treatment in Western Sydney. When the group was examined as a whole it was found that a significant proportion of the group (44%) spent a significant proportion of time in prison (46 terms) and/or drug treatment (37 subjects were admitted 59 times to detoxification units or residential treatment and spent 1,760 in-patient days there). One of the applicants who did not complete assessment and three of those who were rejected died in the period to follow-up. Two each of the two subgroups were considered to be successfully abstinent – a proportion that is to be expected from studies of the natural history of opioid dependence (Wodak, 1985).

The fate of the individuals followed over time in this study raises two issues. For those who were rejected, Bell *et al.* (1990) argue that the main consequence of rejection was a 16-month delay in their entry to methadone maintenance and their subjection in the intervening period to the risk of imprisonment and death. For the applicants who did not complete the assessment process, the question arises as to whether the assessment process itself discouraged them from entering methadone maintenance. This issue is examined in the next section.

TIME BETWEEN ASSESSMENT AND COMMENCEMENT OF TREATMENT

It is often claimed that a protracted assessment process will select out the unmotivated applicants from those who wish to change. This proposition was investigated by Woody *et al.,* (1975) who compared the retention rates of patients who went through a one- to three-day assessment process and those who were accepted or rejected after a first assessment interview. The patients who went through the minimal assessment procedure had significantly better retention rates at two and five months suggesting that, rather than selecting out the more motivated individuals, the protracted assessment procedure had negative consequences.

In another study that examined the relationship between assessment and subsequent retention during treatment, Bell, Caplehorn and McNeil (1994) compared the retention rates of two groups of patients, one of which had virtually no assessment at a private methadone clinic and another which went through a long assessment process (up to nine weeks) at a nearby public methadone clinic. This natural experiment was made possible when the private methadone clinic was closed because it was thought that the patients were not being assessed properly. The patients attending the private clinic were then referred to the public methadone clinic where they received the same treatment as the public patients who had been subjected to the protracted assessment. Analysis of the retention data revealed that individuals who had been carefully screened through the protracted assessment were more likely to leave treatment or be discharged for non-compliance during the first 400 days of treatment, although it should be noted that this relationship was reversed after the first 400 days of treatment, with those receiving virtually no assessment being more likely to leave. When heroin use, as measured by urinalysis, was examined, it was found that individuals who received the protracted assessment at the public methadone clinic were almost twice as likely to have used heroin compared with their minimal assessment counterparts.

Maddux, Desmond and Esquivel (1995) examined similar issues in a randomised controlled trial designed to evaluate the influence of immediate (within 24 hours of first assessment) versus delayed (up to 14 days) commencement of methadone treatment on pre-treatment attrition and retention during the first year of treatment. They found that those dosed within 24 hours of their first assessment were more likely to commence treatment than those who had to wait up to 14 days. This finding is consistent with the findings of Dennis and colleagues (1994) who similarly found pre-treatment attrition to be reduced when the waiting time for admission to methadone treatment was reduced. When Maddux *et al.* examined subsequent retention during the first year of treatment they found no difference between the immediate and delayed admission groups, although there was a trend for the immediate admission group to stay longer. There were no discernible differences between the two study groups in terms of illicit drug use and other rehabilitation criteria. The authors concluded that there appeared to be no advantage to a protracted assessment process and suggested that a brief initial assessment to establish suitability should be followed by the commencement of opioid administration. A more detailed assessment of the patient's history and current circumstances would then be carried out during the first days or weeks of treatment.

On the basis of the studies reviewed in this section, it is concluded that there is no evidence that a protracted assessment process for opioid replacement therapy results in the selection of a more motivated group of patients. On the contrary, the evidence indicates that an assessment of an individual's suitability for opioid maintenance should be done briefly and medication administered as quickly as possible. A more thorough clinical assessment could then be carried out, as Maddux *et al.* (1995) suggest, on subsequent days when the patient attends for medication. These conclusions are consistent with evidence from other areas of treatment, including general medical treatment, outpatient psychotherapy and treatment for alcohol problems which suggests that reducing the waiting time between treatment seeking and the first appointment decreases pre-treatment attrition (Baekeland & Lundwall, 1975; Stark, 1992).

ASSESSMENT AS THE FIRST MOMENT IN A THERAPEUTIC RELATIONSHIP

Assessment is an important part of most long-term treatments and can have a range of purposes (Miller & Rollnick, 1991). It can be used for evaluating the needs of the applicant, for diagnosis, for devising a treatment plan, and for determining suitability. Bell *et al.* (1992) have argued that policy concerning assessment has been dominated by the perceived necessity to prevent iatrogenic physical dependence at all costs. They go on to suggest – and this is consistent with the evidence reviewed above – that this concern is misplaced as it does not take account of the compulsive nature of opioid use.

According to Miller and Rollnick (1991), in the worst case the assessment process becomes a set of hoops that the applicant has to jump through in order to be allowed to receive treatment. The assessment process described by Bell *et al.* (1990; 1992) seems typical of this type of assessment. In order to be accepted for methadone maintenance, applicants had to attend two interviews at each of which they had to provide a urine specimen. If the patient was suspected of not being dependent, he or she was asked to attend for a naloxone test. Owing to the low numbers of applicants turning up for these tests, they were soon dropped. A set of procedures like these, with relatively long delays before methadone is dispensed, consists of a set of tests that the applicant has to pass in order to gain entry.

An applicant's first contact with a treatment agency is very important and has a strong influence in defining the nature of the future therapeutic relationship (Bell, *et al.*, 1992; Kauffman & Woody, 1995; Langrod, 1993; Miller & Rollnick, 1991; Woody, *et al.*, 1975). Opioid-dependent people who feel in need of help for their drug problems are not unusual in often being reluctant to seek out treatment (Gerstein & Harwood, 1990; Woody, *et al.*, 1975). Methadone maintenance, in particular, has a poor image among the drug-using subculture and many patients remain ambivalent about methadone while in treatment (Hunt *et al.*, 1985-86; Rosenblum *et al.*, 1991). The motivational interviewing technique of dealing with ambivalence about drug use could usefully be applied in such cases by helping the applicant/patient to think about the positive and negative aspects of being 'on' or 'off' methadone (see Miller & Rollnick, 1991).

Bell *et al.* (1994) emphasise the need to be aware of the ambivalence of applicants for opioid replacement therapy.

> Rather than attempting to determine whether the applicant 'really' wants to change, and trying to discourage "precipitate" entry into treatment, clinicians should take the opportunity to demonstrate the benefits of methadone maintenance treatment (p. 469).

Bell and colleagues (1992) also suggest that rather than screening people out, assessment for opioid replacement therapy would be more usefully seen as a procedure in which the applicant is assisted to make an informed, rational decision about whether he or she would benefit from treatment, thus shifting the responsibility for the decision on to the applicant. It is also important to assist the applicant to try and understand what they expect and want from a treatment program. At the same time, it is important to orient new patients by explaining to them how the treatment system works, what is expected of them and what alternative treatments are available should they find opioid replacement therapy is not meeting their needs and expectations (Langrod, 1993).

While one of the major purposes of assessment is to decide about the suitability of the applicant for opioid replacement therapy, the process itself is also important in defining a therapeutic relationship and might also be a potentially important moment in reconfiguring the patient's motivation to change their drug use and their attitudes to treatment (Miller & Rollnick, 1991). Assessing dependence and suitability for opioid replacement therapy need not be in contradiction with these goals.

SUMMARY

Admission criteria for opioid replacement programs reflect concerns about maintaining individuals in a drug-dependent state, the extent to which they are treatable, and the safe management of patients once they are in treatment. Over the three decades since the introduction of opioid replacement therapy there has been a tendency to relax the criteria for entry.

Physical dependence refers to the adaptive changes that take place in the body due to the chronic administration of a drug. Its presence is indicated by the onset of a withdrawal syndrome when the use of the drug is abruptly terminated. In the case of opioid dependence, these physiological changes are primarily thought to involve the adaptation of neurones (neuroadaptation) to drug effects. Physical dependence is an imprecise term because some individuals may be neuroadapted to opioids but not dependent in the usual sense of this term, for example patients who are administered morphine for pain relief and who experience a withdrawal syndrome when it is stopped but who do not then experience any impulse to take morphine again or exhibit drug-seeking behaviour.

The requirement that patients show evidence of physical dependence as a criteria for admission to opioid replacement therapy is inconsistent with contemporary conceptions of the nature of opioid dependence. According to the drug dependence syndrome as formulated by Edwards *et al.* (1981), opioid dependence consists of some or all of the following: neuroadaptation (marked tolerance and withdrawal); a compulsive desire to use opioids; a loss of control over opioid use; an habitual and routine pattern of opioid use; the use of opioids (and other drugs) to prevent withdrawal; a preoccupation with drug use to the exclusion of other activities; and rapid relapse after withdrawal. Neuroadaptation is neither necessary nor sufficient for a diagnosis of opioid dependence.

Neuroadaptation to opioids can be assessed by three methods: abrupt cessation of the drug of dependence and observation of the ensuing withdrawal syndrome; the use of naloxone to induce an immediate withdrawal syndrome; and by measuring the extent of pupil constriction in response to a low dose of methadone. Although there is a demonstrable quantitative relationship between chronic opioid dose and the severity of a naloxone-induced withdrawal syndrome, the procedure is not useful for assessing prospective patients for opioid replacement therapy because at lower dose levels it is unreliable. Furthermore, obvious neuroadaptation is not always a necessary feature of opioid dependence and the procedure is unpleasant which may have negative consequences for the future relationship between the treatment program and the patient. Bringing assessment procedures for methadone maintenance into line with contemporary thinking about opioid dependence means abandoning the reliance on the single criterion of neuroadaptation (physical dependence) and assessing applicants for all the syndrome elements listed above.

When used for the purposes of assessment, urinalysis demonstrates recent drug use but not extent or pattern of use. It provides no information about the presence or extent of dependence, and therefore serves no useful purpose in the assessment of dependence. The ICD-10 and the DSM-IV, on the other hand, provide useful guidelines for the assessment of the opioid dependence syndrome by establishing criteria for diagnosis based on the Edwards *et al.* model. At present, a clinical assessment by an experienced clinician probably remains the best, albeit imperfect, method of assessing opioid dependence in replacement therapy programs.

Illicit drug use is associated with a range of medical, legal and psychosocial problems that entail serious costs to both the individual and society. A person is suitable for opioid replacement therapy if the individual and social harms associated with illicit opioid use are likely to be reduced by entry to treatment.

Assessment for methadone maintenance should be more than a series of barriers that the applicant has to pass through in order to be allowed entry to the program. An assessment interview is the applicant's first experience of the program and probably lets the applicant know what to expect as a patient in the future. As well as a process in which the applicant's suitability for therapy is assessed, assessment may also be seen as an opportunity to establish the beginnings of a working relationship. There is a need to shift the emphasis away from exclusion criteria to viewing assessment as an initiation of the treatment process.

REFERENCES

American Psychiatric Association (1994). *Diagnostic and Statistical Manual of Mental Disorders (DSM-IV)* (4th ed.). Washington: American Psychiatric Association.

Baekeland, F., & Lundwall, L. (1975). Dropping out of treatment: A critical review. *Psychological Bulletin, 82,* 738-783.

Bell, J., Caplehorn, J. R. M., & McNeil, D. R. (1994). The effect of intake procedures on performance in methadone maintenance. *Addiction, 89,* 463-471.

Bell, J., Digiusto, E., & Byth, K. (1992). Who should receive methadone maintenance? *British Journal of Addiction, 87,* 689-694.

Bell, J., Fernandes, D., & Batey, R. (1990). Heroin users seeking methadone treatment. *Medical Journal of Australia, 152,* 361-364.

Blachly, P. H. (1973). Naloxone for diagnosis in methadone programs. *Journal of the American Medical Association, 224,* 334-335.

Burgess, P. M., Stripp, A. M., Pead, J., & Holman, C. P. (1989). Severity of opiate dependence in an Australian sample: Further validation of the SODQ. *British Journal of Addiction, 84,* 1451-1459.

Cooper, J. R., Altman, F., & Keeley, K. (1983). Discussion summary [of Judson & Goldstein, Uses of naloxone in the diagnosis and treatment of heroin addiction]. In J. R. Cooper, F. Altman, B. S. Brown, & D. Czechowicz (Eds.), *Research on the treatment of narcotic addiction: State of the art* (pp. 17-18). Rockville, MD: National Institute on Drug Abuse

Darke, S., Hall, W., Wodak, A., Heather, N., & Ward, J. (1992). Development and validation of a multi-dimensional instrument for assessing outcome of treatment among opiate users: The Opiate Treatment Index. *British Journal of Addiction, 87,* 733-742.

Dennis, M. L., Ingram, P. W., Burks, M. E., & Rachal, J. V. (1994).

Effectiveness of streamlined admissions to methadone treatment: A simplified time-series analysis. *Journal of Psychoactive Drugs,* **26,** 207-216.

Dole, V. P., & Nyswander, M. (1965). A medical treatment for diacetylmorphine (heroin) addiction: A clinical trial with methadone hydrochloride. *Journal of the American Medical Association,* **193,** 80-84.

Edwards, G., Arif, A., & Hodgson, R. (1981). Nomenclature and classification of drug-and alcohol-related problems: A WHO memorandum. *Bulletin of the World Health Organization,* **59** (2), 225-242.

Feingold, A., & Rounsaville, B. (1995). Construct validity of the dependence syndrome as measured by DSM-IV for different psychoactive substances. *Addiction,* **90,** 1661-1669.

Gerstein, D. R., & Harwood, H. J. (Ed.). (1990). *Treating drug problems, Vol. I. A study of the evolution, effectiveness, and financing of public and private drug treatment systems.* Washington: National Academy Press.

Ghodse, H., Taylor, D. R. S., Greaves, J. L., Britten, A. J., & Lynch, D. (1995). The opiate addiction test: A clinical evaluation of a quick test for physical dependence on opiate drugs. *British Journal of Clinical Pharmacology,* **39,** 257-259.

Gossop, M., & Grant, M. (1991). A six country survey of the content and structure of heroin treatment programmes using methadone. *British Journal of Addiction,* **86,** 1151-1160.

Higgins, S. T., Stitzer, M. L., McCaul, M. E., Bigelow, G. E., & Liebson, I. A. (1985). Pupillary response to methadone challenge in heroin users. *Clinical Pharmacology and Therapeutics,* **37,** 460-463.

Hunt, D. E., Lipton, D. S., Goldsmith, D. S., Strug, D. L., & Spunt, B. (1985-86). "It takes your heart": The image of methadone maintenance in the addict world and its effect on recruitment into treatment. *International Journal of the Addictions,* **20,** 1751-1771.

Jacobsen, L. K., & Kosten, T. R. (1989). Naloxone challenge as a biological predictor of treatment outcome in opiate addicts. *American Journal of Drug and Alcohol Abuse,* **15,** 355-366.

Jaffe, J. H. (1990). Drug addiction and drug abuse. In A. G. Gilman, T. W. Rall, A. S. Nies, & P. Tayler (Eds.), *The pharmacological basis of therapeutics* (pp. 522-573). USA: Pergamon.

Jaffe, J. H., & Martin, W. R. (1990). Opioid analgesics and antagonists. In A. G. Gilman, T. W. Rall, A. S. Nies, & P. Tayler (Eds.), *The pharmacological basis of therapeutics* (pp. 485-521). USA: Pergamon.

Judson, B. A., & Goldstein, A. (1983). Uses of naloxone in the diagnosis and treatment of heroin addiction. In J. R. Cooper, F. Altman, B. S. Brown, & D. Czechowicz (Eds.), *Research on the treatment of narcotic addiction: State of the art* (pp. 1-13). Rockville, MD: National Institute on Drug Abuse

Judson, B. A., Himmelberger, D. U., & Goldstein, A. (1980). The naloxone test for opiate dependence. *Clinical Pharmacology and Therapeutics, 27*, 492-501.

Kanof, P. D., Aronson, M. J., Ness, R., Cochrane, K. J., Horvath, T. B., & Handelsman, L. (1991). Levels of opioid physical dependence in heroin addicts. *Drug and Alcohol Dependence, 27*, 253-262.

Kauffman, J. F., & Woody, G. E. (1995). *Matching treatment to patient needs in opioid substitution therapy.* Rockville, MD: Centre for Substance Abuse Treatment, U.S. Department of Health and Human Services.

Kosten, T. A., Jacobsen, L. K., & Kosten, T. R. (1989). Severity of precipitated opiate withdrawal predicts drug dependence by DSM-III-R criteria. *American Journal of Drug and Alcohol Abuse, 15*, 237-250.

Kosten, T. R., Rounsaville, B. J., Babor, T. F., Spitzer, R. L., & Williams, J. B. W. (1987). Substance-use disorders in DSM-III-R. *British Journal of Psychiatry, 151*, 834-843.

Langenbucher, J., Morgenstern, J., Labouvie, E., & Nathan, P. E. (1994). Lifetime DSM-IV diagnosis of alcohol, cannabis, cocaine, and opiate dependence: Six-month reliability in a multi-site clinical sample. *Addiction, 89*,1115-1127.

Langrod, J. (1993). Admissions policies and procedures. In M. W. Parrino (Eds.), *State methadone treatment guidelines* (pp. 33-40). Rockville, MD: Centre for Substance Abuse Treatment, U.S. Department of Health and Human Services.

Levine, D. P., & Sobel, J. D. (Ed.). (1991). *Infections in intravenous drug abusers.* New York: Oxford University Press.

Maddux, J. F., Desmond, D. P., & Esquivel, M. (1995). Rapid admission and retention on methadone. *American Journal of Drug and Alcohol Abuse, 21*, 533-547.

Mattick, R. P., & Hall, W. (Ed.). (1993). *A treatment outline for approaches to opioid dependence.* Canberra, Australia: Australian Government Publishing Service.

McLellan, A. T., Luborsky, L., Woody, G. E., & O'Brien, C. P. (1980). An improved evaluation instrument for substance abuse patients. *Journal of Nervous and Mental Diseases, 168*, 26-33.

Miller, W. R., & Rollnick, S. (1991). *Motivational interviewing: Preparing people to change addictive behavior.* New York: Guilford.

O'Brien, C. P., Greenstein, R., Ternes, J., & Woody, G. E. (1978). Clinical pharmacology of narcotic antagonists. *Annals of the New York Academy of Sciences, 311*, 232-239.

Peachey, J. E., & Lei, H. (1988). Assessment of opioid dependence with naloxone. *British Journal of Addiction, 83*, 193-201.

Phillips, G. T., Gossop, M. R., Edwards, G., Sutherland, G., Taylor, C., & Strang, J. (1987). The application of the SODQ to the measurement of the severity of opiate dependence in a British sample. *British Journal of*

Addiction, **82,** 691-699.

Resnick, R. (1983). Methadone detoxification from illicit opiates and methadone maintenance. In J. R. Cooper, F. Altman, B. S. Brown, & D. Czechowicz (Eds.), *Research on the treatment of narcotic addiction: State of the art* (pp. 160-167). Rockville, MD: National Institute on Drug Abuse.

Rosenblum, A., Magura, S., & Joseph, H. (1991). Ambivalence towards methadone treatment among intravenous drug users. *Journal of Psychoactive Drugs,* **23,** 21-27.

Rounsaville, B. J., Bryant, K., Babor, T., Kranzler, H., & Kadden, R. (1993). Cross system agreement for substance use disorders: DSM-III-R, DSM-IV and ICD-10. *Addiction,* **88,** 337-348.

Rounsaville, B. J., Kosten, T. R., Williams, J. B. W., & Spitzer, R. L. (1987). A field trial of DSM-III-R psychoactive substance dependence disorders. *American Journal of Psychiatry,* **144,** 351-355.

Rounsaville, B. J., Spitzer, R. L., & Williams, J. B. W. (1986). Proposed changes in DSM-III substance use disorders: Description and rationale. *American Journal of Psychiatry,* **143,** 463-468.

Sanchez-Ramos, J. R., & Senay, E. C. (1987). Ophthalmic naloxone elicits abstinence in opioid-dependent subjects. *British Journal of Addiction,* **82,** 313-315.

Stark, M. J. (1992). Dropping out of substance abuse treatment: A clinically oriented review. *Clinical Psychology Review,* **12,** 93-116.

Sutherland, G., Edwards, G., Taylor, C., Phillips, G., Gossop, M., & Brady, R. (1986). The measurement of opiate dependence. *British Journal of Addiction,* **81,** 485-494.

Sutherland, G., Edwards, G., Taylor, C., Phillips, G. T., & Gossop, M. R. (1988). The opiate dependence syndrome: Replication study using the SODQ in a New York clinic. *British Journal of Addiction,* **83,** 755-760.

Uchtenhagen, A. (1990). Policy and practice of methadone maintenance: An analysis of worldwide experience. In A. Arif & J. Westermeyer (Eds.), *Methadone maintenance in the management of opioid dependence: An international review* (pp. 55-74). New York: Praeger.

van Ameijden, E. J. C., van den Hoek, A. A. R., van Haastrecht, H. J. A., & Coutinho, R. A. (1992). The harm reduction approach and risk factors for Human Immunodeficiency Virus (HIV) seroconversion injecting drug users, Amsterdam. *American Journal of Epidemiology,* **136,** 236-243.

Wang, R. I. H., Wiesen, R. L., Lamid, S., & Roh, B. L. (1974). Rating the presence and severity of opiate dependence. *Clinical Pharmacology and Therapeutics,* **16,** 653-658.

WHO (1992). *The ICD-10 classification of mental and behavioural disorders: Clinical descriptions and diagnostic guidelines.* Geneva: World Health Organisation.

Wodak, A. (1985). The treatment of heroin dependence: An overview. *Proceedings of the Institute of Criminology, 65,* 27-44.

Woody, G., O'Hare, K., Mintz, J., & O'Brien, C. (1975). Rapid intake: A method for increasing retention rate of heroin addicts seeking methadone treatment. *Comprehensive Psychiatry, 16,* 165-169.

Woody, G. E., Cottler, L. B., & Cacciola, J. (1993). Severity of dependence: Data from the DSM-IV field trials. *Addiction, 88,* 1573-1579.

Zilm, D. H., & Sellers, E. M. (1978). The quantitative assessment of physical dependence on opiates. *Drug and Alcohol Dependence, 3,* 419-428.

9

THE USE OF METHADONE DURING MAINTENANCE TREATMENT: PHARMACOLOGY, DOSAGE AND TREATMENT OUTCOME

JEFF WARD, RICHARD P. MATTICK
AND WAYNE HALL

INTRODUCTION

In this chapter, we develop a rational framework for the management of methadone dosing during maintenance treatment. This framework strives for clarity in terms of what is trying to be achieved by a given dose of methadone while taking into account what is known at present about the pharmacology of methadone. In developing this framework, we assume two principles for regulating our own conclusions that we suggest should also be used to regulate clinical decision making, namely that the role of the medical practitioner and other health workers involved in the care of opioid-dependent individuals should be to act in the best interests of the patient, and that harm minimisation be used to define what is or is not in the interests of the patient. This means that in initiating treatment and setting dosage levels, clinical decision making should aim to alleviate suffering and improve the health of the individual. In acting in the best interests of the individual, broader social goals such as reduced heroin use, drug-related crime and the spread of infectious diseases associated with drug injecting will also be achieved, but these goals should not override the interests of the patient (Blum, 1984; Newman, 1977). Setting methadone doses on the basis of these principles and the evidence reviewed in this chapter involves individualising the dosage to suit the needs and aspirations of each patient.

In this chapter, an initial review of what is known about the pharmacology of methadone is followed by a discussion of dosage schedules during the initiation of treatment. The history of low- and high-dose models of methadone treatment is then discussed, along with a consideration of these two models in the light of research. Other issues discussed include the value of monitoring blood concentrations of methadone in predicting outcome and managing patients with special difficulties; the relationship between methadone dose levels and psychopathology; and the issue of whether patients should be allowed to regulate their own methadone dose.

THE PHARMACOLOGY OF METHADONE

In order to understand issues that arise concerning appropriate methadone dosing, it is necessary to review what is known about the pharmacology of methadone and the shorter-acting opioids (usually heroin) on which applicants for methadone maintenance are usually dependent. In this section, we consider the way methadone is absorbed, its fate after absorption and the factors that influence this process.

Methadone is a synthetic opioid agonist that has effects on humans similar to those observed with morphine (Jaffe & Martin, 1990; Kreek, 1979; Säwe, 1986). It differs from morphine in that it has a high level of bioavailability when ingested orally. Specifically, 80-90% of methadone is absorbed through the gastro-intestinal tract, as against 40% for orally administered morphine. Once absorbed into the bloodstream, most of the methadone (90%) is bound to blood proteins and after repeated administration accumulates in various tissues in the body, including the brain. The elimination half-life of methadone has been estimated to be 24 to 36 hours, but most studies show considerable variation across individuals (from 10 to 80 hours, Säwe, 1986). This compares with the relatively short half-life for morphine which has been estimated to be around three hours. The main site in the body for the biotransformation of methadone is the liver. Methadone is eliminated from the body in the form of metabolites resulting from biotransformation and by excretion of the drug itself in urine and faeces.

As the proponents of methadone maintenance treatment have often pointed out, the pharmacological profile of methadone makes it ideal for use as a maintenance drug (e.g., Dole, 1988; Kreek, 1991). The oral route of administration avoids the risks associated with injecting, its long half-life allows for a single daily dosing schedule and the fact that it accumulates in the body means that steady-state plasma levels are easily achieved after repeated administration. As well as these features, methadone has no serious long-term side-effects associated with chronic administration (Novick *et al.*, 1993). In stabilised methadone maintenance patients, methadone does not have the pronounced narcotic effects seen with shorter acting opioids such as heroin (Kreek, 1991).

Factors Influencing the Metabolism of Methadone

A number of factors are classically known to influence the metabolism of most drugs in human beings. These include body weight, age, sex, individual differences in metabolism and excretion rate, certain physiological or pathological states, and the presence of other drugs in the body (Blum, 1984). In this section, we review what is known about such factors and the metabolism of methadone. The main indicator used to estimate the influence of these factors is variations in the concentration of methadone found in plasma.

Individual Differences

Henderson and Harkey (1990), in a review of the literature on monitoring blood concentrations of methadone, noted that one of the most important findings is the marked variation between individuals in the way in which they metabolise and excrete methadone. They note that oral bioavailability has been reported to vary from 41% to 99%, that half-lives have been reported as ranging from 4 to 91 hours, and that the rate of clearance from the body has been reported to vary by a factor of almost 100 from 23 ml/min to 2,100 ml/min.

The clinical implications of this variable response to methadone are evident from a series of case reports of individuals who are said to have a fast, or atypical, methadone metabolism. For these patients the usual dose and dosing schedule may not be sufficient to meet their needs, because most or all of the methadone ingested is eliminated during the 24-hour dosing cycle which results in withdrawal signs and symptoms before the next daily dose is due. For example, Walton, Thornton and Wahl (1978) in a case study of two individuals with apparent atypical methadone metabolism, measured methadone plasma concentrations to develop individually tailored dosing schedules. By using much higher and more frequent doses than usual, patient comfort and satisfaction were achieved. The overall daily dose (i.e., the sum total of the split doses used) needed to achieve this goal for the two patients was 180 mg for one and 260 mg for the other. Kreek (cited in Cooper *et al.*, 1983b) has also suggested that doses in excess of 100 mg may be necessary to achieve successful maintenance with patients who have a fast methadone metabolism.

Physiological and Pathological Status

The most notable physiological state associated with changes in methadone metabolism is pregnancy. Pregnancy is associated with lower than expected methadone plasma levels, especially in the third trimester (Finnegan, 1983; Kreek, 1983a; Pond *et al.*, 1985). The management of methadone maintenance during pregnancy is discussed in detail in Chapter 16.

Since the major site for the biotransformation of methadone in humans is the liver, liver disease may affect methadone metabolism. Disease of the liver is common in methadone maintenance patients due to hepatitis infections and in some cases alcohol abuse. When present, liver disease may result in a slowing down of the elimination of methadone from the body (Kreek, 1983b). Novick *et al.* (1981), in study of the disposition of methadone in 19 methadone patients, 14 of whom had liver disease, found that those patients categorised a priori as having severe disease had a prolonged methadone elimination half-life compared with patients with moderate, mild or no liver disease. There were no other discernible pharmacokinetic differences between the groups. Novick *et al.* concluded that the presence of chronic liver disease was not a contraindication for methadone maintenance treatment and that such individuals can be maintained on the usual dosage regimen. However, in cases where there is a sudden change in disease status, or where the disease status is particularly severe, such individuals should be dosed with care to avoid toxicity (Kreek, 1983a). It is also suspected that renal dysfunction may affect the disposition of methadone in humans (Kreek, 1983a; Säwe, 1986).

Other Drugs

Some drugs have been shown to influence the amount of methadone present in blood plasma by speeding up the elimination of methadone from the body. Most drugs, including methadone, are transformed in the body by the microsomal enzyme systems located in the liver (Benet & Sheiner, 1985). Some drugs are known to induce the activity of these enzymes, thus speeding up the rate at which the elimination of methadone takes place. As in the case of individuals with an atypical methadone metabolism, the effect of this enhanced elimination of methadone is to produce seemingly inexplicable signs and symptoms of withdrawal in patients who are being maintained on an apparently otherwise adequate daily dose.

Rifampin, a drug used in the treatment of tuberculosis, and the anticonvulsant phenytoin, have been associated with withdrawal symptoms in methadone maintenance patients to whom they are administered (Bell *et al.*, 1988; Brockmeyer *et al.*, 1991; Kreek, 1979, 1983a). The concurrent ingestion of phenobarbital (barbiturates) leads to lowered methadone plasma levels and is also associated with the same withdrawal effect (Bell *et al.*, 1988; Kreek, 1983a). Benzodiazepines and another anticonvulsant, carbamazepine, are suspected of producing similar effects (Bell *et al.*, 1990; Bell *et al.*, 1988; Kreek, 1983a; Schall, *et al.*, 1996; Wolff *et al.*, 1991). Another drug suspected of enhancing methadone metabolism is disulfiram, which is sometimes used in the treatment of alcohol dependence (Kreek, 1983a; Wolff *et al.*, 1991). A recent study conducted by Tennant and Shannon (1995) suggests that cocaine may also increase methadone clearance.

While the drugs discussed above induce withdrawal, a recent report has suggested that fluvoxamine, which is a serotonin re-uptake inhibitor used in the treatment of depression, inhibits the metabolism of methadone, resulting in higher than expected blood levels of methadone during fluvoxamine intake and withdrawal symptoms when this antidepressant is stopped (Bertschy *et al.*, 1996). This suggests that the initiation and cessation of treatment for depression with fluvoxamine should be handled with care (Perucca *et al.*, 1994). In an earlier study that examined whether there were any discernible drug interactions between methadone and the tricyclic antidepressant desipramine, Maany *et al.* (1989) reported that serum levels of desipramine were significantly elevated when administered during methadone maintenance, suggesting that care should be taken to avoid toxicity when using desipramine to treat depression among methadone patients. Similarly, the anti-viral agent zidovudine (AZT) has been reported to be associated with a slowing down of the clearance of AZT in some patients (Schwartz *et al.*, 1992). The examples cited above suggest that the concurrent prescription of drugs that enhance or inhibit the microsomal enzyme systems in the liver may lead to alterations in the metabolism of methadone during maintenance treatment, and that in some cases methadone might alter the disposition of other medications.

As well as drugs that enhance or inhibit the metabolism of methadone, opiate antagonists, such as naloxone, and partial agonists, such as buprenorphine and pentazocine, will produce withdrawal signs and symptoms in methadone-maintained individuals. Accordingly, the partial agonists should not be used for pain management in methadone maintenance patients (Kreek, 1983b; Strain *et al.*, 1993a; Walsh *et al.*, 1995). The capacity for buprenorphine to precipitate withdrawal appears to be a dose-related phenomenon in methadone-maintained individuals, with the likelihood of withdrawal increasing as methadone dose increases. Initiating buprenorphine maintenance in methadone-maintained patients is best achieved by reducing the methadone dose to approximately 30 mg per day and increasing the dose of buprenorphine gradually from a low to a maintenance dose (see Chapter 5 for a detailed discussion of buprenorphine maintenance) (Walsh *et al.*, 1995).

COMMENCING METHADONE MAINTENANCE TREATMENT

The initial goal in commencing methadone maintenance treatment is to prevent the onset of withdrawal and to safely achieve an adequate maintenance dose as quickly as possible. In practice, a patient commencing treatment is usually given a relatively low dose of methadone that is increased gradually over a number of weeks until a satisfactory maintenance dose is reached, at which point the patient is said to have been stabilised. A stabilised patient should have no signs or symptoms of withdrawal or intoxication. There has been very little experimental research on this initial period of methadone maintenance because the major pharmacological effects of methadone are well known, and there has been a basic consensus about dosing during the induction phase of methadone treatment. In this section, we summarise the clinical literature about initial dosing procedures. We also consider three reports in which overdosing during induction into methadone maintenance was found to have contributed to death.

Pharmacological Issues for Initial Dosing

The usual oral analgesic dose for non-tolerant individuals is in the range of 2.5-15 mg (Jaffe & Martin, 1990). As already noted, in most individuals methadone has a long half-life in comparison to other narcotics (24 to 26 hours) and, because it accumulates in body tissue, on repeated administration its effects can be cumulative in individuals with little or no tolerance. While it is difficult to specify what a lethal dose for a non-tolerant individual might be (Mattick & Hall, 1993), it is thought to be in excess of 40-60 mg (Drummer *et al.*, 1992). Toxicity is related to blood plasma concentrations and at very high levels, especially in combination with other drugs such as alcohol, may be due to effects other than the narcotic actions of methadone (Wu & Henry, 1994). Some effects, such as respiratory depression, have been found to persist for longer than the usual half-life after one dose in non-tolerant individuals (Olsen *et al.*, 1981).

Cases of Methadone Toxicity During Treatment Induction

Three investigations into deaths associated with the commencement of methadone maintenance are instructive in terms of which aspects of the induction process contributed to the deaths of the individuals concerned. Gardner (1970) inspected coroners' records in London for the period January 1965 to March 1969 and found 12 cases of methadone overdose-induced death. In the cases where the individuals concerned had just commenced treatment and the initial dose was found to have been too high, the following factors were considered to be of concern: seven non-tolerant or minimally tolerant individuals were commenced on methadone doses greater than 70 mg per day; there had been inadequate assessment of applicants for treatment; there had been a lack of understanding on the part of prescribers of the cumulative effects and lethal dose levels of methadone; and there was no evidence that patients who were given prescriptions for several days had been informed about the dangers of overdosing.

Swensen (1988) also concluded that a number of deaths due to methadone toxicity that were reported in the state of Western Australia in the period 1975-1980 were due to liberal access via prescription to the unsupervised ingestion of large quantities of methadone, a situation that was rectified in 1980 when legislation was passed that stipulated that methadone should be consumed under supervision. Since that time there have been few deaths in Western Australia due to methadone poisoning.

The commencement of methadone maintenance was also associated with a number of deaths in the state of Victoria during late 1989 and early 1990 (Drummer *et al.*, 1992; State Coroner of Victoria, 1990). However, unlike the cases reported by Gardner (1970) and Swensen (1988), these cases did not involve any in which self-administration of methadone was a likely cause of death. In a coronial inquest into four of the deaths, methadone toxicity or overdose was found to be the cause of at least two of the deaths (State Coroner of Victoria, 1990). As already noted liver disease can slow down the elimination of methadone and chronic persistent hepatitis was present in 10 of the 12 cases examined in detail by Drummer *et al.* (1992). Even though chronic hepatitis is not unusual in the injecting drug-using population, it was noted as a matter for concern as it may have led to slower than expected clearance (Drummer *et al.*, 1992; Wu & Henry, 1994).

The coroner found that at the time of the deaths there was little information easily available to guide clinicians in selecting starting doses of methadone and that consequently there was a need for a more careful assessment of potential methadone maintenance patients and subsequent monitoring of new patients' responses to methadone, especially during the first week of treatment (State Coroner of Victoria, 1990). Since that time, training courses have been developed for medical practitioners who manage methadone patients and comprehensive training manuals have been written to guide clinicians in their decision making (e.g., Bell & O'Connor, 1994; Bolton *et al.*, 1994; Drug and Alcohol Services Council, 1994; Gill *et al.*, 1992).

Initial Dosing

There is considerable agreement that initial doses should be somewhere in the range of 10-40 mg (e.g., Aylett, 1982; Blum, 1984; Dole & Nyswander, 1967; Gardner, 1970; Goldstein, 1971; Holman & Brown, 1989; Institute of Medicine, 1995; Lowinson & Millman, 1979; Payte & Khuri, 1993). Those authors who recommend lower first doses tend to encourage serial or split dosing on the first day based on a careful observation of the reaction of the patient. For example, Lowinson and Millman (1979) suggest that a starting dose should not exceed 40 mg unless the patient has been transferred from another program. Split or divided daily dosing is often found to be useful where 10-20 mg is administered and the patient is observed for three to four hours to see what the response to the initial dose is. New patients should be carefully monitored for sedation. Given that methadone usually reaches peak plasma concentrations within two to six hours after oral administration (Kreek, 1979), careful assessment for withdrawal or intoxication based on this time frame can be used to ensure patient comfort with a measure of safety. Because of the possibility of cumulative effects, the dose should be increased with care. Lowinson and Millman (1979) suggest that after patient comfort has been achieved, increases of 10 mg every three to four days until maintenance dose level is achieved should be sufficient.

To summarise, the first dose of methadone at the commencement of maintenance treatment should be based on a careful assessment of the patient, which should be carried out by a medical practitioner experienced in working with opioid addicts (see Chapter 8). Important factors concerning the effect of methadone are that it has a long elimination half-life of 24 to 36 hours, that a lethal dose for non-tolerant individuals may occur with doses in excess of 40-60 mg, and that methadone can accumulate in the body over successive doses and result in overdosing, even though each single dose may not be toxic. The first dose should be between 10-40 mg. Split or serial dosing may be useful where there is doubt about the degree of tolerance. Patients with severe liver dysfunction should be dosed with care.

HIGH AND LOW DOSAGE TREATMENT PHILOSOPHIES

In this section, the question of what is an appropriate dose range for adequately maintaining individuals on methadone will be examined.

In order to place the discussion in context, we will review some aspects of the history of methadone maintenance as a treatment modality before examining the research evidence on the role of dosage in delivering effective methadone maintenance treatment. We suggest that the two outcome measures of direct relevance to this issue are retention in treatment and the suppression of heroin use. They are the two measures most commonly reported across the studies that we will review.

Retention in treatment is an accepted indicator of program functioning, given that it is important to keep patients in treatment in order for change to occur. Successful maintenance on methadone is also *the* goal of treatment, according to some practitioners (e.g., Dole & Nyswander, 1965; Kreek, 1992; Newman, 1991). The amount of heroin use is an important outcome that might be expected to exhibit a dose – response relationship to methadone dose given. The provision of an 'adequate' dose of methadone should therefore lead to the cessation of, or a dramatic reduction in, heroin use. The debate about high versus low dose methadone maintenance has revolved around the definition of the term 'adequate'.

Rationales for High and Low Dose Maintenance

As explained in Chapter 8, tolerance to a drug is said to occur when repeated, chronic ingestion at the same dose leads to a reduction in the drug's effects on the body. A person who is tolerant to a drug will require increasing doses of that drug to achieve the sought-after effect. Cross-tolerance refers to the phenomenon in which tolerance to one drug produces tolerance to another drug of the same type (Blum, 1984). For opioid drugs such as heroin, morphine and methadone, developing tolerance to the effects of one means that the person concerned is tolerant to the effects of others.

Dole and Nyswander (1965) argued that one of the reasons why methadone maintenance is effective at reducing illicit opioid use is because when high doses (>80 mg) are used, the substantial level of tolerance to methadone that develops induces sufficient cross-tolerance to heroin, preventing it from producing its desired effects should a patient use heroin. They referred to this high level of cross-tolerance as 'narcotic blockade' (see also Dole *et al.,* 1966). Dole and Nyswander (1967) believed that opioid dependence was a metabolic disease and argued that high, blockading maintenance doses of methadone for long periods of time were a necessary component of successful methadone maintenance.

The high dose model of methadone maintenance treatment proposed by Dole and Nyswander was shown to be effective in a series of case reports and observational studies (e.g., Dole & Nyswander, 1965; Dole *et al.*, 1968), and was subsequently supported in the randomised controlled trials reviewed in detail in Chapter 2. The rationale for using such high doses of methadone is also supported by three published reports which suggest that a daily dose of methadone in the vicinity of 80-100 mg should be sufficient to induce a substantial level of cross-tolerance to heroin in the majority of individuals (Dole *et al.*, 1966; Jones & Prada, 1975; Martin *et al.*, 1973). Further empirical support is provided by Volavka *et al.*, (1978), who found that cross-tolerance to heroin increased as a function of increasing methadone dose. The metabolic disease hypothesis was given impetus with the discovery of the opiate receptors and their associated endogenous opioids in the early 1970s and the mechanism involved in this metabolic disease process is now seen as an opiate receptor disorder (Dole, 1988; Goldstein, 1991; Kreek, 1990).

During the 1960s, Dole and Nyswander developed protocols for an opioid maintenance program using high dose methadone. By the end of the decade, other practitioners began to question the necessity for such high doses of methadone for a number of reasons and lower doses (around 30-40 mg) were experimented with. There were a number of reasons put forward for changing what had been shown to be an effective treatment. First, the metabolic disease model of opioid dependence was viewed as being implausible and hence the necessity for long periods of blockade methadone maintenance was questioned. Second, it was believed that lower doses of methadone sufficient to prevent withdrawal and craving for heroin would serve most patients' needs and that lower doses of methadone would be just as effective as higher doses in suppressing heroin use, with fewer side-effects (e.g., Berry, 1972; Goldstein & Judson, 1973). Third it was thought that effective lower doses of methadone might allow easier withdrawal at the end of treatment which would be possible after relatively brief periods of methadone maintenance (Berry, 1972; see also Jaffe, 1970). Fourth, the use of lower doses was seen as consistent with the pharmacological principle of the least effective dosage being the best (Berry, 1972; Goldstein & Judson, 1983). Fifth, there was also concern about the morality of prescribing a drug of dependence to dependent individuals which was translated into a concern about the dose that was being prescribed (Attewell & Gerstein, 1979; D'Amanda, 1983; Schuster, 1989).

Because of the controversy about the necessity for high doses of methadone, a significant amount of research effort in the 1970s addressed the question of what might be the optimum dose for methadone maintenance. Unfortunately, this question was primarily addressed by research that evaluated the relative effectiveness of 'high' and 'low' *fixed*-dose methadone regimens. The researchers who undertook this work perceived the issue as one of whether a *fixed*-low dose regimen was equivalent in effectiveness to a fixed high dose regimen. When they failed to find a difference in treatment outcome (measured by treatment retention and heroin use) they usually concluded that high and low dose regimens were of equivalent effectiveness. In so doing they were trying, in statistical terms, to prove the null hypothesis.

There are circumstances in which it is reasonable to act as if a null hypothesis was true (Hall & Einfeld, 1990). In the case of high and low dose methadone regimens this would require: a) there was no statistically significant difference between the two dose regimens, and b) alternative explanations of a failure to find such a difference had been ruled out. When the research design was a randomised controlled trial, the most plausible alternative explanation that needs to be excluded is that insufficient numbers of cases were observed to ensure a reasonable chance of detecting a difference of the expected magnitude.

The second of these conditions has rarely been addressed in the research on methadone dose because researchers have not posed the question of what the expected size of the difference would be between high and low fixed-dose regimens, and so have not designed studies with a specified sample size to detect the nominated difference. Judged by the relatively small sample sizes that have typically been used in these studies and the categorical outcome measures used to assess outcome, many of these researchers have implicitly assumed that the difference would be a large one. This seems a doubtful assumption when a fixed-dose regimen is used – a dosing practice that bears little resemblance to clinical practice. It is perhaps all the more remarkable then that many of these studies have found differences in outcome in favour of higher dose regimens.

METHADONE DOSE AND TREATMENT OUTCOME

The research literature on the relationship between methadone dose and treatment outcome has been reviewed in detail previously by Hargreaves (1983), Mattick and Hall (1993) and Ward *et al.* (1992). The review by Hargreaves (1983) was considered at the Research on the Treatment of Narcotic Addiction: State of the Art symposium held by the United States National Institute on Drug Abuse (Cooper *et al.*, 1983b; Goldstein & Judson, 1983). These reviews and the participants at the State of the Art symposium all concluded that a better response to treatment is observed when doses in excess of 50 mg are used, when compared with routine dosing at lower levels. They also concluded that there was no evidence from treatment outcome studies to suggest that routine dosing at levels in excess of 100 mg per day resulted in any benefit for the majority of patients.

In this section, we review the best available evidence, including studies that have been published since the publication of the aforementioned reviews. Immediately below we consider the randomised controlled trials that have been conducted which, as already noted, examine the question of whether routine dosing at a higher fixed level confers any benefit when compared to routine fixed dosing at a lower level. We then consider the evidence from observational studies that examine whether there is a relationship between methadone dose level set, according to routine clinical practice, and treatment retention and heroin use during treatment. We also consider two studies that have examined the relationship between methadone dose and the likelihood of HIV seroconversion. Finally, we consider one study that has examined the relationship between clinic policy on dosage and retention. We conclude from this evidence that there is a relationship between methadone dose and retention and heroin use regardless of whether a fixed or individualised dosing schedule is used.

Randomised Controlled Trials

There have been eleven studies comparing high and low dosage methadone treatments that have employed a randomised design and some form of blinding (Banys *et al.*, 1994; Berry & Kuhn, 1973; Garbutt & Goldstein, 1972; Goldstein & Judson, 1973; Jaffe, 1970; Johnson *et al.*, 1992; Kosten *et al.*, 1993; Ling *et al.*, 1976; Ling *et al.*,

Table 9.1
Randomised controlled trials comparing various methadone dosage schedules

Study	N	Design	Study period	Groups (mg)	Retention[a]	Heroin use[a]	Comments
Jaffe (1970)	63	Double-blind	14 weeks	(100-110) vs (<45)	(100-110) = (<45)	(100-110) = (<45)	Low power due to attrition. Trend in expected direction for heroin use.
Garbutt & Goldstein (1972)	180	Single-blind	12 weeks	100 vs 50 vs 30	–	100=50>30	
	120		26 weeks	"	100=50>30	100>50>30	Trend in expected direction for heroin use at 52 weeks (i.e., 100>50>30).
	60		52 weeks	"	–	100=50>30	
Berry & Kuhn (1973)	52	Double-blind, matched for time in treatment	26 weeks	100 vs 50	100=50	100=50	Heroin use was very low (<6% of all urine samples). Attrition and low level of drug use resulted in low statistical power.
Goldstein & Judson (1973)	120	Single-blind	26 weeks	160 vs 80 vs 40	160>80>40	160=80=40	Attrition in low dose group may have obscured effect for heroin.
Ling et al. (1976)	288	Double-blind	40 weeks	100 vs 50	50=100	100>50	
Johnson et al. (1992)	109	Double-blind	25 weeks	60 vs 20	60 > 20	60>20	
Strain et al. (1992)	212	Double-blind, matched for gender and race	26 weeks	50 vs 20 vs 0	50>20>0	50>20>0	Long-term detoxification treatment. Stable doses for 14 weeks.
Strain et al. (1993b)	247	Double-blind, placebo control	25 weeks	50 vs 20 vs 0	50>20>0	50>20=0	
Kosten et al. (1993)	125	Double-blind	24 weeks	65 vs 35	65 = 35	65 = 35	
Banys et al. (1994)	38	Double-blind	26 weeks	80 vs 40	80 = 40	80 = 40	Expected trend for heroin use (80>40). Small sample/low power. Stable dose for 12 weeks.
Ling et al. (1996)	150	Double-blind	52 weeks	80 vs 30	80 > 30	80 > 30	

[a] For retention and heroin use, "=" implies equivalence, "<" suggests a poorer outcome, and ">" suggests a better outcome.

1996; Strain *et al.,* 1992; Strain *et al.,* 1993b). These studies are summarised in Table 9.1, which shows the nature of design employed (single- or double-blind, form of subject matching if any), the length of the study period, the methadone dosing groups established for the study, the results for retention and heroin use expressed in terms of the equivalence or otherwise of the dosing groups, and any comments pertinent to the interpretation of the results. Two of these studies (Banys *et al.,* 1994; Strain *et al.,* 1992) were of long-term methadone detoxification procedures, but have been included because they both included at least 3 months of stable dosing which could be viewed as maintenance for that period.

Two features of the results presented in Table 9.1 are worth noting: the preponderance of the results suggests that higher doses (>50 mg) result in better retention and less heroin use than the low dose comparisons employed. With the exception of Garbutt and Goldstein (1972) who found that 100 mg led to less heroin use than the 50 mg and 30 mg comparison groups, these findings are apparent for high doses in the range of 50-80 mg. While the effect is not always present, in all cases except one (Kosten *et al.,* 1993), there was either a trend in the expected direction or there was insufficient statistical power to determine if there was an effect or not.

The general import of the randomised controlled trials of methadone maintenance is, therefore, that a general policy of maintaining patients on doses in the range of 50-80 mg results in better retention and less heroin use than maintaining them on lower levels. However, with regard to doses above that range, there are too few studies to draw any conclusions about where the ceiling of this dose-response effect might be.

Observational Studies

Whereas randomised controlled trials compare arbitrarily defined groups of patients who are maintained on a priori specified dose levels, observational studies examine the relationship between methadone dose and heroin use and retention in the setting of the routine treatment delivered in methadone clinics. Those studies that employ statistical adjustment to control for bias in the analysis of data are more powerful than studies that have not adjusted for such factors. The review below provides an overview of the available observational research, but focuses on the best available studies.

Numerous observational studies published over the past two decades have found an association between methadone dose and heroin use and treatment retention (Ball & Ross, 1991; Caplehorn & Bell, 1991; Caplehorn *et al.*, 1993; Caplehorn *et al.*, 1994; Handal & Lander, 1976; Hartel *et al.*, 1995; Joe *et al.*, 1991; Joe *et al.*, 1994; Maremmani *et al.*, 1994; McGlothlin & Anglin, 1981; Reynolds & Magro, 1976; Siassi *et al.*, 1977; Simpson & Joe, 1993; Swensen *et al.*, 1993; Torrens *et al.*, 1996; White *et al.*, 1994). By contrast there are few studies that have failed to find this association (Brown *et al.*, 1982-83; Maddux *et al.*, 1991; Seow *et al.*, 1980).

McGlothlin and Anglin (1981) conducted a retrospective study of patients graduating from three methadone maintenance programs in California. Two of the programs were high dose, long retention programs and the other was a low dose, abstinence-oriented program. As expected, given the difference in retention policy, the high dose programs retained their patients in treatment for longer periods than the low dose programs. However, as Hargreaves (1983) has pointed out, when program termination types are examined, the results consistently favour the high dose programs. In the high dose programs, more patients completed their treatment course, fewer dropped out and fewer were expelled for illicit drug use. While it is difficult to disentangle the effects of dose and policy on retention and discharge in this study, the finding is consistent with the other findings. The findings concerning retention were mirrored by self-reported heroin use, with patients attending the high dose clinics reporting significantly less heroin use than those attending the low dose clinic.

In the influential Three Cities Study reported by Ball and Ross (1991), a key finding was that as methadone dose increased the rate of current heroin use during methadone maintenance decreased (see Chapter 2 for details of this study). Some indication of the size of this effect is given by the estimate that patients maintained on low doses of methadone (45 mg or less) were approximately five times more likely to have used heroin in the past 30 days compared with patients who were on higher doses (>45 mg; Relative Risk = 5.2). Results of the regression analyses reported in Ball and Ross (1991) confirm this finding, with the results suggesting that patients maintained on lower doses of methadone were more likely to have used heroin in the past 30 days than patients maintained on higher doses of methadone. This relationship remained when patient and other treatment variables were statistically controlled for.

In a further series of studies that have employed multivariate statistical modelling to predict retention and heroin use, Caplehorn and colleagues have consistently found methadone dose to be a predictor of treatment outcome. In the first study in this series, Caplehorn and Bell (1991; see also Caplehorn & Bell, 1993) inspected the records of 238 patients admitted to two Sydney methadone units during 1986 and 1987 to determine if there was any evidence of a relationship between maximum daily dose of methadone recorded for a patient and retention in treatment. Methadone dose was found to be significantly associated with retention in a regression analysis that controlled for clinic and a range of patient variables. Compared to patients who received a maximum dose of less than 60 mg, the relative risk of leaving treatment was almost halved for those whose maximum dose was between 60 and 79 mg (Relative Risk = 0.6, 95% confidence interval 0.4-0.7), and almost halved again for those whose maximum dose was over 80 mg (Relative Risk = 0.3, 95% confidence interval 0.2-0.5). That is, patients who always received less than 60 mg were twice as likely to leave treatment as those in the mid-range quoted above, and four times as likely to leave treatment as those in the highest range. This relationship between methadone dose and retention was confirmed in a further study reported by Caplehorn *et al.* (1994). In this study, the statistical model developed to predict leaving treatment indicated that for each 40 mg increase in maximum methadone dose received during treatment, the risk of leaving treatment was again almost halved (Relative Risk = 0.6, 95% confidence interval 0.5-0.8).

A further independent replication of the findings of Caplehorn and Bell (1991), has been reported from Spain by Torrens *et al.* (1996) who investigated the relationship between methadone dose and other predictors of retention among 370 patients attending for methadone treatment in Barcelona. Methadone dose was found to be the most important predictor of retention, with patients maintained on less than 80 mg of methadone per day being more than three times likely to leave treatment than those maintained on doses greater than 80 mg per day (Relative Risk = 3.6, 95% confidence interval 3.0-4.2).

In another study, which examined the relationship between methadone dose and heroin use as indicated by routine urine testing, Caplehorn *et al.* (1993) found that after controlling for patient characteristics and time in treatment, the odds of using heroin were reduced by 2% for every milligram increase in methadone dose. To give some indication of what this might imply in terms of usual dosing practices, Caplehorn *et al.,* (1993) estimated that the odds of an individual maintained on 40 mg per day using heroin were twice those of an individual maintained on 80 mg per day (odds ratio = 2.2. 95% confidence interval 1.3-3.8). Similar findings are reported by Hartel *et al.* (1995), who found that after statistically adjusting for other predictors of heroin use that the odds of using heroin for individuals maintained on less than 70 mg per day were twice those of individuals maintained on higher doses (odds ratio = 2.1, 95% confidence interval 1.3-3.4). The role of methadone dose in the suppression of heroin use is further supported by a number of reports of reductions in heroin use being associated with increases in methadone dose (Gossop *et al.,* 1982; Ling *et al.,* 1980; Strain *et al.,* 1994).

In addition to these studies of the relationship between methadone dose and retention and heroin use, there have been two studies, one from Italy and one from the United States, which have found that higher methadone doses appear to protect against HIV infection in areas where the HIV seroprevalence is high among opioid injectors (Brown *et al.,* 1989; Serpelloni *et al.,* 1994). While one would prefer more replications before drawing strong conclusions about this relationship, the findings of these two studies are plausible and consistent with what is known about methadone dose, injecting opioid use and HIV infection.

The results of these observational studies confirm the findings of the randomised controlled trials and indicate that there is a linear dose-response relationship between methadone dose and the two outcomes of retention and heroin use. The likelihood of using heroin and leaving treatment decreases as methadone dose increases, and for the doses examined in the studies there is no evidence of plateau in the relationship, although one would expect this to occur at very high doses.

Flexibility in Dosage Policy

Only one study was retrieved after searches which has examined whether a flexible or individualised dosing protocol has an influence on retention during methadone treatment. Brown *et al.* (1982-83) surveyed 113 methadone clinics that responded from a random sample of 154 clinics situated in 11 states of the USA. The 113 clinics participating in the study had 13,177 patients on stabilised doses in their programs. Patients were classified as being on a high (60 mg or more), medium (30-59 mg), or low (0-29 mg) dose. The differences in the States' policies concerning dose were reflected in marked State differences in numbers of patients in different dose ranges. Methadone units were classified into four categories of dosage policy according to the percentage of patients found in each dosing range. This resulted in high, medium or low dose policy programs and, in cases where there seemed to be no specific concentration of patients in any one range, flexible dosage policy programs.

In terms of patient characteristics, low dose policy programs tended to have younger patients than high dose programs. These low dose patients had less years of heroin use than patients in either medium or high dose programs. Low dose patients had less prior treatment episodes than all the other groups, and medium dose patients had less than their high dose counterparts. Dose setting policy was significantly related to treatment retention, with clinics classified as having a flexible dosage policy retaining patients longer in treatment than fixed dose policy programs. Dose itself, as categorised in this study, was found to be unrelated to retention. Brown *et al.* (1982-83) concluded that individualising treatment was associated with retaining patients in treatment.

High and Low Dose Maintenance: Conclusions

The evidence from both randomised controlled trials and observational studies suggests that the appropriate range for methadone dosing during maintenance treatment should be 50-100 mg per day for the majority of individuals. Doses in this range result in longer stays in treatment and less heroin use while the patient remains in treatment. Some individuals can be maintained successfully on lower doses of methadone and they tend to be more highly motivated to change and more psychologically stable than others (Schut *et al.*, 1973; Williams, 1971). In setting methadone doses, it is important to avoid two forms of fallacious reasoning, namely, drawing inferences from exceptional cases and applying them to the majority, and the reverse fallacy of applying principles applicable to the majority to exceptional cases (Ward, 1994). Advocates of low dose methadone maintenance tend to commit the former fallacy, while a literal-minded reading of the evidence could result in the latter. Taking into account the evidence concerning individuals with a fast methadone metabolism and the similar effect found with microsomal enzyme-inducing drugs such as phenytoin, it is important to also keep in mind that some individuals may require doses in excess of 100 mg per day. Thus, the most reasonable conclusion to draw from the evidence is that doses should be individualised to suit the needs of the patient and that, for most patients, this can be achieved with a daily dose in the vicinity of 50-100 mg per day.

THERAPEUTIC DRUG MONITORING

Therapeutic drug monitoring refers to the use of measurements of drug concentrations in the blood to optimise therapeutic effect. This practice is based on the reasoning that the concentration of the therapeutic agent in the blood is a more valid indicator of the amount of drug available at the site of action than the actual dose administered (Henderson & Harkey, 1990; Tonkin & Bochner, 1994). In the case of methadone, this implies that the concentration of methadone in the blood is a better measure of the amount of methadone available to the opiate receptors than is the oral dose ingested. As Henderson and Harkey (1990) point out, therapeutic drug monitoring is especially useful for the management of drug therapy where there is some danger of toxicity at doses near to therapeutic ranges, or where there is wide variation in the disposition of the drug across individuals or across time. In this section, we consider the practice of therapeutic drug monitoring during methadone maintenance treatment. In so doing, we review the literature on the relationship between oral dose ingested and methadone blood levels, and the literature on the relationship between methadone blood levels and treatment outcome and withdrawal signs and symptoms.

Methadone Plasma Levels and Dosage

The wide inter-individual variability in methadone metabolism would seem to indicate a role for therapeutic drug monitoring in the management of methadone maintenance patients. However, the evidence concerning the relationship between oral dose ingested and methadone plasma concentrations suggests that dose may be a reliable indicator of plasma concentrations for the majority of methadone patients. For example, some consistency of the relationship between dose and methadone plasma concentrations has been reported in a number of well-controlled studies (Bell *et al.*, 1990; Bell *et al.*, 1988; Loimer & Schmid, 1992; Verebely *et al.*, 1975; Wolff *et al.*, 1991). As

Bell *et al.* (1988) have argued, while a number of other studies have failed to find such a relationship (e.g., Goldstein & Judson, 1973; Horns & Goldstein, 1975), these were studies of outpatients where there was no control over illicit methadone ingestion, diversion of methadone dose, and other perhaps influential but unknown factors that might have affected methadone levels (e.g., barbiturate use). A plausible confounding influence on the relationship between dose and methadone plasma concentrations of methadone may be the presence of a dispositional tolerance in some individuals (Holmstrand *et al.,* 1978; Verebely *et al.,* 1975). This refers to the tendency for plasma levels to fall over time in some patients who have been maintained on a constant dose of methadone. While the exact mechanism is not clear, dispositional tolerance is likely to be due to either increased clearance or to an increase in the amount of methadone being stored in body tissue (Holmstrand *et al.,* 1978).

Methadone Plasma Levels and Treatment Outcome

While the relationship between dose and blood concentrations is an important one, the measurement of blood concentration is only of use if it has a stronger relationship to treatment outcome than dose. This has yet to be demonstrated for methadone as used in the treatment of opioid dependence, although few studies have been published which have examined this issue. Holmstrand *et al.* (1978) found that high plasma levels were associated with less illicit drug use and more successful rehabilitation. They concluded that patients on high doses (65 to 85 mg), who also had trough plasma levels greater than 200 ng/ml have a better chance of good outcome. Tennant *et al.,* (1984), in another study, found an association between heavy drinking and illicit drug use and lower mean plasma levels among a group of 24 subjects on a standard high dose (80 mg) of methadone. Although these two studies are suggestive it would be difficult to conclude that plasma levels are a useful predictor of treatment outcome for most patients without further research. We therefore conclude that the *routine* use of therapeutic drug monitoring is unwarranted until there is reasonable evidence that blood concentration is a better predictor of treatment outcome than dosage for most individuals.

A number of commentators have remarked that in their opinion a minimum trough plasma level is necessary for successful methadone maintenance (e.g. Dole, 1988 150 to 600 ng/ml; Loimer *et al.,* 1991 >400 ng/ml). While two studies have failed to find a relationship between plasma levels and subjective perceptions of withdrawal (e.g., Horns & Goldstein, 1975; Tennant *et al.*, 1984), two other studies have found that withdrawal symptoms are likely when methadone plasma levels fall below 50 ng/ml (Bell *et al.*, 1988; Wolff, 1990 cited in Wolff *et al.*, 1991). The most sensible clinical inference to draw from this evidence is that therapeutic drug monitoring may be of most use in patients who complain of withdrawal, despite being maintained on an otherwise adequate dose of methadone.

PSYCHOPATHOLOGY AND METHADONE DOSE

As well as preventing withdrawal and providing a protective cross tolerance to other opioids, a given dose of methadone may also play a role in the management of psychopathology (Jaffe, 1992; Martin *et al.*, 1991; Verebey, 1982). According to Jaffe (1992): "For some individuals, opioids appear to have the capacity to ameliorate certain varieties of depression, to control anxiety, to reduce anger, and to blunt paranoid feelings and ideation (p. 187)." There is suggestive evidence from two studies supporting the clinical lore that this effect of methadone is dose-related.

Descriptive evidence gathered so far suggests that patients who tend to receive higher doses are those with certain kinds of psychiatric disorders and those who are in greater psychological distress (independent of psychiatric diagnosis) than other patients. For example, Treece and Nicholson (1980) have reported finding a relationship between personality disorder and dose level using DSM-III criteria. The three groups of subjects of interest for this discussion were Type A patients, classified as having schizoid, schizotypal, or paranoid personality disorder and generally described by the authors as appearing withdrawn, odd and eccentric; Type B patients, classified as having histrionic, narcissistic, antisocial, or borderline personality and described by the DSM-III as appearing dramatic and emotional; and a group with no diagnosed personality disorder. On a small sample of subjects (n = 31), the authors found that Type A subjects were more likely to be on a high dose (75 mg or more) than either Type B or the group with no personality disorder. The group with no personality disorder was more likely to be on a low dose (45 mg or less). On a larger group of subjects (n = 75), the frequency of Type A subjects increased as dose increased. This study suggests though that certain types of personality disorder may be associated with higher doses.

Roszell and Calsyn (1986) also set out to test the hypothesis that patient characteristics explain why certain patients end up on certain dose levels. While acknowledging that individual differences in methadone metabolism are an important determinant of maintenance dose, they chose to examine the importance of a range of demographic, drug use, and psychological variables. The sample consisted of 106 male veterans on a program with a flexible-dose policy. Stabilised dose, which was a result of negotiation between patients and program staff, was classified using a priori categories as either high (60 mg or more), medium (36-59 mg), or low (35 mg or less). In comparison to the low dose group, the high dose group was found to be less stable and to be in greater 'psychological turmoil'; to exhibit greater anxiety; to have been prescribed psychoactive medications more frequently; to have more illicit drug use as indicated by urinalysis during the first months of treatment; and to have had a history of barbiturate, sedative, and amphetamine use.

PATIENT SELF-REGULATION OF DOSE

A matter of some contention is who should set and control methadone doses. There are three simple alternative answers to this question: the prescribing doctor, either alone or in consultation with unit staff; the prescribing doctor and/or unit staff in negotiation with the patient; and finally, within certain constraints, the patient without the aid or interference of clinic staff. The first two options may have negative therapeutic consequences in that they perpetuate the patient's belief that ingesting a drug will solve their problems. It can also result in a great deal of conflict with unit staff when the patient claims that his or her dose is not 'holding' (i.e., sufficient to prevent withdrawal). Goldstein *et al.* (1975) claimed that when these conflicts result in an increased dose, the patient was often satisfied with the increase, but that the same increase when made 'blind' had no effect on patient satisfaction, suggesting that non-pharmacological factors are an important determinant of a satisfactory dose, at least for some patients.

Goldstein *et al.* (1975) decided to investigate the effect of giving patients some control over their own dose on dose levels and illicit drug use as measured by urinalysis. Fifty-nine subjects, who were attending a methadone unit that operated on a single-blind basis in which only staff knew and controlled dose, were studied for five weeks to provide a baseline. Then an open-dose, self-regulation policy was instituted for 25 weeks. Patients could change their dose up or down once a week by 5 mg, the maximum possible dose being 120 mg. If their dose at any time exceeded 50 mg their take-home privileges were withdrawn. The important finding was that patients did not opt for the highest dose possible. Moreover, patients who increased their dose had significantly less drug use as measured by urinalysis than at baseline, and both patients and staff were satisfied with the policy changes and the limitations imposed on self-adjustment of dose. The findings of this study suggest that if patients are allowed to control their dose (within certain constraints), they will do so responsibly, and that this may have a positive effect on their drug use and on clinic life in general.

The issue of self-regulation was tested more thoroughly in a randomised controlled trial by Havassy and Hargreaves (1979, 1981). Of interest are the comparisons between a group of patients who had control over their dose (with limitations similar to the Goldstein *et al.* study) and a group who were constrained under the usual program conditions of having to negotiate their dose. The self-regulating group, consistent with the Goldstein *et al.* study, did not increase their dose to any great degree. After initially increasing the dose slightly, this group tended subsequently to stabilise. On the whole, except for a significant improvement for a four-week period early in the study, there was no change in the amount of illicit drug use as measured by urinalysis for the self-regulating group compared to baseline.

The findings of these earlier studies were confirmed in a recently published report by Maddux, Desmond and Vogtsberger (1995) who randomised 300 patients attending for methadone treatment in Texas to a group who received standard treatment, a group in which patients could regulate their own methadone dose and a group where counselling was optional. When compared to the standard treatment group, the self-regulated dose group had equivalent rates of retention and illicit drug use. When methadone doses in the two groups were compared it was found that the average dose of the self-regulated group was slightly higher than that for the standard treatment group (58 mg versus 53 mg per day), but this difference was not statistically significant.

In conclusion, there seems little basis to the fear that if patients are given control over their own methadone dose they will raise it irresponsibly in an attempt to achieve intoxication. It has to be emphasised, however, that these studies had constraints in place to guard against the possibility of overdose. With regard to illicit drug use, it appears that self-regulation is no better or worse that standard procedures for the setting of doses. Self-regulation may, however, independent of its effect on illicit drug use, contribute to the process of methadone maintenance by enhancing patient trust and responsibility and this outcome is worthwhile in and of itself (Havassy & Tschann, 1983).

SUMMARY

Methadone maintenance is initiated by administering an oral dose of 10-40 mg of methadone which may be followed up on the same day by further dose(s) if withdrawal is still apparent after 4 to 6 hours. A maintenance dose can then be safely reached by increasing the initial dose at a rate of approximately 10 mg per day. Research suggests that the majority of individuals will require 50-100 mg per day, although some individuals can be successfully maintained at lower doses. On average, a heroin-dependent individual will use less heroin, and stay in treatment longer, if maintained on a higher rather than a lower dose of methadone. In cases where 50-100 mg does not prevent withdrawal for the full 24-hour dosing cycle, an attempt should be made to determine if enzyme-inducing drugs are being taken concurrently or if the individual metabolises methadone at a faster rate than average. For these purposes therapeutic drug monitoring is indicated, but the procedure is unnecessary for most patients. Individuals with high levels of emotional distress, or who exhibit schizophrenic-like personality disorder pathology, may benefit from being maintained on higher rather lower doses of methadone. Finally, it has been demonstrated that (within certain constraints) patients can responsibly manage their own methadone dose levels and that this may have positive effects in terms of how they feel about their treatment.

REFERENCES

Attewell, P., & Gerstein, D. R. (1979). Government policy and local practice. *American Sociological Review, 44*, 311-327.

Aylett, P. (1982). Methadone dose assessment in heroin addiction. *International Journal of the Addictions, 17*, 1329-1336.

Ball, J. C., & Ross, A. (1991). *The effectiveness of methadone maintenance treatment: Patients, programs, services, and outcome.* New York: Springer-Verlag.

Banys, P., Tusel, D. J., Sees, K. L., Reilly, P. M., & Delucchi, K. L. (1994). Low (40 mg) versus high (80 mg) dose methadone in a 180-day heroin detoxification program. *Journal of Substance Abuse Treatment,* 11, 225-232.

Bell, J., Bowron, P., Lewis, J., & Batey, R. (1990). Serum levels of methadone in maintenance clients who persist in illicit drug use. *British Journal of Addiction,* 85, 1599-1602.

Bell, J., & O'Connor, D. (1994). *New South Wales methadone prescribers manual.* Sydney: Australian Professional Society on Alcohol and Other Drugs.

Bell, J., Seres, V., Bowron, P., Lewis, J., & Batey, R. (1988). The use of serum methadone levels in patients receiving methadone maintenance. *Clinical Pharmacology and Therapeutics,* 43, 623-629.

Benet, L. Z., & Sheiner, L. B. (1985). Pharmacokinetics: The dynamics of drug absorption, distribution, and elimination. In A. G. Gilman, L. S. Goodman, & F. Murad (Eds.), *The pharmacological basis of therapeutics* (7th Edition ed., pp. 3-34). USA: Macmillan.

Berry, G. J. (1972). Dose-related responses to methadone, including placebo therapy. *Proceedings of the Fourth National Conference on Methadone Treatment* (pp. 409-410). New York: National Association for the Prevention of Addiction to Narcotics.

Berry, G. J., & Kuhn, K. L. (1973). Dose-related response to methadone: Reduction of maintenance dose. *Proceedings of the Fifth National Conference on Methadone Treatment* (pp. 972-979). New York: National Association for the Prevention of Addiction to Narcotics.

Bertschy, G., Baumann, P., Eap, C.B., & Baettig, D. (1996). Probable metabolic interaction between methadone and fluvoxamine in addict patients. *Therapeutic Drug Monitoring,* 16, 42-45.

Blum, K. (1984). *Handbook of abusable drugs.* USA: Gardner Press.

Bolton, M., Reynolds, A., & Biggs, L. (1994). *Queensland methadone program: Policies and procedures manual.* Brisbane, Australia: Queensland Health.

Brockmeyer, N. H., Mertins, L., & Goos, M. (1991). Pharmacokinetic interaction of antimicrobial agents with levomethadon in drug-addicted AIDS patients. *Klinische Wochenschrift,* 69, 16-18.

Brown, B. S., Watters, J. K., & Iglehart, A. S. (1982-83). Methadone maintenance dosage levels and program retention. *American Journal of Drug and Alcohol Abuse,* 9, 129-139.

Brown, L. S., Chu, A., Nemoto, T., Ajuluchukwu, D., & Primm, B. J. (1989). Human immunodeficiency virus infection in a cohort of intravenous drug users in New York City: Demographic, behavioral, and clinical features. *New York State Journal of Medicine,* 89, 506-510.

Caplehorn, J. R. M., & Bell, J. (1991). Methadone dosage and retention of patients in maintenance treatment. *Medical Journal of Australia,* 154,

195-199.

Caplehorn, J. R. M., & Bell, J. (1993). Correction of error: Methadone dosage and retention of patients in maintenance treatment [Letter]. *Medical Journal of Australia,* **159,** 640.

Caplehorn, J. R. M., Bell, J., Klein, D. G., & Gebski, V. J. (1993). Methadone dose and heroin use during maintenance treatment. *Addiction,* **88,** 119-124.

Caplehorn, J. R. M., Dalton, M. S. Y. N., Cluff, M. C., & Petrenas, A. (1994). Retention in methadone maintenance and heroin addicts' risk of death. *Addiction,* **89,** 203-207.

Cooper, J. R., Altman, F., Brown, B. S., & Czechowicz D. (Eds.). (1983a) *Research on the treatment of narcotic addiction: State of the art.* Rockville, MD: National Institute on Drug Abuse.

Cooper, J. R., Altman, F., & Keeley, K. (1983b). Discussion summary [of W.A. Hargreaves, Methadone dosage and duration for maintenance treatment]. In J. R. Cooper, F. Altman, B. S. Brown, & D. Czechowicz (Eds.), *Research on the treatment of narcotic addiction: State of the art* (pp. 92-94). Rockville, MD: National Institute on Drug Abuse.

D'Amanda, C. (1983). Program policies and procedures associated with treatment outcome. In J. R. Cooper, F. Altman, B. S. Brown, & D. Czechowicz (Eds.), *Research on the treatment of narcotic addiction: State of the art* (pp. 637-679). Rockville, MD: National Institute on Drug Abuse.

Dole, V. P. (1988). Implications of methadone maintenance for theories of narcotic addiction. *Journal of the American Medical Association,* **260,** 3025-3029.

Dole, V. P., & Nyswander, M. (1965). A medical treatment for diacetylmorphine (heroin) addiction: A clinical trial with methadone hydrochloride. *Journal of the American Medical Association,* **193,** 80-84.

Dole, V. P., & Nyswander, M. (1967). Heroin addiction: A metabolic disease. *Archives of Internal Medicine,* **120,** 19-24.

Dole, V. P., Nyswander, M., & Warner, A. (1968). Successful treatment of 750 criminal addicts. *Journal of the American Medical Association,* **206,** 2708-2711.

Dole, V. P., Nyswander, M. E., & Kreek, M. J. (1966). Narcotic blockade. *Archives of Internal Medicine,* **118,** 304-309.

Drug and Alcohol Services Council. (1994). *South Australian methadone prescribers manual.* Adelaide, Australia: Drug and Alcohol Services Council of South Australia.

Drummer, O. H., Opeskin, K., Syrjanen, M., & Cordner, S. M. (1992). Methadone toxicity causing death in ten subjects starting on a methadone maintenance program. *American Journal of Forensic Medicine and Pathology,* **13,** 346-350.

Finnegan, L. P. (1983). Clinical perinatal and development effects of methadone. In J. R. Cooper, F. Altman, B. S. Brown, & D. Czechowicz (Eds.), *Research on the treatment of narcotic addiction: State of the art* (pp. 392-443). Rockville, MD: National Institute on Drug Abuse.

Garbutt, G. D., & Goldstein, A. (1972). Blind comparison of three methadone dosages in 180 patients. In *Proceedings of the Fourth National Conference on Methadone Treatment* (pp. 411-14). New York: National Association for the Prevention of Addiction to Narcotics.

Gardner, R. (1970). Methadone misuse and death by overdosage. *British Journal of Addiction, 65*, 113-118.

Gill, A., Pead, J., & Mellor, N. (1992). *Methadone prescribers' manual for general practitioners.* Melbourne, Australia: Drug Services Victoria.

Goldstein, A. (1971). Blind dosage comparisons and other studies in a large methadone program. *Journal of Psychedelic Drugs, 4*, 177-181.

Goldstein, A. (1991). Heroin addiction: Neurobiology, pharmacology, and policy. *Journal of Psychoactive Drugs, 23*, 123-133.

Goldstein, A., & Judson, B. (1973). Efficacy and side effects of three widely different methadone doses. *Proceedings of the Fifth National Conference on Methadone Treatment* (21-44). New York: National Association for the Prevention of Addiction to Narcotics.

Goldstein, A., & Judson, B. A. (1983). Critique [of W.A. Hargreaves, Methadone dosage and duration for maintenance treatment]. In J. R. Cooper, F. Altman, B. S. Brown, & D. Czechowicz (Eds.), *Research on the treatment of narcotic addiction: State of the art* (pp. 80-91). Rockville, MD: National Institute on Drug Abuse.

Goldstein, A., Hansteen, R.W., & Horns, W.H. (1975). Control of methadone dosage by patients. *Journal of the American Medical Association, 234*, 734-737.

Gossop, M., Strang, J., & Connell, P. H. (1982). The response of out-patient opiate addicts to the provision of a temporary increase in their prescribed drugs. *British Journal of Psychiatry, 141*, 338-343.

Hall, W., & Einfeld, S. (1990). On doing the "impossible": Inferring that a putative causal relationship does not exist. *Australian and New Zealand Journal of Psychiatry, 24*, 217-226.

Handal, P. J., & Lander, J. J. (1976). Methadone treatment: Program evaluation and dose response relationships. *International Journal of the Addictions, 11*, 363-375.

Hargreaves, W. A. (1983). Methadone dosage and duration for maintenance treatment. In J. R. Cooper, F. Altman, B. S. Brown, & D. Czechowicz (Eds.), *Research on the treatment of narcotic addiction: State of the art* (pp. 19-79). Rockville, MD: National Institute on Drug Abuse.

Hartel, D. M., Shoenbaum, E. E., Selwyn, P. A., Kline, J., Davenny, K., Klein, R. S., & Friedland, G. H. (1995). Heroin use during methadone maintenance treatment: The importance of methadone dose and cocaine use. *American Journal of Public Health, 85*, 83-88.

Havassy, B. & Hargreaves, W.A. (1979). Self-regulation of dose in methadone maintenance with contingent privileges. *Addictive Behaviors,* 4, 31-38.

Havassy, B. & Hargreaves, W.A. (1981). Allowing methadone clients control over dosage: A 48-week controlled trial. *Addictive Behaviors,* 6, 283-288.

Havassy, B.E. & Tschann, J.M. (1983). Client initiative, inertia, and demographics: More powerful than treatment interventions in methadone maintenance? *International Journal of the Addictions,* 18, 617-631.

Henderson, G. L., & Harkey, M. R. (1990). *The use of therapeutic drug monitoring to improve the effectiveness of methadone treatment programs.* Sacramento, CA: Department of Alcohol and Drug Programs.

Holman, C. P., & Brown, J. P. (Eds.). (1989). *The Pleasant View manual on addiction.* Melbourne, Australia: Pleasant View Publications.

Holmstrand, J., Änggård, E., & Gunne, L.-M. (1978). Methadone maintenance: Plasma levels and therapeutic outcome. *Clinical Pharmacology and Therapeutics,* 23, 175-180.

Horns, W. H., & Goldstein, A. (1975). Plasma levels and symptom complaints in patients maintained on daily dosage of methadone hydrochloride. *Clinical Pharmacology and Therapeutics,* 17, 636-649.

Institute of Medicine (1995). *Federal regulation of methadone treatment.* Washington: National Academy Press.

Jaffe, J. H. (1970). Further experience with methadone in the treatment of narcotics users. *International Journal of the Addictions,* 5, 375-389.

Jaffe, J. H. (1992). Opiates: Clinical aspects. In J. H. Lowinson, P. Ruiz, R. B. Millman, & J. G. Langrod (Eds.), *Substance abuse: A comprehensive textbook* (2nd ed., pp. 186-194). Baltimore: Williams & Wilkins.

Jaffe, J. H., & Martin, W. R. (1990). Opioid analgesics and antagonists. In A. G. Gilman, T. W. Rall, A. S. Nies, & P. Tayler (Eds.), *The pharmacological basis of therapeutics* (8th ed., pp. 485-521). USA: Pergamon.

Joe, G. W., Simpson, D. D., & Hubbard, R. L. (1991). Treatment predictors of tenure in methadone maintenance. *Journal of Substance Abuse,* 3, 73-84.

Joe, G. W., Simpson, D. D., & Sells, S. B. (1994). Treatment process and relapse to opioid use during methadone maintenance. *American Journal of Drug and Alcohol Abuse,* 20, 173-197.

Johnson, R. E., Jaffe, J. H., & Fudala, P. J. (1992). A controlled trial of buprenorphine treatment for opioid dependence. *Journal of the American Medical Association,* 267, 2750-5.

Jones, B. E., & Prada, J. A. (1975). Drug-seeking behavior during methadone maintenance. *Psychopharmacologia,* 41, 7-10.

Kosten, T. R., Schottenfeld, R., Ziedonis, D., & Falcioni, J. (1993). Buprenorphine versus methadone maintenance for opioid dependence.

Journal of Nervous and Mental Disease, **181**, 358-364.

Kreek, M. J. (1979). Methadone in treatment: Physiological and pharmacological issues. In R. I. Dupont, A. Goldstein, J. O'Donnell, & B. Brown (Eds.), *Handbook on drug abuse* (pp. 57-86). Rockville, MD: National Institute on Drug Abuse.

Kreek, M. J. (1983a). Factors modifying the pharmacological effectiveness of methadone. In J. R. Cooper, F. Altman, B. S. Brown, & D. Czechowicz (Eds.), *Research on the treatment of narcotic addiction: State of the art* (pp. 95-114). Rockville, MD: National Institute on Drug Abuse.

Kreek, M. J. (1983b). Health consequences associated with the use of methadone. In J. R. Cooper, F. Altman, B. S. Brown, & D. Czechowicz (Eds.), *Research on the treatment of narcotic addiction: State of the art* (pp. 456-491). Rockville, MD: National Institute on Drug Abuse.

Kreek, M. J. (1990). Immune function in heroin addicts and former heroin addicts in treatment: Pre- and post-AIDS epidemic. In P. T. K. Pham & K. Rice (Eds.), *Drugs of abuse: Chemistry, pharmacology, immunology, and AIDS* (NIDA Research Monograph 96, pp. 192-219). Rockville, MD: National Institute on Drug Abuse.

Kreek, M. J. (1991). Using methadone effectively: Achieving goals by application of laboratory, clinical, and evaluation research and by development of innovative programs. In R. W. Pickens, C. G. Leukefeld, & C. R. Schuster (Eds.), *Improving drug abuse treatment* (NIDA Research Monograph 106, pp. 245-66). Rockville, MD: National Institute on Drug Abuse.

Kreek, M. J. (1992). Rationale for maintenance pharmacotherapy of opiate dependence. In C. P. O'Brien & J. H. Jaffe (Eds.), *Addictive states* (Research publications: Association for Research in Nervous and Mental Disease Vol. 70, pp. 205-230). New York: Raven Press.

Ling, W., Blakis, M., Holmes, E. D., Klett, C. J., & Carter, W. E. (1980). Restabilization with methadone after methadyl acetate maintenance. *Archives of General Psychiatry,* **37**, 194-196.

Ling, W., Charuvastra, C., Kaim, S. C., & Klett, C. J. (1976). Methadyl acetate and methadone as maintenance treatments for heroin addicts. *Archives of General Psychiatry,* **33**, 709-720.

Ling, W., Wesson, D. R., Charuvastra, C., & Klett, J. (1996). A controlled trial comparing buprenorphine and methadone maintenance in opioid dependence. *Archives of General Psychiatry,* **53**, 401-407.

Loimer, N., & Schmid, R. (1992). The use of plasma levels to optimize methadone maintenance treatment. *Drug and Alcohol Dependence,* **30**, 241-246.

Loimer, N., Schmid, R., Grünberger, J., Jagsch, R., Linzmayer, L., & Presslich, O. (1991). Psychophysiological reactions in methadone maintenance patients do not correlate with methadone plasma levels. *Psychopharmacology,* **103**, 538-540.

Lowinson, J. H., & Millman, R. B. (1979). Clinical aspects of methadone treatment. In R. I. Dupont, A. Goldstein, J. O'Donnell, & B. Brown (Eds.), *Handbook on drug abuse* (pp. 49-56). Rockville, MD: National Institute on Drug Abuse.

Maany, I., Dhopesh, V., Arndt, I. O., Burke, W., Woody, G., & O'Brien, C. P. (1989). Increase in desipramine serum levels associated with methadone treatment. *American Journal of Psychiatry, 146,* 1611-1613.

Maddux, J. F., Esquivel, M., Vogtsberger, K. N., & Desmond, D. P. (1991). Methadone dose and urine morphine. *Journal of Substance Abuse Treatment, 8,* 195-201.

Maddux, J.F., Desmond, D.P., & Vogtsberger, K.N. (1995). Patient-regulated methadone dose and optional counseling in methadone maintenance. *American Journal of the Addictions, 4,* 18-32.

Maremmani, I., Nardini, R., Zolesi, O., & Castrogiovanni, P. (1994). Methadone dosages and therapeutic compliance during a methadone maintenance program. *Drug and Alcohol Dependence, 34,* 163-166.

Martin, J., Payte, J. T., & Zweben, J. E. (1991). Methadone maintenance treatment: A primer for physicians. *Journal of Psychoactive Drugs, 23*(2), 165-76.

Martin, W. R., Jasinski, D. R., Haertzen, C. A., Kay, D. C., Jones, B. E., Mansky, P. A., & Carpenter, R. W. (1973). Methadone: A reevaluation. *Archives of General Psychiatry, 28,* 286-295.

Mattick, R. P., & Hall, W. (Eds.). (1993). *A treatment outline for approaches to opioid dependence.* Canberra, Australia: Australian Government Publishing Service.

McGlothlin, W. H., & Anglin, M. D. (1981). Long-term follow-up of clients of high- and low-dose methadone programs. *Archives of General Psychiatry, 38,* 1055-1063.

Newman, R. G. (1977). *Methadone treatment in narcotic addiction: Program management, findings and prospects for the future.* New York: Academic Press.

Newman, R. G. (1991). What's so special about methadone maintenance? *Drug and Alcohol Review, 10,* 225-232.

Novick, D. M., Kreek, M. J., Fanizza, A. M., Yancovitz, S. R., Gelb, A. M., & Stenger, R. J. (1981). Methadone disposition in patients with chronic liver disease. *Clinical Pharmacology and Therapeutics, 30,* 353-362.

Novick, D. M., Richman, B. L., Friedman, J. M., Friedman, J. E., Fried, C., Wilson, J. P., Townley, A., & Kreek, M. J. (1993). The medical status of methadone maintenance patients in treatment for 11-18 years. *Drug and Alcohol Dependence, 33,* 235-245.

Olsen, G. D., Wilson, J. E., & Robertson, G. E. (1981). Respiratory and ventilatory effects of methadone in healthy women. *Clinical Pharmacology and Therapeutics, 29,* 373-380.

Payte, J. T., & Khuri, E. T. (1993). Principles of methadone dose determination. In M. W. Parrino (Ed.), *State methadone treatment guidelines* (pp. 47-58). Rockville, MD: U.S. Department of Health and Human Services.

Perucca, E., Gatti, G., & Spina, E. (1994). Clinical pharmacokinetics of fluvoxamine. *Clinical Pharmacokinetics, 27*, 175-190.

Pond, S. M., Kreek, M. J., Tong, T. G., Raghunath, J., & Benowitz, N. L. (1985). Altered methadone pharmacokinetics in methadone-maintained pregnant women. *Journal of Pharmacology and Experimental Therapeutics, 233*, 1-6.

Reynolds, I., & Magro, D. (1976). The use of methadone as a treatment tool for opiate addicts: A two-year follow-up study. *Medical Journal of Australia, 2*, 560-562.

Roszell, D.K., & Calsyn, D.A. (1986). Methadone dosage: Patient characteristics and clinical correlates. *International Journal of the Addictions, 21*, 1233-46.

Säwe, J. (1986). High-dose morphine and methadone in cancer patients: Clinical pharmacokinetic considerations of oral treatment. *Clinical Pharmacokinetics, 11*, 87-106.

Schall, U., Pries, E., Katta, T., Klöppel, A., & Gastpar, M. (1996). Pharmacokinetic and pharmacodynamic interactions in an outpatient maintenance therapy of intravenous heroin users with levomethadone. *Addiction Biology, 1*, 105-113.

Schuster, C. R. (1989). Methadone maintenance: An adequate dose is vital in checking the spread of AIDS. *NIDA Notes* 4(2), pp. 3,33.

Schut, J., Wohlmuth, T. W., & File, K. (1973). Low dosage maintenance: A re-examination. *International Journal of Clinical Pharmacology and Toxicology, 7*, 48-53.

Schwartz, E.L., Brechbühl, A-B., Kahl, P., Miller, M.A., Selwyn, P.A., & Friedland, G.H. (1992). Pharmacokinetic interactions with zidovudine and methadone in intravenous drug-using patients with HIV infection. *Journal of Acquired Immune Deficiency Syndromes, 5*, 619-626.

Seow, S. S. W., Swensen, G., Willis, D., Hartfield, M., & Chapman, C. (1980). Extraneous drug use in methadone-supported patients. *Medical Journal of Australia, 1*, 269-271.

Serpelloni, G., Carrieri, M. P., Rezza, G., Morganti, S., Gomma, M., & Binkin, N. (1994). Methadone treatment as a determinant of HIV risk reduction among injecting drug users: A nested case control study. *AIDS Care, 16*, 215-220.

Siassi, I., Angle, B. P., & Alston, D. C. (1977). Comparison of the effect of high and low doses of methadone on treatment outcome. *International Journal of the Addictions, 12*, 993-1005.

Simpson, D. D., & Joe, G. W. (1993). Motivation as a predictor of early dropout from drug abuse treatment. *Psychotherapy, 30*, 357-368.

State Coroner of Victoria. (1990). *Records of investigation into deaths: Case Nos. 623/89, 3273/89, 4439/88.* Melbourne, Australia: State Coroner's Office.

Strain, E. C., Preston, K. L., Liebson, I. A., & Bigelow, G. E. (1993a). Precipitated withdrawal by pentazocine in methadone-maintained volunteers. *Journal of Pharmacology and Experimental Therapeutics, 267*, 624-634.

Strain, E. C., Stitzer, M. L., Bigelow, G. E., & Liebson, I. (1992). Methadone dosing level: Effects on treatment outcome. In L. Harris (Ed.), *Problems of drug dependence 1991. Proceeding of the 53rd Annual Scientific Meeting. The Committee on Problems of Drug Dependence, Inc.* (NIDA Research Monograph 119, p. 357). Rockville, MD: National Institute on Drug Abuse.

Strain, E. C., Stitzer, M. L., Liebson, I. A., & Bigelow, G. E. (1993b). Dose-response effects of methadone in the treatment of opioid dependence. *Annals of Internal Medicine, 119*, 23-27.

Strain, E. C., Stitzer, M. L., Liebson, I. A., & Bigelow, G. E. (1994). Comparison of buprenorphine and methadone in the treatment of opioid dependence. *American Journal of Psychiatry, 151*, 1025-1030.

Swensen, G. (1988). Opioid drug deaths in Western Australia: 1974-1984. *Australian Drug and Alcohol Review, 7*, 181-185.

Swensen, G., Ilett, K. F., Dusci, L. J., Hackett, L. P., Ong, R. T. T., Quigley, A. J., Lenton, S., Saker, R., & Caporn, J. (1993). Patterns of drug use by participants in the Western Australian methadone program, 1984-1991. *Medical Journal of Australia, 159*, 373-376.

Tennant, F. S., Rawson, R. A., Cohen, A., Tarver, A., & Clabough, D. (1984). Methadone plasma levels and persistent drug abuse in high dose maintenance patients. In L. S. Harris (Ed.), *Problems of drug dependence, 1983: Proceedings of the 45th Annual Scientific Meeting, The Committee on Problems of Drug Dependence Inc.* (NIDA Research Monograph 49, pp. 262-268). Rockville, MD: National Institute on Drug Abuse.

Tennant, F. & Shannon, J. (1995). Cocaine abuse in methadone maintenance patients is associated with low serum methadone concentrations. *Journal of Addictive Diseases, 14*, 67-74.

Tonkin, A. L., & Bochner, F. (1994). Therapeutic drug monitoring and patient outcome: A review of the issues. *Clinical Pharmacokinetics, 27*, 169-174.

Torrens, M., Castillo, C., & Pérez-Solá, V. (1996). Retention in a low-threshold methadone maintenance program. *Drug and Alcohol Dependence, 41*, 55-59.

Treece, C., & Nicholson, B. (1980) DSM-III Personality type and dose levels in methadone maintenance patients. Journal of *Nervous and Mental Disease, 168*, 621-628.

Verebely, K., Volavka, J., Mulé, S., & Resnick, R. (1975). Methadone in man: Pharmacokinetic and excretion studies in acute and chronic treatment. *Clinical Pharmacology and Therapeutics, 18,* 180-190.

Verebey, K. E. (Ed.), (1982). Opioids in mental illness: Theories, clinical observations, and treatment possibilities. *Annals of the New York Academy of Sciences, 398.*

Volavka, J., Verebey, K., Resnick, R., & Mulé, S. (1978). Methadone dose, plasma level, and cross-tolerance to heroin in man. *Journal of Nervous and Mental Disease, 166,* 104-109.

Walsh, S. L., June, H. L., Schuh, K. J., Preston, K. L., Bigelow, G. E., & Stitzer, M. L. (1995). Effects of buprenorphine and methadone in methadone-maintained subjects. *Psychopharmacology, 119,* 268-276.

Walton, R. G., Thornton, T. L., & Wahl, G. F. (1978). Serum methadone as an aid in managing methadone maintenance patients. *International Journal of the Addictions, 13,* 689-694.

Ward, J. (1994). Methadone doses: Adequate and otherwise. Comments on Wolff and Hay's "Plasma methadone monitoring with methadone maintenance treatment." *Drug and Alcohol Dependence, 36,* 73-75.

Ward, J., Mattick, R. P., & Hall, W. (1992). *Key issues in methadone maintenance treatment.* Sydney: New South Wales University Press.

White, J. M., Dyer, K. R., Ali, R. L., Gaughwin, M. D., & Cormack, S. (1994). Injecting behaviour and risky needle use amongst methadone maintenance clients. *Drug and Alcohol Dependence, 34,* 113-119.

Williams, H. R. (1971). Low and high methadone maintenance in the outpatient treatment of the hard core heroin addict. In S. Einstein (Ed.), *Methadone maintenance* (pp. 93-101). New York: Marcel Dekker.

Wolff, K., Sanderson, M., Hay, A. W. M., & Raistrick, D. (1991). Methadone concentrations in plasma and their relationship to drug dosage. *Clinical Chemistry, 37,* 205-209.

Wu, C., & Henry, J. A. (1994). Interaction between ethanol and opioids in a protozoan assay. *Human and Experimental Toxicology, 13,* 145-148.

10

THE USE OF URINALYSIS DURING OPIOID REPLACEMENT THERAPY

JEFF WARD, RICHARD P. MATTICK
AND WAYNE HALL

INTRODUCTION

The terms "urine testing" and "urinalysis" describe methods used to determine if any given drug or its metabolites are present in a sample of urine. According to De Angelis (1972), large-scale urine testing for illicit drug use was developed during the occupation of Japan after World War II, because American military personnel serving there began to use opiates in substantial numbers. The need to develop reasonably inexpensive and accurate urine tests resulted in paper chromatography procedures that were able to detect small amounts of opiates in urine. Derivatives of this procedure – for example, thin layer chromatography – are still in use today.

Since its inception, opioid replacement therapy has played a pivotal role in the development of urine testing to detect illicit drug use. After World War II, urinalysis was first used regularly on a reasonably large scale by Dole and his colleagues in New York in the first methadone program (De Angelis, 1972). Since that time, urinalysis has been a familiar and important component of methadone treatment. As Trellis, Smith, Alston and Siassi (1975) have pointed out, for much of the past three decades most clinical and administrative decisions in methadone maintenance programs have been based in part on urinalysis results. In this chapter, we assess the role urinalysis has played in methadone maintenance treatment and discuss what role it might play in the future on the basis of what has been learnt after nearly three decades of its use. Although the discussion focuses on methadone maintenance treatment, the conclusions are readily translatable to other opioid replacement therapies.

THE USE OF URINALYSIS IN METHADONE PROGRAMS

Patients in methadone maintenance treatment have been traditionally tested for drug use using urinalysis for two reasons: to ensure that they are ingesting the methadone they are being dispensed, and to detect the use of other non-prescribed drugs. Urinalysis results are also sometimes used to establish daily heroin use during assessment for methadone maintenance (although its usefulness in this regard is debatable – see Chapter 8). When patients are tested, they are asked to provide a sample of their urine and the act of urination is often observed to ensure that the sample provided is the patient's own and has not been tampered with (e.g., diluted with water to reduce the concentration of any drug that may be present). The sample is then sent to a laboratory to be tested for the presence of the prescribed opioid (e.g., methadone) and a range of other drugs. A report is returned after the urinalysis has been completed. In some countries (e.g., USA) urinalysis is stipulated as a necessary component of methadone maintenance treatment by government regulations (Calsyn *et al.*, 1991; Marion, 1993).

Urinalysis results are essentially used for two purposes: as part of patient management and for program evaluation and research. In terms of patient management, drug-positive urine results are responded to in a variety of ways. They might lead to: a counselling session in which a staff member expresses concern that the patient has relapsed; an increase or decrease in methadone dose; the loss of take-home methadone privileges; extra individual counselling; or the drawing up and signing of a contract promising not to relapse again, which may eventually lead to discharge from treatment (Barthwell & Gastfriend, 1993; Calsyn *et al.*, 1991). Urinalysis results are also often used for program evaluation by unit managers, government officials and researchers. Historically, this has been important in establishing the effectiveness of methadone maintenance as an intervention to reduce heroin use. Urinalysis results provide politicians and other interested parties with the data they need to convince sceptics that methadone maintenance is a worthwhile intervention despite its controversial status.

THE ACCURACY OF URINALYSIS

The immediate goal of urinalysis is to determine whether or not a drug, or its metabolites, are present in a urine sample (Blanke, 1986). However, like most scientific procedures, urine testing is subject to a variety of sources of error. Because of the possible serious consequences of a positive result in the case of testing for illicit drug use, the way in which error is controlled for tends to favour the production of true positive results. This allows for the occurrence of false negative results in which the outcome of the test is negative even though the drug concerned was taken and is present in the sample. The usual procedure is to screen all samples by an inexpensive and relatively insensitive method and then to confirm positive results by using more sensitive and more expensive procedures.

Apart from the sensitivity of the testing procedures, other factors also affect the interpretation of urinalysis results (Manno, 1986a). These factors include the type of drug being tested for, the dose taken, the number of times the drug has been taken recently, the delay between last ingestion and the taking of the urine, and the quality of the procedures used by the laboratory doing the tests. Different drugs are eliminated from the body at different rates, and so, depending upon the drug, the time between ingestion and taking urine will affect test results. For example, cocaine is eliminated from the body very quickly and will only be detected in a sample of urine taken within a day of ingestion, whereas a drug like methadone can be detected for much longer periods. Higher doses and frequent use both increase the likelihood of detection by increasing the time period during which the drug will be present in urine. Finally, in the USA, different laboratories have been shown to have more or less likelihood of detecting drugs in a specimen because of differences in the quality control of laboratory procedures (Hansen *et al.*, 1985).

A negative test result, therefore, does not mean that the subject being tested has not taken the drug. He or she may not have used the drug concerned; they may have used the drug recently but not recently enough to still have traces in their urine; they may have interfered with the sample by substituting other urine for it, by drinking excessive amounts of water before urinating, or by adulterating the specimen with a diluent or some other substance (Manno, 1986a; 1986b; Montalvo *et al.,* 1972). A positive result has more confidence associated with it and, in nearly all cases, means that the person has recently taken the drug detected.

ADVANTAGES AND DISADVANTAGES OF URINALYSIS

In this section, we assess the arguments for and against the use of urinalysis to monitor drug use in methadone maintenance programs. Because many of the issues concerned with urinalysis are not amenable to research, the advantages and disadvantages of urinalysis have to be considered when deciding what role urinalysis should play in methadone maintenance treatment.

The advantages and disadvantages of urinalysis that have been suggested are listed below.

Advantages:

- Objective measurement of drug use on which to base clinical decisions
- Monitoring of illicit drug use for program evaluation
- Monitoring of patient compliance in taking methadone
- Reduction in illicit drug use
- Suitability of results for legal purposes
- Increased patient contact with the treatment program
- Provision of a basis for staff–patient bond

Disadvantages:

- Implied distrust of patients
- Humiliation of patients and staff
- Inaccuracy as an indicator of drug use
- Expense

The most important advantage of urinalysis is its objectivity in providing information about patients' drug use. Urinalysis results provide an objective index for monitoring the success of programs in reducing illicit drug use and for making clinical decisions concerning methadone dose, take-home privileges and treatment termination for continued illicit drug use (Magura & Lipton, 1988). One of the important advantages claimed for urinalysis is that it reduces drug use. Urinalysis results also allow program staff to ensure that patients are actually taking the methadone dispensed to them and they have also been used for legal purposes as evidence of compliance with treatment goals (De Angelis, 1972). De Angelis has also proposed that urinalysis keeps patients in contact with the program and that the inability to deceive staff about drug use fosters respect and honesty among patients.

The disadvantages of urinalysis fall into three categories: the negative effect it has on patients and treatment; the relative inaccuracy of the procedure; and the economic cost involved. It has been claimed that urinalysis has a negative impact on patients and treatment by conveying to patients that they are not to be trusted. The humiliation involved in having to urinate while being watched by staff members is also thought to affect staff–patient relationships and patients' attitudes to treatment (Gottheil *et al.*, 1976). Proponents of this view argue that time and money would be better spent in trying to construct more cooperative relationships with clients in order to deal with their drug use.

A second disadvantage of urinalysis is the relative inaccuracy of the procedure. Although positive results indicate that a person is using a specified drug, the possibility of false negatives is quite high due to the insensitivity of the tests used, the short elimination half-life of many of the drugs being tested for, and the proven unreliability of some laboratories in blind studies (Gottheil *et al.*, 1976; Hansen *et al.*, 1985; Trellis *et al.*, 1975). Attewell and Gerstein (1979) found, in a study of methadone maintenance clinics in California, that the inconsistent detection rate of urine monitoring also had adverse consequences on patients' attitudes to treatment. Rather than seeing urinalysis as an objective, scientific procedure, they viewed it as a game of luck that depended on whether they would be caught out on a 'bad' day and, if so, a further round in the game as to whether the result would come back negative or not. According to Attewell and Gerstein (1979) patients:

tended to respond to being caught with a dirty urine by becoming angry. Indeed, anger is a rational response to a situation where a series of low-probability outcomes (day urine requested, metabolism, accuracy of urinalysis, etc.) all coincide causing the addict to be caught. Yet anger was seen by staff as addicts' refusal to take personal responsibility for their actions (p. 322).

A third major disadvantage of urinalysis is the substantial cost involved. Cost, as will be seen in the section below, has always been an important factor in determining the frequency of urine testing in methadone maintenance programs. Urinalysis is a major component in the overall cost of methadone maintenance, although in Australia, for example, this seems to vary between public clinics that have access to relatively cheap government laboratories and private clinics that often test elsewhere (Baldwin, 1987; Swensen, 1989; Wells & McKay, 1989). In government programs, the annual cost for regular testing was estimated during the 1980s to be roughly equivalent to that of the methadone syrup itself (Baldwin, 1987; Swensen, 1989). However, more recently the overall cost of testing has fallen below that of the syrup due to a general reduction in the frequency of urine testing that has occurred in recent years (Ward, *et al.*, 1996).

URINE SAMPLING SCHEDULES AND SUPERVISION

Given the short elimination half-life of most opioids and most of the other drugs used by patients in opioid replacement therapy (e.g., cocaine), the most reliable method of detecting drug use is to have a daily schedule of urine specimen collection. This was the option adopted in the first methadone maintenance program (Dole & Nyswander, 1965). A daily testing schedule removes the possibility that patients will have safe periods where they can risk drug use because they do not expect to be tested in the near future (Harford & Kleber, 1978). However, daily testing is not feasible for a number of reasons. First, the cost of daily testing is prohibitive (e.g., laboratory, transportation, etc.). Second, the daily testing of all patients takes up considerable staff time in supervising the collection of samples and filling out the requisite forms in preparation for sending them to the laboratory, time which otherwise could be spent on other clinical tasks. Finally, providing a sample every day is inconvenient and irritating for patients (Harford & Kleber, 1978).

Fixed-day Collection Schedules

In order to avoid the difficulties associated with daily collection, a number of collection schedules have been developed that seek to collect the minimum number of samples possible while at the same time retaining a reasonable likelihood of detecting patients' drug use (Harford & Kleber, 1978). A fixed collection schedule, where urine is taken on fixed days known in advance to the patients, is not thought to be an appropriate method for reliably detecting most drugs because the patients know when they can and cannot engage in drug use without being detected. In order to avoid this problem, a variety of collection procedures have been developed that rely on some random factor to determine on which day any given patient will be required to provide a sample.

Random Collection Schedules

Random Selection of Daily Collected Samples

One possible solution to the cost involved in daily testing is to take samples daily but to select randomly from those samples one or more specimens to be tested each week. While this solves the problem of the cost involved in daily testing, it does not alleviate the considerable burden to staff and patients of having samples taken daily (Goldstein & Judson, 1974). More widely practised are a variety of collection procedures that randomly select patients to be tested each day. Harford and Kleber, (1978) have described three possible random urinalysis collection schedules.

Fixed-Interval Schedules

The first and, according to Harford and Kleber (1978), the most widely-used schedule for collecting urine samples is what they term a 'fixed-interval schedule'. According to this procedure, each patient is tested a specified number of times within a pre-determined period. For example, if the period is one week and each patient has to be tested once during that interval, then each week each patient is tested on a day that is randomly chosen for them. The problem with this method is that if the period is a calendar week beginning on Sunday and the patient is tested on Monday they will very quickly learn that they are free to take whatever drugs they like until approximately 24 hours before the time they show up for the first methadone dose of the next week. Harford and Kleber argue that such a schedule might encourage drug use by signalling the periods when the patient will not be tested.

Goldstein and Brown (1970) proposed a possible solution to the problems set out above. They tried to provide an answer to the question 'If testing is less than daily, how often does it need to be done to adequately monitor drug use?' Using statistical procedures they devised a probability model to determine the consequences for a truly random schedule (i.e., the patients would neither know the time interval, nor be able to predict when a test would be). According to this model, for any time period, if there were 20 consecutive negative results, it would be reasonably certain that the patient had not used drugs on more than 13% of the days in the time period. The actual number of days would depend on the frequency of the tests. In the case of one test every five or so days, 20 negative test results would mean that the patient has used illicit drugs on less than 12 days out of 90 (i.e., 13% of 90). Harford and Kleber (1978) argue that this procedure still allows for relatively long periods without testing (e.g., if the patient is tested on the first day of a testing interval and the last day of the following interval it will mean that there will be an extended period when they will not be tested), so as an alternative they proposed random-interval testing.

Random-Interval Schedules

The solution to the latter problem, according to Harford and Kleber, is to be found in what they call a random-interval schedule. This schedule was originally proposed by Kleber and Gould (1971). Long periods without testing are eliminated by having a maximum period during which a patient will not be tested. For example, if a sample is taken on a Monday in a weekly testing schedule then the next testing period begins the next day (i.e., on Tuesday). The patient will then be tested again during the next week beginning Tuesday. Using this procedure, no more than six days can elapse without testing on a weekly schedule. Kleber and Gould point out that patients at different levels of functioning (doing well, doing poorly, etc.) can be managed on different testing schedules to accommodate their progress in treatment. New patients could be tested on a three-day schedule and stabilised patients could be tested on a more infrequent schedule (e.g., fortnightly or monthly). All that this procedure requires is a table of random numbers that includes the numerals for their period (i.e., one to three for the new patients and one to 14 for the well-stabilised group). The next number in the table would determine on which day in the next period the patient would be tested.

Harford and Kleber (1978) conducted a study to determine the impact of random-interval testing on unsanctioned drug use in a methadone maintenance program. They assessed the change from a fixed-interval to a random-interval schedule by looking at the rates of opiate-positive samples before and after the change. The authors interpreted the data which showed an initial increase in detected drug use and then a permanent decline as showing that the random-interval schedule was more successful at detecting illicit drug use and, therefore, in controlling it. However, this conclusion is difficult to support on the basis of this study, because of the retrospective single-group design used in the study which makes it impossible to rule out that the decrease in detected drug use may have been due to some other factor. The possibility that the decrease may have been due to some other factor is supported by the fact that there was a similar increase in detected use in the year before the beginning of the study. Such increases may be due to influences such as fluctuations in the availability and price of heroin on the streets. Another likely confounding influence is that simultaneous with the introduction of the new testing schedules was the adoption of a stricter policy concerning illicit drug use. Patients who gave drug-positive urine samples were punished by withdrawal of privileges and threatened with expulsion from the program. The fall in drug use may have been due to this stricter policy rather than the testing schedule itself. However, if prolonged periods without testing are of concern when using random schedules, then, as Harford and Kleber argue, the adoption of random-interval collection would alleviate that concern.

Supervised Specimen Collection

It has become common practice to supervise the collection of urine samples in methadone maintenance programs to prevent patients from subverting the process (Calsyn *et al.*, 1991). A variety of procedures have been employed to make sure that patients do not interfere with or provide a substitute for their sample, including close observation of the act of urination, observing the client through a one-way mirror and monitoring the act by means of a video camera placed in the toilet. Goldstein and Brown (1970) suggested that every sample collected should be supervised and, where this is not done, there is no point in collecting the sample at all. According to this argument, if the taking of the sample is not supervised, the cost involved might as well be saved and patients simply asked whether they had recently used any drugs or not. While not all patients will interfere with the collection procedure, it does seem to be the case that some patients will go to extraordinary lengths to avoid providing a proper sample of their urine if they know that it will return a positive result, especially if there will be negative consequences as a result.

One alternative to observing the act of urination is taking the temperature of the sample (Judson *et al.,* 1979; Moran *et al.,* 1995). If the sample is around body temperature (37°C), then it can be assumed that it has not been diluted with water. However, as Manno (1986b) points out this does not solve the problem of adulteration. Ordinary table salt, detergent and many other household cleansing products can affect the sample and return a false negative result. Other solutions are to remove all soap and any other possible adulterants from the toilet room and dye the water in the cistern so that adding it to the sample will change its colour. Manno (1986b) warns that these measures are only suitable if there is a low possibility that the persons to be tested will bring other substances (e.g., salt) to the testing room. As Judson *et al.* (1979) point out, it is impossible to conduct a foolproof sample collection procedure and the only real way to stop interference in the long term would be in cases where there were no negative consequences to handing in drug-positive samples. Supervised collection is, then, probably a necessary part of monitoring drug use by means of urinalysis, because a proportion of patients will not provide a true sample of their urine under other circumstances; but it has to be acknowledged that it is probably impossible to devise a tamper-proof collection system.

Although deemed a necessary part of urine testing, supervision remains one of the most controversial aspects of the procedure. According to critics of the practice, supervised urine collection essentially means that in order to receive treatment, methadone patients have to regularly humiliate themselves by urinating in front of clinic staff. According to Lewis *et al.,* (1972), in summarising the results of a study of male ex-addicts' attitudes to urine testing as part of parole surveillance:

For the subject, urinalysis represents on the average a demeaning procedure designed by the state to determine with a certain accuracy whether or not he has reverted to drug use... For most subjects...the process is a further indication of the absence of control over important parts of their body and their existence. Given the shame associated with the evacuative functions in American society, such a finding should not be surprising (p. 306).

The most frequent responses reported by the participants in the Lewis *et al.* study of ex-addicts to supervised urine sample collection were: they were embarrassed; they felt angry and upset; they could not urinate while being observed; and the supervising officer was usually just as embarrassed as they were. It has also been suggested that the usual response to the procedures employed to ensure proper urine collection is that those being tested come to see the collection procedure as a 'game' that they attempt to win. This has been shown to occur with American soldiers in Vietnam and ex-addict parolees, as well as with methadone maintenance patients (Gottheil *et al.*, 1976). The extent to which the negative effects of supervision on patients are worthwhile has to be weighed against the need for accurate urinalysis results.

URINALYSIS AND DRUG USE

In 1977, Goldstein, Horns and Hansteen remarked that even though urinalysis was almost universal, there were no answers to the simple question of whether it played a useful role in methadone maintenance treatment or not. Subsequently, in a brief review of the literature in 1983, D'Amanda (1983) observed that little had changed since 1977 and that there was not much more information available with which to answer this question. There has, however, since that time, been a substantial research program that has examined the application of behaviour modification principles to the use of urinalysis results in managing the illicit drug use of methadone maintenance patients.

Does urinalysis reduce or control illicit drug use?

Three early experiments attempted to answer the question of whether urinalysis reduces illicit drug use. In the first of these studies, 64 stabilised patients in a San Francisco methadone maintenance program were randomly allocated to receive or not receive feedback about their urinalysis results (Grevert & Weinberg, 1973). Feedback consisted of a preliminary discussion with a staff member and could result in revocation of take-home privileges, being put on 'probation', or finally being placed on a withdrawal regimen as a precursor to having treatment terminated. The study assessed the impact of feedback about urinalysis results on the incidence of unsanctioned drug use. The main finding was that there was no difference between the two groups in terms of drug-positive test results. Interestingly, unit staff were more likely to attribute drug use to patients in the feedback condition than in the no feedback condition. This finding was contrary to the initial expectations of the unit staff, who thought that not responding to urinalysis results would result in an increase in drug use. This study provides evidence against the notion that negative consequences contingent upon handing in a drug-positive urine sample lead to a reduction in illicit drug use among methadone patients.

In a subsequent study that also employed a randomised design, Goldstein and Judson (1974) assigned new methadone maintenance patients to monitored and unmonitored groups in a series of three experiments at three different methadone maintenance units to examine whether urinalysis monitoring had an effect on drug use. In the monitored group, take-home methadone privileges could be revoked if positive urinalysis results were returned (no other details of clinical response to positive results are given, nor is it stated whether there were differences in response across the three clinics). After three months, on a date unknown to patients and unit staff, the researchers appeared at the clinic and took a urine sample from each of the subjects in both groups. In the first experiment, a significant difference was found showing that the monitored group had less heroin use than the unmonitored group, but in the subsequent two experiments no differences in heroin use were observed. Taken overall, these three experiments failed to consistently refute the hypothesis that the presence of urine testing results in a reduction in heroin use during methadone maintenance treatment.

Havassy and Hall (1981) argue that Goldstein and Judson's (1974) results only *suggested* that urinalysis does not deter drug use among methadone patients because the study was flawed by a high drop-out rate that resulted in small final sample sizes, by marked variation between the three clinics used in the study, and by too brief a study period. They conducted a further study that tried to overcome these flaws by randomly allocating 431 methadone patients in stratified blocks to a monitored and an unmonitored condition for a year at five methadone clinics in northern California. The effect of monitoring was measured by two surprise collections of urine specimens at four and eight months after the commencement of the experiment. The data were analysed in two ways. First, by not including subjects who refused to provide a specimen and, secondly, by including refusals as being drug-positive, which is the usual method employed in such cases. The only significant difference between the two groups was for the eight-month test when subjects who did not return a specimen were excluded from the analysis. The monitored group returned slightly more drug-free specimens than the unmonitored group and this difference was statistically significant. However, when refusals were included as drug-positive this difference was diminished and no longer significant. The latter result is the stronger evidence. Havassy and Hall concluded that urinalysis does not reduce or control drug use for methadone patients as whole, nor for any definable subgroup of patients. The only other relevant finding was that being monitored was associated with a higher treatment drop-out rate, suggesting that there may be a cost for the use of urinalysis in terms of patients dropping out of treatment.

The above three studies suggest that there is little to be gained by using urinalysis to monitor drug use, if the main purpose of the procedure is to deter patients from using illicit drugs. Unmonitored patients do not, according to these three studies, return more positive urine test results than patients who are monitored. On the basis of the *available* evidence, it has to be concluded that there is no compelling evidence that the absence of urinalysis leads to an increase in illicit drug use.

Are there ways to make urinalysis more effective at reducing drug use?

The three studies discussed in the previous section suggest that urinalysis does not reduce unsanctioned drug use during methadone maintenance treatment. However, perhaps the reasons why there are no discernible effects of urinalysis monitoring is because the test results are not being used in an optimal fashion to intervene with patients. More studies have tried to resolve this issue than the more general one of whether having urinalysis *per se* makes a difference or not in terms of patients' drug use. All of these studies have investigated ways of using urinalysis results that are based on behaviour modification principles.

Two studies have found that immediate feedback on urinalysis results is no more effective than delayed feedback in reducing unsanctioned drug use (Goldstein *et al.*, 1977; Schwartz *et al.*, 1987). The studies were based on the principle that immediate reinforcement is more effective than delayed reinforcement. In both studies, on-site testing (immediate feedback condition) was done using the EMIT system and off-site testing (delayed feedback condition) was done by thin layer chromatography. Neither Goldstein *et al.* (1977) nor Schwartz *et al.* (1987) found any discernible differences between the EMIT and thin layer chromatography groups. On the basis of the results of these two studies, it is concluded that evidence for the efficacy of immediate versus delayed feedback about urinalysis results is lacking.

By far the most intensively researched and widely practised set of procedures for applying behaviour modification techniques to the management of illicit drug use during methadone maintenance treatment are what are known as contingency management procedures. According to the theoretical model on which such techniques are based, behaviour is determined by reinforcement contingencies found in the environment. Changing behaviour in any given environment, therefore, requires taking control of these reinforcement contingencies (Hall, 1983). In methadone maintenance clinics, such contingencies include the use of positive reinforcers such as increases in dose and take-home privileges contingent upon drug-free urine samples, and negative consequences such as dose reduction and expulsion from treatment in response to drug-positive samples. Proponents of this view argue that most methadone clinics employ an informal contingency management system, though the way in which the system is applied is neither well thought out, nor well enacted, according to the behaviourist model about the relationship between reinforcement and behaviour (e.g., Calsyn & Saxon, 1987; Grabowski *et al.*, 1993). The proponents of this view also argue that the three tests of urinalysis described in the previous section attract this same criticism. However, we would dispute this because, in at least two of the three trials (Goldstein & Judson, 1974; Grevert & Weinberg, 1973), there were clearly stipulated consequences to continued illicit drug use and, given that the practice is almost universal, it seems likely that this was also the case in the third study (Havassy & Hall, 1981).

Stitzer *et al.* have reviewed the literature on a number of occasions (e.g., 1985; 1993) and have concluded that although there is suggestive evidence that supports the use of dose increases and decreases in reducing illicit drug use among methadone patients, only the use of take-home methadone as a reward had been widely evaluated and found to be effective. Other procedures that have individual studies in support of them are findings such as those of McCarthy and Borders (1985) who found that threatened expulsion is effective with some patients in reducing drug use, and those of Stitzer and colleagues (1986) who found that dose increases (positive reinforcement) contingent upon drug-negative urine samples were just as effective as dose decreases (punishment) in response to drug-positive samples.

However, it is now widely recognised that there is a price to be paid for the relatively small reductions in drug use achieved by programs that employ negative consequences in contingency management programs and this is high treatment drop-out rates (Iguchi *et al.,* 1988; Stitzer *et al.,* 1986; Stitzer *et al.,* 1993). As a number of commentators have pointed out, the discovery of the HIV and hepatitis epidemics among injecting drug users has revealed the potential risk for patients not receiving treatment and this brings into question any treatment practice that entails an increase in the numbers of patients dropping out of treatment (e.g., Iguchi *et al.,* 1988; Kleber, 1994; Kolar *et al.,* 1990; Nolimal & Crowley, 1990; Zweben, 1993). The use of expulsion from treatment in response to relapse also attracts the same criticism. The evidence overall suggests that patients respond in an 'all or none' fashion to contingency management with only a small proportion stopping their illicit drug use and the rest not responding positively at all (Iguchi *et al.,* 1988; Magura *et al.,* 1988; Stitzer *et al.,* 1986; Stitzer *et al.,* 1993). No patient variables have been identified as being associated with a positive response to contingency management, so it is not possible to avoid a high drop-out rate by predicting which patients will respond well. A final problem with contingency management systems is that clinic staff are often concerned about the fate of patients who leave or are expelled from treatment and, for this reason, they will refuse to comply with or will actively subvert the system (Calsyn & Saxon, 1987).

Although popular in the past, the use of negative consequences and expulsion from treatment as a response to drug-positive urine samples has little experimental support and may have serious public and individual health consequences. The reduction of methadone doses as part of such systems is especially contraindicated given the importance of dosage to successful treatment (see Chapter 9; Kreek, 1993; Payte & Khuri, 1993; Stitzer *et al.*, 1993). However, the use of take-home methadone as a reward for drug-free urine samples does not seem to have any negative features associated with it and seems to be no less effective than punishment. It is important to add a patient perspective to the overall assessment of contingency management systems, because it brings into relief the dissonance that at times exists between what treatment providers think they are doing and how patients experience these actions. As we have already noted, Attewell and Gerstein (1979) found that patients view urine surveillance for illicit drug use as an arbitrary system not that different from a game of chance. In addition to this, Attewell and Gerstein found that patients in the methadone maintenance programs they surveyed regarded the ultimate punishment of mandatory detoxification not as the termination of treatment but as inflicting upon them the pain of withdrawal. Programs that readmit patients after a stipulated period of time reinforce this view among patients.

Is urinalysis more accurate than self-report?

One important reason for using urinalysis to monitor drug use is the assumption that patients will lie about their drug use when asked about it. This assumption is confirmed often in clinics where urinalysis results will reveal drug use in the face of the vehement denial of some patients. Nevertheless, it could be argued that the use of urinalysis itself is partly responsible for a climate in which patients feel they have to lie about their drug use. If the consequences of telling the truth are perceived to be some form of punishment, then it is highly likely that most patients will lie if asked about their drug use. The belief that patients will not be truthful may be a self-fulfilling prophecy based upon the experience that methadone maintenance clinic staff create the conditions within which such beliefs are always confirmed. There is some indirect support for such a proposition from the research literature on the veracity of self-report by methadone maintenance patients when interviewed by independent interviewers.

The veracity of self-reported drug use has been investigated by Magura and colleagues (Magura *et al.*, 1987; Magura & Lipton, 1988) who reviewed and reanalysed nine studies that reported on either former or current drug treatment patients and that compared self-report with urinalysis data. They concluded that this evidence suggests that under certain conditions many patients will tell the truth about their drug use. Under these conditions, self-report reveals as much drug use as does urinalysis. However, Magura *et al.* suspected that one possible confounding influence on the results of these studies was the relatively inaccurate urinalysis method (thin layer chromatography) used. A low rate of detection would perhaps have produced spurious correlations between the self-report and the urinalysis results. To test this they conducted a study comparing self-reported drug use and urinalysis results using the more sensitive EMIT system, as well as the usual thin layer chromatography procedure.

As suspected, the number of detected drug-positive samples was much higher when analysed by EMIT than by thin layer chromatography. In one of the studies, the latter method detected only 27% of the samples identified as drug positive by EMIT (Magura *et al.,* 1987). However, a fall in correspondence between self-report and the urinalysis data was not observed as expected when the more sensitive EMIT method was used (15% of self-reported opioid use was detected by thin layer chromatography: kappa = 0.17, p .01; and 34% by EMIT: kappa = 0.23, p .01). Despite the consistent concordance with the more sensitive method, it was still the case that some subjects who had not admitted their drug use were found to be drug positive through urinalysis (3% of opioid-negative self-reports were detected as positive by thin layer chromatography and 12% were detected as positive by EMIT). Magura *et al.* (1987) concluded that self-report reveals as much drug use as does urinalysis, but that both methods together reveal more than either method when used alone.

The review conducted by Magura *et al.* and their subsequent study suggest that under certain conditions, a majority of methadone maintenance patients will give reasonably accurate accounts about their drug use. However, these conditions have not traditionally been found in methadone treatment programs. Magura *et al.* (1988) point out that there are no non-controversial ways of resolving the problems associated with the use of urinalysis in methadone maintenance programs. One alternative they propose is the abandonment of scheduled urinalysis, pointing out that many clinical staff believe that if the treatment environment was oriented towards developing more cooperative relationships with patients, then the patients would be able to be honest about their drug use without fearing punishment and, in the end, would also be more amenable to change. In the next section, we consider the advantages and disadvantages of the various options available for the use of urine testing during opioid replacement therapy.

OPTIONS FOR THE USE OF URINALYSIS DURING OPIOID REPLACEMENT THERAPY

Routine Urinalysis

Although there is no evidence to support the view that urinalysis controls or reduces the illicit drug use of methadone maintenance patients, this is not the only reason for its traditional place in methadone programs. Urinalysis is also thought by some to be worthwhile as a clinical aid in guiding treatment and as an objective source of data for program evaluation and research. These benefits should be weighed against the personal and economic costs involved in frequent, routine testing.

If urinalysis continues to be employed in methadone maintenance programs, then there are a number of measures that can be taken to reduce costs and to ensure that the results obtained are the best possible indicator of patients' drug use. Having different schedules for patients at different stages of treatment, which is a common practice in many methadone clinics, is one way to reduce the overall frequency of tests and therefore the cost involved. New patients are monitored frequently in the first few weeks of treatment and the frequency of tests reduced as they become stabilised.

Testing stabilised patients who have responded well to treatment too frequently (more than once a month) may be of limited value considering the cost involved. There is perhaps no reason why such patients need to be tested at all except for program evaluation; behavioural signs of use or intoxication could be used as an indication of when testing is needed for clinical purposes. While this proposal does not remove the negative aspects associated with the use of urinalysis (such as the humiliation and lack of trust involved), it does allow for the development of trust and the possibility of graduating beyond a treatment practice that many patients dislike.

Two important conditions must be met if urinalysis is used to monitor patients' drug use. Every sample should be randomly taken at a time unknown to the patient concerned and its collection should be observed, or the temperature of the sample taken to ensure that it has not been tampered with in any way. If these two conditions are not met, then testing is a waste of time and money.

Infrequent Urinalysis

This option involves the abandonment of regular testing and would retain infrequent, random tests unmatched to individual patients for the purposes of program evaluation. It does not preclude the option of on-the-spot testing for any patient showing signs of intoxication or any other indications of relapse to chronic illicit drug use. This option would save a substantial amount of money and may have positive benefits on staff–patient relationships.

OTHER METHODS OF MONITORING DRUG USE

If urinalysis were abandoned as a means of monitoring drug use, then other means might be employed to assess programs and make clinical decisions. A number of authors have suggested this option (Goldstein & Judson, 1974; Gottheil *et al.*, 1976; Magura & Lipton, 1988). Goldstein and Judson (1974) have proposed that if equivalent treatment success rates could be achieved for the same or less expense by emphasising other aspects of treatment, then there is no justifiable reason to continue using urinalysis. Gottheil *et al.* (1976) suggested using the substantial money spent on urinalysis for expanding counselling services. Finally, Magura and Lipton (1988) reiterated this proposal when they argued that if urinalysis no longer became a part of methadone maintenance treatment, then better staff–patient ratios and a different conception of methadone maintenance programs would have to be developed.

However, if treatment delivery remains contingent upon abstinence from illicit drug use, then the reliance on self-report that these measures would ultimately depend upon would not be possible. Put simply, no patient is going to be honest about their drug use if there is a possibility that they will be dropped from treatment for doing so.

Hair Analysis

Another way of monitoring drug use and one that has attracted considerable attention is the toxicological analysis of samples of body hair (Magura *et al.*, 1992; Strang *et al.*, 1993). Traces of drugs ingested by an individual can be identified in hair within a few days of any given use episode, and one strand of hair will contain a living record of the subject's recent drug use history. This history may be as long or as short as the length of any given person's hair (5 cm = approximately four months' growth). Hair analysis may also provide information on the amount as well as the pattern of consumption, although the reliability and validity of the procedure is yet to be fully established (Cone *et al.*, 1995).

Clearly, hair analysis has the potential to be useful for both clinical and research purposes and it avoids many of the shortcomings of urinalysis. The taking of a sample does not involve the unpleasant features that are associated with the taking of a supervised urine sample. Hair retains traces of drugs used for much longer than they are present in urine, and ways in which the subject might interfere with a sample are not apparent, although the effect of hair treatments and dyes is not as yet known. As well as the usual uses of urinalysis as a measure of drug use both during and after treatment, hair analysis, unlike urinalysis, would be useful for establishing the history and extent of drug use at assessment for treatment. The one important qualification to this list of advantages is that hair analysis is, at the time of writing, expensive (A$30 per drug) and is not at a stage of development where it is suitable for routine use.

Magura *et al.* (1992) and Strang *et al.* (1993) also caution about the possibility that new technology such as hair analysis might lead to an over-enthusiastic spate of drug surveillance within drug treatment programs. According to Magura *et al.*, referring as much to urinalysis as any other form of drug testing:

> ...for patients who otherwise are 'doing well' (e.g., complying with therapy, employed), continuous testing to identify minimal illicit drug use or periodic 'slips' might actually do more harm than good if the clinician is (or feels) obligated to make a strong punitive response. It is important not to allow drug testing to become an end in itself during drug abuse treatment, but to consider carefully the rationale and value of any planned testing protocol for the program, the clinicians, and the individual patients (p. 66).

CONCLUSION

The economic and other costs involved in the use of urinalysis to monitor drug use during opioid replacement therapy has led to its reassessment as a useful clinical tool over recent years. In Australia, for example, the frequency of testing has been reduced in most methadone clinics as a result of the widespread adoption of a harm reduction treatment philosophy. This approach is consistent with the research reviewed in this chapter. The research that has been done suggests that a reduction in the frequency of testing, or its abandonment, does not lead to widespread illicit drug use among patients attending for opioid replacement therapy. It may, however, have positive consequences in terms of reducing those aspects of treatment that the patients experience as being unnecessarily controlling and confrontational. No matter what method is used to monitor illicit drug use in methadone maintenance programs, the reduction or elimination of drug use is only one way in which a beneficial treatment outcome might be measured. Improvements in health, social and psychological functioning, and reductions in involvement with crime are also important.

SUMMARY

Urinalysis is used in methadone maintenance treatment to monitor patients' unsanctioned drug use and to ensure that they are ingesting the methadone prescribed to them. The advantages of urinalysis are that it provides an objective means of monitoring drug use that can be used for program evaluation, making clinical decisions about patients, monitoring methadone ingestion, and as evidence in court. Urinalysis is also thought to reduce illicit drug use. The disadvantages of urinalysis are: the procedure communicates to patients from the outset that they are not to be trusted; it is humiliating for both patients and staff to either be observed urinating or to observe the act of urination; it is a relatively inaccurate measure of drug use; and, in the light of the former shortcoming, it is an expensive procedure.

Unless samples are taken every day, urinalysis is not a reliable method of monitoring drug use. Because daily testing is prohibitively expensive, tests are usually done less frequently but on a random basis to try to retain a reasonable chance of detecting illicit drug use while at the same time keeping costs down. Testing less than daily without adopting a random schedule allows patients safe periods for illicit drug use and is probably a waste of resources. Random schedules can be devised in a number of ways. The most efficient is when patients neither know the day they will be tested nor the period of time around which the schedule is conducted. To ensure that samples are not interfered with, the act of urination should be observed or the temperature of each sample tested.

Research that has examined the ability of urinalysis to reduce illicit drug use has found that it is not reliably effective. Attempts to increase the effectiveness of urinalysis results by using contingency management procedures have not demonstrated any enhanced impact over usual procedures. Few patients seem to respond to such interventions and any benefit that might be involved is offset by losing substantial numbers of patients from treatment. By way of contrast, research has consistently demonstrated that under conditions where methadone patients do not have to be concerned about being punished for doing so, they will be truthful about their drug use.

REFERENCES

Attewell, P., & Gerstein, D. R. (1979). Government policy and local practice. *American Sociological Review, 44*, 311-327.

Baldwin, R. (1987). The cost of methadone maintenance programs: A comparison between public hospital clinics and private practitioner programs in New South Wales. *Australian Drug and Alcohol Review, 6*, 185-193.

Barthwell, A., & Gastfriend, D. R. (1993). Treating multiple substance abuse. In M. W. Parrino (Ed.), *State methadone treatment guidelines* (pp. 73-84). Rockville, MD: Centre for Substance Abuse Treatment, U.S. Department of Health and Human Services.

Blanke, R. V. (1986). Accuracy in urinalysis. In R. L. Hawks & C. N. Chiang (Eds.), *Urine testing for drugs of abuse* (NIDA Research Monograph 73, pp. 43-53). Rockville, MD: National Institute on Drug Abuse.

Calsyn, D. A., & Saxon, A. J. (1987). A system for uniform application of contingencies for illicit drug use. *Journal of Substance Abuse Treatment, 4*, 41-47.

Calsyn, D. A., Saxon, A. J., & Barndt, D. C. (1991). Urine screening practices in methadone maintenance clinics: A survey of how the results are used. *Journal of Nervous and Mental Disease, 179*, 222-227.

Cone, E. J., Welch, M. J., & Babecki, M. B. G. (Eds.). (1995). *Hair testing for drugs of abuse: International research on standards and technology.* Rockville, MD: National Institute on Drug Abuse.

D'Amanda, C. (1983). Program policies and procedures associated with treatment outcome. In J. R. Cooper, F. Altman, B. S. Brown, & D. Czechowicz (Eds.), *Research on the treatment of narcotic addiction: State of the art* (pp. 637-679). Rockville, MD: National Institute on Drug Abuse.

De Angelis, G. G. (1972). Testing for drugs: Advantages and disadvantages. *International Journal of the Addictions, 7,* 365-385.

Dole, V. P., & Nyswander, M. (1965). A medical treatment for diacetylmorphine (heroin) addiction: A clinical trial with methadone hydrochloride. *Journal of the American Medical Association, 193,* 80-84.

Goldstein, A., & Brown, B. W. (1970). Urine testing schedules in methadone maintenance treatment of heroin addiction. *Journal of the American Medical Association, 214,* 311-315.

Goldstein, A., Horns, W. H., & Hansteen, R. W. (1977). Is on-site urine testing of therapeutic value in a methadone treatment program? *International Journal of the Addictions, 12,* 717-728.

Goldstein, A., & Judson, B. A. (1974). Three critical issues in the management of methadone programs. In P. G. Bourne (Ed.), *Addiction* (pp. 129-148). New York: Academic Press.

Gottheil, E., Caddy, G. R., & Austin, D. L. (1976). Fallibility of urine drug screens in monitoring methadone programs. *Journal of the American Medical Association, 236,* 1035-1038.

Grabowski, J., Rhoades, H., Elk, R., Schmitz, J., & Creson, D. (1993). Clinicwide and individualized behavioral interventions in drug dependence treatment. In L. S. Onken, J. D. Blaine, & J. J. Boren (Eds.), *Behavioral treatments for drug abuse and dependence* (NIDA Research Monograph 137, pp. 37-71). Rockville, MD: National Institute on Drug Abuse.

Grevert, P., & Weinberg, A. (1973). A controlled study of the clinical effectiveness of urine test results in a methadone maintenance program, *Proceedings of the 5th National Conference on methadone treatment* (pp. 1052-1059). New York: National Association for the Prevention of Addiction to Narcotics.

Hall, S. M. (1983). Methadone treatment: A review of the research findings. In J. R. Cooper, F. Altman, B. S. Brown, & D. Czechowicz (Eds.), *Research on the treatment of narcotic addiction: State of the art* (pp. 575-632). Rockville, MD: National Institute on Drug Abuse.

Hansen, H. J., Caudill, S. P., & Boone, J. (1985). Crisis in drug testing: Results of CDC blind study. *Journal of the American Medical Association, 253,* 2382-2387.

Harford, R. J., & Kleber, H. D. (1978). Comparative validity of random-interval and fixed-interval urinalysis schedules. *Archives of General Psychiatry, 35,* 356-359.

Havassy, B., & Hall, S. (1981). Efficacy of urine monitoring in methadone maintenance. *American Journal of Psychiatry, 138*, 1497-1500.

Iguchi, M. Y., Stitzer, M. L., Bigelow, G. E., & Liebson, I. A. (1988). Contingency management in methadone maintenance: Effects of reinforcing and aversive consequences on illicit poly drug use. *Drug and Alcohol Dependence, 22*, 1-7.

Judson, B. A., Himmelberger, D. U., & Goldstein, A. (1979). Measurement of urine temperature as an alternative to observed urination in a narcotic treatment program. *American Journal of Drug and Alcohol Abuse, 6*, 197-205.

Kleber, H. D. (Ed.). (1994). *Assessment and treatment of cocaine-abusing methadone-maintained patients.* Rockville, MD: Center for Substance Abuse Treatment, U.S. Department of Health and Human Services.

Kleber, H. D., & Gould, L. C. (1971). Urine testing schedules in methadone maintenance. *Journal of the American Medical Association, 215*, 2115-2116.

Kolar, A. F., Brown, B. S., Weddington, W., & Ball, J. C. (1990). A treatment crisis: Cocaine use by clients in methadone maintenance programs. *Journal of Substance Abuse Treatment, 7*, 101-107.

Kreek, M. J. (1993). Epilogue - A personal retrospective and prospective viewpoint. In M. W. Parrino (Ed.), *State methadone treatment guidelines* (pp. 133-143). Rockville, MD: Center for Substance Abuse Treatment, U.S. Department of Health and Human Services.

Lewis, V. S., Petersen, D. M., Geis, G., & Pollack, S. (1972). Ethical and social-psychological aspects of urinalysis to detect heroin use. *British Journal of Addiction, 67*, 303-307.

Magura, S., Casriel, C., Goldsmith, D. S., Strug, D. L., & Lipton, D. S. (1988). Contingency contracting with polydrug-abusing methadone patients. *Addictive Behaviors, 13*, 113-118.

Magura, S., Freeman, R. C., Siddiqi, Q., & Lipton, D. S. (1992). The validity of hair analysis for detecting cocaine and heroin use among addicts. *International Journal of the Addictions, 27*, 51-69.

Magura, S., Goldsmith, D., Casriel, C., Goldstein, P. J., & Lipton, D. S. (1987). The validity of methadone clients' self-reported drug use. *International Journal of the Addictions, 22*, 727-749.

Magura, S., & Lipton, D. S. (1988). The accuracy of drug use monitoring in methadone treatment. *Journal of Drug Issues, 18*, 317-326.

Manno, J. E. (1986a). Interpretation of urinalysis results. In R. L. Hawks & C. N. Chiang (Eds.), *Urine testing for drugs of abuse* (NIDA Research Monograph 73, pp 54-61). Rockville, MD: National Institute on Drug Abuse.

Manno, J. E. (1986b). Specimen collection and handling. In R. L. Hawks & C. N. Chiang (Eds.), *Urine testing for drugs of abuse* (NIDA Research Monograph 73, pp. 24-29). Rockville, MD: National Institute on Drug Abuse.

Marion, I. J. (1993). Urinalysis as a clinical tool. In M. W. Parrino (Ed.), *State methadone treatment guidelines* (pp. 59-65). Rockville, MD: Center for Substance Abuse Treatment, U.S. Department of Health and Human Services.

McCarthy, J. J., & Borders, O. T. (1985). Limit setting on drug abuse in methadone maintenance patients. *American Journal of Psychiatry, 142,* 1419-1423.

Montalvo, J.G., Scrignar, C. B., Alderette, E., Harper, B., & Eyer, D. (1972). Flushing, pale-colored urines, and false negatives: Urinalysis of narcotic addicts. *International Journal of the Addictions, 7,* 355-364.

Moran, J., Mayberry, C., Kinniburgh, D., & James, D. (1995). Program monitoring for clinical practice: Specimen positivity across urine collection methods. *Journal of Substance Abuse Treatment, 12,* 223-226.

Nolimal, D., & Crowley, T. J. (1990). Difficulties in a clinical application of methadone-dose contingency contracting. *Journal of Substance Abuse Treatment, 7,* 219-224.

Payte, J. T., & Khuri, E. T. (1993). Principles of methadone dose determination. In M. W. Parrino (Ed.), *State methadone treatment guidelines* (pp. 47-58). Rockville, MD: Center for Substance Abuse Treatment, U.S. Department of Health and Human Services.

Schwartz, B., Lauderdale, R. M., Montgomery, M. L., Burch, E. A., & Gallant, D. M. (1987). Immediate versus delayed feedback on urinalyses reports for methadone maintenance patients. *Addictive Behaviors, 12,* 293-295.

Stitzer, M. L., Bickel, W. K., Bigelow, G. E., & Liebson, I. A. (1986). Effect of methadone dose contingencies on urinalysis test results of polydrug-abusing methadone-maintenance patients. *Drug and Alcohol Dependence, 18,* 341-348.

Stitzer, M. L., Bigelow, G. E., & McCaul, M. E. (1985). Behavior therapy in drug abuse treatment: Review and evaluation. In R. J. Asherry (Ed.), *Progress in the development of cost-effective treatment for drug abusers* (NIDA Research Monograph 58, pp. 31-49). Rockville, MD: National Institute on Drug Abuse.

Stitzer, M. L., Iguchi, M. Y., Kidorf, M., & Bigelow, G. E. (1993). Contingency management in methadone treatment: The case for positive incentives. In L. S. Onken, J. D. Blaine, & J. J. Boren (Eds.), *Behavioral treatments for drug abuse and dependence* (NIDA Research Monograph 137, pp. 19-35). Rockville, MD: National Institute on Drug Abuse.

Strang, J., Black, J., Marsh, A., & Smith, B. (1993). Hair analysis for drugs: Technological breakthrough or ethical quagmire? *Addiction, 88,* 163-166.

Swensen, G. (1989). The cost of the Western Australian methadone program. *Australian Drug and Alcohol Review, 8,* 35-37.

Trellis, E. S., Smith, F. F., Alston, D. C., & Siassi, I. (1975). The pitfalls of urine surveil-lance: The role of research in evaluation and remedy. *Addictive Behaviors,* 1, 83-88.

Ward, P., Sutton, M. & Mattick, R.P. (1996). *Cost analysis of the public methadone program in New South Wales.* Unpublished manuscript, National Drug and Alcohol Research Centre, University of New South Wales, Australia.

Wells, R., & McKay, B. (1989). *Review of funding of methadone programs in Australia.* Report to the Australian Department of Community Services and Health.

Zweben, J. E. (1993). Review of clinical issues. In M. W. Parrino (Ed.), *State methadone treatment guidelines* (pp. 25-32). Rockville, MD: Center for Substance Abuse Treatment, U.S. Department of Health and Human Services.

11

THE ROLE OF COUNSELLING AND PSYCHOLOGICAL THERAPY

RICHARD P. MATTICK, JEFF WARD
AND WAYNE HALL

INTRODUCTION

The role and value of counselling in methadone maintenance treatment has been an issue that has attracted conflicting views, partly because of a lack of clear evidence of its impact on drug use and associated behaviours. It is true that most of the randomised controlled trials of methadone maintenance reviewed in Chapter 2 included provision of psychosocial services in addition to methadone (Dole *et al.*, 1969; Gunne & Grönbladh, 1981; Newman & Whitehill, 1979), and many authors suggest that counselling is important in determining treatment outcome (Grönbladh & Gunne, 1989). On the other hand, programs with minimal counselling and other ancillary services have been advocated as a way of making methadone maintenance available to more people due to the lower cost involved. These low intervention programs are run in a number of countries, and it is apparent that for some countries the provision of intensive counselling and ancillary services may be unachievable without markedly restricting the availability of the opioid replacement therapy. Given the public health impact of methadone treatment in terms of its protective effects on health through the reduction of needle sharing and infectious disease spread, the maximum distribution of the scarce treatment resource of methadone dosing must be balanced with the benefits that accrue from more expensive and less freely accessible treatment. The issue of the appropriateness of ancillary services is essentially one of the cost-effectiveness of methadone maintenance with and without different levels of ancillary services (see Chapter 5).

This chapter attempts to throw some light on the role that counselling has in methadone maintenance treatment by examining the accumulated evidence with regard to the contribution of counselling to patient outcome. Research on the related issue of the effectiveness and appropriateness of psychotherapy is also reviewed, along with evidence on the characteristics of effective therapists and counsellors. The role of urinalysis is reviewed in Chapter 10.

COUNSELLING

Introduction

Counselling, along with other ancillary services, was originally conceived as assisting the rehabilitative goals of methadone maintenance treatment. Put simply, it was thought that the provision of methadone would stabilise patients physically and psychologically, while counselling would address the adjustment problems that can accrue from long-term illicit heroin use. The early practitioners of methadone treatment rejected the view that dependent individuals have pre-existing psychological problems of some sort, arguing strongly that most of their patients' problems were a result of having to maintain a heroin habit, or were due to the socio-economic conditions under which they had grown up (Dole & Nyswander, 1967; Newman, 1974). The form of counselling that the opioid dependent were thought to require, therefore, was focused on the practicalities of organising their lives, including assistance with housing, job-seeking, and sorting out their legal problems and family relationships. However, the exact constituents of counselling as delivered in methadone maintenance programs are sometimes unclear. The next section considers the nature of the activities that fall under the rubric of counselling.

What Does Counselling Involve?

Although occasional articles have been published over the past three decades describing particular models of methadone maintenance treatment (Kaufman & Blaine, 1974), until relatively recently little has been known about the day-to-day activities of methadone programs, what services they deliver, and how those services affect their patients. Counselling is in some ways exemplary in this regard. Fortunately, Ball and Ross's (1991) in-depth account of six methadone clinics in three cities in the north-east of the USA has provided an account of what counsellors actually do on a day-to-day basis in methadone programs. A further US report (General Accounting Office, 1990) has also provided information about counselling services offered in 24 public methadone maintenance programs across the USA, and Calsyn and colleagues (Calsyn *et al.*, 1990) have published the results of a 1984 national survey of the staffing patterns of USA methadone units which provides some insight into the services being offered to patients. The account of the findings of the Treatment Outcome Prospective Study (TOPS) has also provided some information on counselling services delivered in the 17 methadone maintenance units that participated in the study (Hubbard *et al.*, 1989). In Australia, comparable information has been provided by a report on 17 public methadone maintenance clinics (Australian Social Issues Research, 1991) and a national survey of treatment practices (Baillie *et al.*, 1992).

What does a counsellor in a methadone maintenance clinic do? U.S. research (Ball & Ross, 1991) has found that most of what counsellors do can be described by ten activities: case management; liaising with other social service agencies; assessing new applicants; one-to-one counselling; brief contacts; group therapy; family and couples therapy; assessment for psychological problems; vocational counselling; and education. Case management refers to the ongoing documentation and care of the clients that make up a counsellor's case-load. This involves keeping records, representing the client at case meetings, and disciplining the client for misbehaviour and drug-positive urinalysis results. Ball and Ross (1991) emphasised the importance of the 'brief contact' – a term that refers to the brief communications between a counsellor and their client when they meet in the hallway, or when the client drops in to ask a question. Though all of the above listed activities were offered at one or other of the participating methadone maintenance programs, by far the majority of the counselling activity was taken up by brief contacts, one-to-one counselling and group work, in that order.

Nearly all patients in the six programs had regular (on average fortnightly) one-to-one counselling sessions, a pattern that was also found in the study conducted by the General Accounting Office (1990). The topics dealt with in these sessions ranged from current problems related to work, health and the law, and to case management issues such as clinic attendance and ongoing drug use. One important topic early in treatment was helping the patient to understand and comply with the program rules. The general focus, both in terms of time spent on the issue and in terms of the overall goal of treatment, was on what Ball and Ross described as rehabilitation. The way in which counsellors 'rehabilitated' their clients varied considerably, with the approach being determined by training and/or program philosophy and goals, as well as the individual needs of their clients. Whereas some counsellors took a more active approach in terms of giving advice and focusing on behaviour modification, other counsellors took a more traditional counselling approach and focused on their clients' psychological problems rather than their drug use alone.

Group sessions accounted for much less of the face-to-face contact between patients and counsellors and tended to be topic-oriented rather than generally therapeutic. This result is consistent with that from the TOPS study where 78% of the patients surveyed received mostly individual counselling and only 7% reported any group therapy (Hubbard *et al.*, 1989). Ball and Ross (1991) found that groups were usually convened for special purposes, such as dealing with cocaine or alcohol problems, and were attended by individuals with those problems. Other interventions, such as family therapy, were offered to only a few patients, as was psychological assessment, both being based on the needs of the patient. Vocational guidance and education, though available throughout the study period, were only taken advantage of by a minority of patients, a disinterest noted by others (Brewington *et al.*, 1990).

One important role that methadone maintenance programs fulfil for their patients is crisis intervention. Ball and Ross (1991) found that counsellors were not the only staff members who were involved in this activity, although in some programs at least one counsellor was always available on a roster basis. Medical, nursing and administrative staff also helped patients with urgent problems. These crises involved a range of problems from serious trauma through to less serious matters. Ball and Ross (1991) cite the following examples:

> . . . suicide attempts, acute depression, auto accident, arrest, fear of gang violence, rape, assault, bereavement, loss of place to live, discharge from program, recognition of HIV positivity, end of welfare payments for family, and so forth (p. 142).

It is generally the consensus that a methadone clinic should provide a point of contact where patients' problems can be assessed, and from where they could be referred elsewhere if they were found to need specialist treatment (Hagman, 1994). If referrals are to be successful, however, special effort is necessary to ensure that the patient being referred arrives at their destination and is welcome when they arrive there – methadone maintenance patients are often not welcome in other sectors of the health care system. One way that has been suggested to ensure more successful referrals is for a member of the referring clinic to accompany the patient to the place of referral and to personally introduce their patient to the specialist concerned.

Is Counselling Necessary?

The answer to this question has been unclear for some time. Commenting on the area, some (Newman & Peyser, 1991) have argued that there is a pervasive belief that ancillary services are the most important components of effective methadone maintenance treatment (see Burgess *et al.*, 1990; Renner, 1984), even though there had been relatively little research evidence to support this proposition. They contrast this belief with what they see as a reluctance to acknowledge the potency of methadone in bringing about the changes that have been associated with maintenance therapy. The evidence presented in this book that addresses the efficacy of methadone, the dose of methadone and the duration of methadone, argues for the central role of the drug substitution in bringing about reductions in drug use. Additionally, the results of the study by Yancovitz and colleagues (1991) on interim methadone maintenance dosing have shown the potential of methadone maintenance devoid of ancillary services to reduce illicit opiate use (see Chapter 2). The randomised research reviewed in Chapter 2 suggests that methadone treatment, with or without counselling, brings about behavioural change, but the reverse is not true. Counselling without drug substitution is not effective.

There has been limited evidence that methadone maintenance without ancillary services (such as counselling) would be as effective as methadone maintenance with more intensive ancillary services. Yet, Newman and Peyser's point remains valid: it is reasonable to assume that the replacement of heroin with an adequate daily dose of methadone would have a substantial impact on the life of a person whose day-to-day activities are dominated by the pursuit of heroin and the money necessary to buy it.

An early attempt to address the issue was reported by Ramer and colleagues (1971) who set out to test high dose methadone maintenance with and without ancillary services. The study was quickly abandoned in response to the requests of unit staff who felt that it was unethical to deny patients the benefit of counselling services, especially when they were experiencing crises in their lives. However, the study did provide some pertinent information. One important finding that arose was that patients with psychiatric diagnoses had the worst outcome of the patients participating in the study. In a subsequent comparative observational (non-randomised) study that attempted to examine the issue, Longwell and colleagues (1978) compared the urinalysis results of two groups of patients in a methadone maintenance program in Arizona: those seeing a counsellor, and those who were not seeing a counsellor. They found that patients who received no counselling had significantly more opiate-positive urinalysis results compared to those who did. This result is consistent with the view that counselling has a positive effect on illicit drug use; yet it is difficult to be confident that the apparent difference is attributable to counselling, since the patients in the Longwell study were not randomly allocated to receive counselling or not, and no statistical procedures were used to assess whether those patients in the counselling groups differed in any way from those in the non-counselling group.

The extent to which counselling is an important part of methadone maintenance treatment was also addressed by Ball and Ross (1991) in their correlational study. They note that both the staff and patients at the methadone units that participated in their study viewed counselling as the most important component of the rehabilitative aspect of methadone treatment. Ball and Ross provided some evidence that programs providing 'a high level of treatment services to patients' were associated with less heroin use, less cocaine use, less injecting drug use and less criminal behaviour among their patients. The high level treatment services included: (a) patients being regularly counselled, in (b) adequate counselling services, and receiving (c) a high rate of attendance for medication, along with (d) a long-term maintenance and rehabilitation policy. The Ball and Ross (1991) finding is consistent with the recent report of others (Joe *et al.*, 1991). Joe *et al.* (1991) found an increase in retention as measured survival rate for more intense 'psychological' services. The survival rate increased by 13% for each unit of a six-category measure of frequency of contact which went from none through to daily. For a full description of the Treatment Outcome Prospective Study (Joe *et al.*, 1991) see Chapter 3. These two findings suggest that more intense counselling services lead to a better outcome – reduced drug use, injecting, and crime – and retention for methadone maintenance treatment, respectively.

More recently, U.S. research has addressed these issues in randomised research trials and has thrown some light on the value of counselling. The VA-Penn group foreshadowed the need to address the issue of ancillary services (Childress *et al.*, 1991), and described a three-group randomised controlled trial comparing "minimum methadone maintenance", "basic methadone maintenance" and "enhanced methadone maintenance". The full study results were reported on two years later (McLellan *et al.*, 1993). The content of the three levels of intervention is important:

- Minimum methadone maintenance involved 60-90 mg methadone daily plus emergency counselling and referral services, but no "regular counselling, no privilege or service contingencies based on urine results, and no... family or employment counselling" (p. 172) (Childress *et al.*, 1991).

- Basic methadone maintenance also involved 60-90mg methadone daily plus "regular, supervised counselling and referral services using weekly urine screens as the basis for contingency management... but no... family or employment counselling" (p. 172) (Childress *et al.*, 1991).

- Enhanced methadone maintenance offered the same services as the basic approach, but added regular medical/psychiatric care, social work assistance, family therapy, and employment counselling.

McLellan *et al.* (1993) reported that while the minimum intervention group patients showed reductions in opiate use, they also had a higher rate of opiate-positive urines than the basic counselling group. The enhanced services group showed the greatest reduction in opiate-positive urines. The authors concluded that methadone alone may only be effective for a minority of patients (although they do not specify the size of the "minority"), and argued that the addition of counselling, medical, and psychosocial services dramatically enhanced the efficacy of methadone alone. It does appear, however, that the minimum methadone patients achieved reductions in illicit opioid use, although the full extent of the reduction is not clear as the research report focuses on opioid positive urine results, rather than extent of reduction in injecting of opiates, overall. Yet, on balance, provision of counselling did produce a better outcome than minimal counselling intervention.

Anglin and colleagues (1993) have also addressed the relative value of standard and enhanced methadone dosing for illicit opioid users at high risk of contracting or transmitting HIV. They described these interventions as incorporating the following components:

- Standard methadone maintenance involved two hourly sessions of counselling each month plus crisis intervention counselling as requested, medical examinations at entry and annually, and take-home doses contingent on "acceptable performance" in treatment.

- Enhanced methadone maintenance added counsellor and case manager training to maximise counsellor effectiveness, an intensive first-month contract, incentives contingent on the provision of opiate-free urines, and further enhanced services including case management, crisis management, psychiatric care, incentives such as redeemable restaurant coupons to reduce illicit drug use, additional urinalysis, and group meetings.

These researchers (Grella *et al.*, 1994; Hasson *et al.*, 1994) reported that the patients randomised to the enhanced methadone program had difficulty taking advantage of the services offered. They argued that the "demonstration project" had shown significant barriers to the widespread implementation of the enhanced program. In particular, they found that an "inordinate" amount of counsellor time was spent assisting the clients of the enhanced program to obtain basic services and necessities, while the patients were unwilling to involve themselves in the support services, and there was a reluctance on the part of service providers to work with methadone patients. Others have also noted the reluctance of methadone patients to be involved in rehabilitative efforts (Brewington *et al.*, 1990). Anglin's group did, however, report that the enhanced counselling condition was associated with better retention in treatment, being predictive of a lowered rate of discharge from the program (Grella *et al.*, 1994). As retention in treatment is an important feature of methadone maintenance treatment, these results do suggest some advantage for enhanced services over the standard level of intervention. However, there were no other advantages for the enhanced intervention.

A further study showing little advantage for enhanced services over standard counselling also found little benefit. Saxon and colleagues (1996) randomly allocated over 300 methadone patients to receive:

- Medication only without counselling (pharmacological treatment with no psychosocial services);

- Standard methadone maintenance involving regular sessions of counselling each month plus drug education classes and psychiatric evaluation and care if required;

- Enhanced methadone maintenance that added a sixteen-session relapse prevention skills training program plus weekly group therapy involving anger management, vocational workshops, and "self-awareness groups and process groups".

They reported that the provision of medication alone (pharmacological treatment with no psychosocial services) predicted more frequent opiate use compared with the standard counselling condition, but that there was no advantage for the enhanced services.

Another disappointing result for enhanced services came from a study of pregnant methadone-maintained women (Carroll *et al.*, 1995). In a randomised trial, 20 women were allocated to receive:

- Standard methadone maintenance involving methadone dosing, weekly group counselling, and regular urinalysis;

- Enhanced methadone maintenance involving weekly midwife pre-natal care visits, weekly relapse prevention groups, positive contingencies for abstinence, and child care during treatment visits.

There were no differences between the groups in terms of illicit drug use, but advantages were observed in terms of increased birthweight and longer gestations.

Turning to employment status, there is some evidence of benefit from specific interventions. US researchers (Platt *et al.,* 1993) randomly allocated 130 methadone patients to receive a 10-session vocational problem solving intervention aimed at identifying social and psychological barriers to working, and developing strategies to overcome the barriers. They found that employment rate increased in the intervention participants at short-term follow-up, but were not maintained in the longer term. Preliminary results from another trial has provided similar results, suggestive that specific vocational services are likely to increase employment among methadone patients (Dennis *et al.,* 1993).

DeLeon and colleagues (1995) have reported on the use of therapeutic community methods for the management of methadone patients, and found that patients who entered a therapeutic community and stayed for 6 months had better outcomes than a comparison group of patients who did not enter such treatment. The results are interesting, but the non-randomised non-equivalent design prevents attribution of the benefit to the therapeutic community as such, as motivational factors are not ruled out as explaining the differences obtained.

Counsellor Training

It has been commonplace in the USA to employ 'ex-addict' counsellors in methadone maintenance programs, presumably in the belief that ex-addicts have advantages in this role because of their own experience of being opioid dependent (Siassi *et al.,* 1977). However, there is no reason to assume that an individual's experience of addiction is a ready-made qualification for helping others with their drug dependence. Still, as some claim, it may be the case that ex-addict counsellors are perceived by patients to be more approachable than their 'straight' counterparts, but there is no evidence that this has any significant effect on outcome.

Two findings in the literature suggest that ex-addict counsellors may not be as effective as ordinary counsellors. Siassi and colleagues (1977) compared the performance of ex-addict and other counsellors and found that non-addict counsellors performed better on a range of indicators. Others (McLellan *et al.,* 1988), in a study comparing four counsellors, found that the three trained non-addict counsellors were more effective than their ex-addict counterparts.

In contrast, Longwell and colleagues (1978) found no difference in the effectiveness of ex-addict and non-addict counsellors. An investigation to determine whether professional and non-professional counsellors (ex-addict and non-addict) fulfilled different roles in a range of drug treatment programs across the USA, found that there was little difference in what the various types of counsellors did, or in how they went about it, and few differences in counsellors' or clients' attitudes and expectations concerning each other or treatment (Aiken *et al.*, 1984a). The only exception was that ex-addict counsellors were perceived by clients as being more accessible and better able to understand their clients' lives and problems (LoSciuto *et al.*, 1984). Aiken and her colleagues (1984b) went on to compare the outcome of clients of paraprofessional (ex-addict and non-addict) and professional counsellors and found no differences on a range of outcomes.

The more pertinent question to be answered in relation to the studies reviewed above is whether trained counsellors, no matter what their drug use history, are more effective than untrained counsellors. Moreover, for this question to be answered, it will be necessary to clarify the meaning of the word 'training'. Does it mean that the counsellor concerned has been trained as a general counsellor in a postgraduate course for this purpose? Does it mean that the counsellor concerned has attended training courses while working in a methadone maintenance unit and has developed expertise in this fashion? The fact that there is no clear definition of the role and the goals of counselling in methadone maintenance programs makes this task even more difficult. There is a clear need to define the task of counselling and, on the evidence to date, there is no reason to believe that a person without training would be an effective counsellor. There is also a need to ensure that counsellors implement their interventions faithfully, and evidence that the content of treatment does not always match the label it is given (Baranackie & Crits-Christoph, 1992).

Psychotherapy

According to Kleber (1984) psychotherapy can be distinguished from counselling by the fact that it attempts to influence mental processes which are believed to underlie maladaptive behaviour. In the case of psychodynamic psychotherapy, these mental processes are assumed to consist of unconscious conflicts. For cognitive-behavioural therapy the underlying cognitive processes are believed to be maladaptive negative behaviours, thoughts and emotions. Another way of making the distinction is that suggested by Woody and colleagues (1983), according to whom counselling focuses on external matters that are often resolved by specific and direct assistance of some sort, whereas psychotherapy is concerned with the internal psychological processes of the client. In other words, counselling mainly consists of 'practical problem solving' (Hubbard *et al.*, 1989) or as Kleber (1984) suggested, counselling involves adopting a common sense approach that focuses on support and help.

In this section we examine the more recent research on the use of psychotherapy as an adjunct to methadone maintenance treatment. Early (mainly psychoanalytic) case reports from the pre-methadone maintenance period are not reviewed, except to say that it has long been believed that opioid-dependent individuals are not amenable to psychotherapy.

The New Haven Psychotherapy Study

Rounsaville and his colleagues (1983, 1986) conducted a well-designed, randomised controlled trial that compared six months of weekly interpersonal psychotherapy (IPT) with a low-contact control condition consisting of a brief monthly appointment with a psychiatrist. Interpersonal psychotherapy is an individual therapy in which the focus of discussion is primarily upon interpersonal or relationship issues. According to Rounsaville *et al.* (1983):

> Short-term IPT is based on the concept that psychiatric disorders, including depression and opiate addiction, are intimately associated with disturbances in interpersonal functioning, which may be associated with the genesis and perpetuation of the disorder (p. 630).

In the trial conducted by Rounsaville *et al.*, 72 subjects who had a current psychiatric disorder were assessed on a range of outcomes and psychiatric indicators at the commencement of the study, at four-week intervals until the end of the treatment period, and followed two-and-a-half years later. All subjects also had to attend a 90-minute session of group therapy once a week as part of their methadone maintenance program.

Rounsaville *et al.* (1983) found no indication of an advantage for short-term IPT on any of the assessed outcomes in comparison to the low-contact control condition. In fact, they found support for the long-held clinical wisdom that opioid-dependent individuals will not attend for psychotherapy (Woody *et al.*, 1986), in that patients in the IPT condition were more likely to drop out of the study than were patients in the control condition. Rounsaville *et al.* (1983) point out that the lack of any demonstrable benefit for IPT, and indeed for psychotherapy, in this study is inconsistent with previous research that has shown IPT to be of benefit to depressed patients. It also conflicts with the findings of others (Stanton *et al.*, 1982; Woody *et al.*, 1983; Woody *et al.*, 1987) which indicate that some methadone maintenance patients may benefit from psychotherapy. Rounsaville *et al.* suggest that there may be no discernible benefit for additional psychotherapy in a high intervention methadone maintenance program that offers both counselling on demand and compulsory group therapy on a weekly basis. Substantial attrition from the study may also have made it difficult to demonstrate an effect, although Rounsaville *et al.* point out that the subjects who left IPT did not generally leave the methadone program, suggesting they had lost interest in IPT rather than methadone maintenance treatment.

The VA-Penn Psychotherapy Study

The Philadelphia Veterans Administration Medical Center – University of Pennsylvania (VA-Penn) psychotherapy study was reported by Woody and colleagues (1983, 1987) in an attempt to determine whether psychotherapy could be a useful adjunct to the high intervention, low dose methadone maintenance treatment being delivered at the medical centre to male war veterans. Taking four-and-a-half years to complete, this study remains the largest and most successfully conducted study of psychotherapy with opioid-dependent clients reported to date. In this study, 110 methadone-maintained, male war veterans were randomly assigned to one of three conditions: supportive-expressive psychotherapy (SE – a psychodynamic psychotherapy) plus drug counselling (DC); cognitive-behavioural psychotherapy (CB) plus DC; and DC without additional psychotherapy. Sessions with psychotherapists and counsellors were scheduled weekly and the study period was for six months.

When assessed at seven months from the commencement of psychotherapy (i.e., at one month after the psychotherapy was ceased) the patients who had received psychotherapy in addition to DC made both more and larger improvements than those who received only DC. Statistically significant differences between pre- and post-study assessment scores were observed in 12 of the outcome measures for the SE group, nine for the CB group and seven for the DC group. The SE group made strong gains in the areas of psychiatric symptoms and employment. In terms of drug use, all three groups improved but the SE and DC groups improved more than the CB group. When illicit opiate use was examined, the SE and CB groups had significantly less use than the DC group, even though the DC patients were maintained on higher doses of methadone than the SE and CB groups whose doses declined over the study period. Finally, DC patients were prescribed more ancillary psychotropic medication than the psychotherapy patients; in fact, the number of prescriptions written for the DC patients increased over the study period, whereas they decreased for the psychotherapy patients. Overall, the psychotherapy patients needed less methadone and ancillary medication, and made greater gains in a number of areas, than the DC patients. The two psychotherapy groups only differed significantly in a few areas: SE patients made greater improvements on measures for psychological functioning and employment, while CB patients had significantly less legal problems.

Woody and his colleagues reported the results of the 12-month follow-up assessments in 1987. They found that, in general, scores for the three treatment groups (SE, CB and DC) remained improved when compared with baseline measures. However, significant differences between the two sets of scores were found on 10 measures for the SE group, on 12 for the CB group, but on only two for the DC only group.

When the scores were looked at in more detail, it was evident that the majority of gains observed at seven months were maintained in the SE group, with further improvement being seen in employment, legal status, and psychiatric functioning. For the CB group, most of the gains were still evident at 12 months and further improvements had occurred in drug and alcohol problems and psychiatric condition. The DC-only group maintained improvement in drug use and employment but the previous gains made in psychiatric functioning declined. Legal status in the DC-only group had become significantly worse in the period between 7- and 12-month follow-up. When the records for patients still in methadone maintenance were scrutinised at 12 months it was found that, like at seven months, patients who had the benefit of psychotherapy seemed to require a lower dose of methadone, and fewer psychotropic medications, while maintaining low levels of illicit drug use.

In a further study of cognitive-behavioural psychotherapy at the Veterans Administration methadone program in Philadelphia, subjects who were randomly assigned to cognitive-behavioural therapy did better on a range of outcomes measured one month after the completion of treatment than did subjects who received drug counselling (McLellan *et al.*, 1986). The addition of a procedure to extinguish conditioned responses to drug-related stimuli (e.g., preparing drugs to inject) to cognitive-behavioural psychotherapy did not lead to a better outcome, and the authors concluded that this procedure was therefore unsuitable for patients who were being maintained on methadone, or being treated on an outpatient basis. Woody and his colleagues (1990) foreshadowed a further study in methadone units based in the community to assess the effectiveness of adding SE psychotherapy to methadone maintenance treatment. They found that the results of the randomised trial showed that, compared to drug counselling, SE psychotherapy added to the benefits of drug counselling for psychiatrically symptomatic methadone patients across a broad range of outcome measures (Woody *et al.*, 1995).

Woody *et al.* (1983) argued that the addition of psychotherapy to a traditional methadone maintenance treatment service was successful because the therapy entailed a special kind of relationship – a therapeutic alliance – as well as special knowledge about how to manage that relationship. They observed that although many of the drug counsellors develop very good relationships with their clients, they had difficulty managing the relationship at times, especially when dealing with the more disturbed clients. In order to examine this possibility they went on to analyse the data taking into account the severity of psychiatric problems found among the patients participating in the study.

Psychiatric Severity and Response to Psychotherapy

Methadone maintenance patients suffer from high levels of psychiatric disorders, especially depressive disorders, and the severity with which they suffer from these disorders is predictive of treatment outcome (Chapter 17). Woody and colleagues (1984) examined the seven-month follow-up data collected in the VA-Penn study to determine if the addition of psychotherapy had made any difference to the relationship between psychiatric severity and outcome. A composite psychiatric severity score was calculated on the basis of the ASI psychiatric severity score and the other psychological assessment scales administered at the commencement of the study. Psychiatric severity scores for each patient were then categorised into low, medium and high severity groups and the data reanalysed by treatment group.

Significant improvements were found for low severity patients in all three groups and the addition of psychotherapy of either kind (SE or CB) offered no advantage. However, in the group of patients with medium severity scores, positive change occurred in all three therapy conditions, but the psychotherapy groups showed more changes on psychological assessment scores. Significant differences were observed between the psychotherapy and DC conditions, the majority of them showing an advantage for psychotherapy. The medium severity DC patients were also maintained on significantly higher methadone doses and required more psychotropic medication than the patients who received additional psychotherapy.

A clear benefit for receiving psychotherapy was also apparent for the high severity group. Both the CB and SE groups had improved at seven-month follow-up on most outcome measures and had made large gains on measures for employment, legal status and psychiatric functioning. By comparison, high psychiatric severity patients who received DC only changed little on any of the assessment measures, except for drug use, which showed a significant improvement. When the three groups were compared with each other, it was found that the DC group was poorer on nine out of 10 significant outcome measures. DC patients also required higher mean methadone doses and more psychotropic medicine than the psychotherapy patients. High severity patients, when compared as a group to the other two severity categories, had higher mean doses of methadone, a higher proportion of drug positive urine results, and were prescribed more psychotropic medicine. The low and medium severity groups did not differ on these measures.

As Woody *et al.* (1984) point out, three main points emerge from these data. First, patients in the high severity category had poorer pre-treatment functioning in all of the measures assessed than did medium or low severity patients. This is consistent with previous findings. The most common diagnosis in the high severity group was a depressive disorder. Secondly, high severity patients did not respond in any of the three conditions as well as patients with less severe psychiatric problems. High severity patients gained little from DC by itself. Thirdly, psychotherapy, when added to traditional methadone maintenance, made a difference to the relationship between psychiatric severity and treatment outcome. In this study, high severity patients improved in many areas of functioning and, in comparison with the DC patients, were able to do so on lower doses of methadone and with less psychotropic medication while taking fewer illicit drugs.

One difficulty with the interpretation of the main findings of the study had been that patients overall in the DC condition had less exposure to a counsellor or therapist than had patients in the psychotherapy conditions. This may have led to a treatment effect for the SE and CB conditions simply due to more attention. However, when this matter was examined by level of psychiatric severity, it was found that there were no significant differences in exposure to therapist or counsellor in the medium and high severity groups, suggesting that the observed effect was from therapy type rather than quantity of treatment *per se*. Woody *et al.* (1984) concluded that psychotherapy was a useful addition to methadone maintenance for patients with severe psychiatric symptoms.

Antisocial Personality and Response to Psychotherapy

Woody and his colleagues (1985) used the seven-month follow-up data to examine the traditional belief that individuals with a diagnosis of antisocial personality disorder (ASPD) do not respond well to psychological treatments. The subjects were divided into four categories:

(a) those whose only diagnosis was opioid dependence;

(b) those who had a diagnosis of depression in addition to opioid dependence;

(c) those who were depressed, opioid dependent and diagnosed as having ASPD and

(d) those who were opioid-dependent and had a diagnosis of ASPD but no depressive disorder.

Patients without depressive disorder or ASPD, and those who were depressed, responded well to treatment. The group with ASPD and depression also responded to treatment but not as well as the former groups. By contrast, the group with ASPD and no depression did not respond on most of the outcomes assessed, although they did improve in their drug use and legal status. In comparison to the other three groups, who did benefit from psychotherapy when compared to DC-only patients, the ASPD-only group did not.

Woody *et al.* (1985) concluded that psychotherapy, as has long been believed, does not benefit patients with a diagnosis of ASPD without a concurrent diagnosis of depression. One defining characteristic of ASPD is the inability to form meaningful and enduring relationships with other people. Given that such a relationship is a precondition for effective psychotherapy, it is not surprising that it was found to be of no benefit in individuals with ASPD. However, antisocial behaviour itself is common to the patient population, and by itself is not a contraindication for psychotherapy. Woody *et al.* argue that an additional diagnosis of depression indicates that the individual concerned is capable of an emotional response and is therefore amenable to psychological treatment. Patients with ASPD are amenable to methadone maintenance, however, as is indicated by the observed reduction in drug use and crime.

Other Specific Interventions

A number of specific psychotherapeutic interventions that might be added to counselling procedures to bring about behaviour change have been studied with methadone maintenance patients. Many have been relatively brief approaches that have met with limited success. They are largely unreplicated, and it is not possible to be fully confident of their likely impact. For example, Houston and Milby (1983) attempted to assess the impact of aversion therapy with methadone maintenance patients. They used electric shocks paired with patients' imaginings of drug-seeking behaviour, and (perhaps not surprisingly) found no discernible effect on drug use. In a similarly disappointing and limited study, Goldberg *et al.* (1976) reported four case studies of methadone maintenance patients who were taught 'alpha conditioning' (a relaxation technique using biofeedback), and although the patients reported that the technique induced a pleasant mental state, the authors found no evidence for effects on traditional treatment outcomes such as extent of drug use. Another study using biofeedback techniques to facilitate relaxation found that it reduced measures of anxiety in a small group of methadone maintenance patients; however, the high drop-out rate suggested that the primary difficulty might be getting methadone maintenance patients to participate in sessions at all (Kuna *et al.*, 1976).

In another behaviourally-oriented study of reducing injecting heroin use among methadone maintenance patients, Snowden (1978) found a decline in heroin use in response to covert desensitisation (sessions of imagined negative consequences to injecting heroin) for methadone maintenance patients who were assessed as having an internal locus of control. The finding, in the absence of other research, has to be considered suggestive at best, given that the experiment lasted for only seven weeks, that the subjects were paid to attend sessions, and that the same researcher/therapist conducted all sessions in all three conditions, and therefore could not be considered a disinterested evaluator of success.

More recently, and reflecting developments in the alcohol dependence treatment field, new psychological interventions have been applied to methadone maintenance patients. Specifically, motivational interviewing has been subjected to some study. Motivational interviewing is an approach to drug problems that is based on the reflective listening style of counselling developed by Carl Rogers (Miller & Rollnick, 1991; Rogers, 1957). Saunders and his colleagues (Saunders & Wilkinson, 1990; Saunders *et al.*, 1995) have compared the effect of a two-session motivational interviewing intervention to a two-session educational intervention at the commencement of methadone maintenance. They found that the motivational interviewing subjects complied better with treatment and relapsed less quickly than the control group. The most important contribution that motivational interviewing may make to methadone maintenance treatment might be in improving the general relationship between patients and unit staff as well as counsellors. Future research will clarify this issue. The therapeutic style associated with motivational interviewing is discussed in more detail later in this chapter.

In an investigation of a more global change to methadone maintenance treatment, patients surveyed in an Oregon methadone unit that had developed a 'psychoeducational' approach to ancillary service delivery were found to dislike group activities and life education classes; they preferred individual counselling in the methadone program (Stark & Campbell, 1991). This finding suggests that individual counselling is a form of ancillary intervention that methadone maintenance patients most like, and that a needs analysis approach, in which patients are surveyed to find out what kinds of interventions they need and prefer, is probably a useful step in developing a patient-centred set of services.

Clearly a group format for the counselling of methadone maintenance patients is an attractive option as an intervention because it is cost efficient. However, it does appear that the research evidence and clinical lore agree that methadone maintenance patients do not like to participate in group therapy. Although this may be the case for unstructured therapeutic sessions, recent evidence suggests that special purpose self-help groups may be more attractive if they are presented in the right way. For example, groups for pregnant women and HIV-positive patients and patients with AIDS have been reported as having some success in attracting patients into treatment.

There have, however, been very few studies of group therapy with methadone maintenance patients. An early study (Willet, 1973) compared two types of group therapy (psychoanalytic and T-group) to methadone alone. It failed to find any significant differences in drug use or interpersonal functioning. Unfortunately, a substantial drop-out rate from all three conditions resulted in a very small sample size that rendered the study uninterpretable. A later study compared a cognitive-behavioural group to a non-directive group over a 10-week period on a range of outcomes (Abrahms, 1979). The cognitive-behavioural intervention incorporated an extensive package of skills training which included relaxation, assertion training and how to deal with problem situations. The control group met once a week for the same amount of time and participated in unstructured group discussions with a therapist present. The cognitive-behavioural intervention showed significant improvements on measures for anxiety, depression, and assertiveness. There was no advantage for the cognitive-behavioural group on drug use as measured by urinalysis. This study suggests that the value of group therapy, if patients will comply, may be found in meeting the psychiatric needs of methadone maintenance patients.

Family Therapy

The term 'family therapy' covers a range of interventions that have been developed over the past three decades, all of which have a common theoretical rationale that assumes that behavioural and psychological problems are a function of disordered or maladaptive interpersonal relationships within the family. Each family is understood from a systems theory perspective as a system with rules that govern its functioning (Hazelrigg *et al.*, 1987). Although a family therapist will usually conduct sessions with members of the family and the client together, this is not necessarily a defining feature of the interventions that family therapy covers; some interventions may only involve the individual while others may involve other people in the client's life (e.g., co-workers, drug treatment agency staff, etc.) (Hazelrigg *et al.*, 1987). Family therapy has attracted the interest of counsellors and therapists who work with drug-dependent individuals, including methadone maintenance unit staff. In a national survey of drug and alcohol treatment agencies conducted in the 1970s in the USA, methadone maintenance units expressed the most interest in family therapy (Coleman & Davis, 1978).

According to Hazelrigg *et al.* (1987), family therapies can be classified into two broad types: those that are 'pragmatic', in that they are focused on symptom removal and behaviour change; and those that are 'aesthetic', and have the broader goal of transforming the family system and achieving a holistic integration of the self. Only the pragmatic types of family therapy (structural, strategic, behavioural) have been evaluated using traditional research methods, and these types will be considered here.

Only two controlled studies have looked at the effectiveness of family therapy with an opioid-dependent clientele. The first of these was conducted in the USA (Stanton *et al.*, 1982), while the second, which was intended to be a replication of the USA study, was carried out recently in The Netherlands (Romijn *et al.*, 1990). Both assessed structural family therapy as described by Stanton and his co-workers. This is a goal-directed intervention that requires the client and his or her family of origin (parents and siblings) to be present in the therapy sessions (Stanton *et al.*, 1982). The therapist takes an active role and tries to influence the ways in which family members communicate with each other about the client's drug use. Therapy is time-limited, intense, and focused on the client's drug problems. An important component is that the client's parents have to take an active role in managing their child's treatment.

The Stanton *et al.* (1982) study was a collaboration between the Philadelphia Child Guidance Clinic and the Drug Dependence Treatment Center of the Philadelphia Veterans Administration Hospital. The subjects were all males applying for methadone maintenance who satisfied the eligibility criteria, the most important of which was that they were in more than weekly contact with their parents or parent surrogates. The eligibility criteria were in fact changed a third of the way through the study – subjects had to be living with their parents or parent surrogates. They and their families were randomly allocated to one of three conditions or to a control group if they satisfied the eligibility criteria and there was no therapist available at their time of entry to the program.

This resulted in four conditions being compared:

(a) *paid family therapy* that involved ten therapy sessions in which all members of the family were paid a fee to attend, with the fee increasing if the subject was drug-free for that week (extra money was paid for withdrawing from methadone);

(b) *unpaid family therapy,* which was the same as the paid condition, except that no money was paid for attendance, or for reduced drug use;

(c) *paid family movie condition,* which consisted of an equivalent number of sessions of family movie watching for which family members were paid in the same manner as the paid family therapy condition (for attendance and reduction in drug use); and

(d) *methadone maintenance control condition,* which consisted of subjects who were in methadone maintenance.

Subjects in the movie group and the methadone maintenance control condition had access to a counsellor on demand, whereas in the two family therapy conditions the family therapist assumed the role of drug counsellor and took control of the treatment, including the dispensing of methadone and take-home doses.

This study is unique in the literature for the sophistication of its design in that it includes what is known as a non-specific control group (i.e., a group that received the same amount of exposure to certain basic conditions of therapy but is not exposed to the therapy itself) (Borkovec, 1990). The methadone control condition provided baseline data for what could be expected of a matched group of patients receiving methadone maintenance treatment as usual. The family movie group (non-specific control) provided a control for both payment and the simple effect of the family getting together once a week for ten weeks. The unpaid family therapy group controlled for what might happen when a financial incentive for attendance and reduced drug use was not employed. To summarise, Stanton *et al.* compared a sample of male veteran methadone maintenance patients who were exposed to paid family therapy, unpaid family therapy, paid family movie plus counselling, and counselling.

Stanton *et al.* assessed each of the four groups of subjects on two measures: the percentage of days spent drug free in various drug classes (legal opioids, illegal opioids, other illicit drugs, marijuana and alcohol) and time spent in work or school. Outcome was also measured by the percentage of subjects in each group who were categorised as having a poor, medium or good outcome. Data were collected at six and 12 months after treatment. Differences were found in the direction expected for a family therapy effect for the drug classes other than alcohol (i.e., those who were exposed to family therapy had less drug use). No effect was found for employment or schooling. The differences in favour of family therapy were, however, only statistically significant for illicit drug use other than opiates, while the findings for the two classes of opioids were marginally significant (p<0.06).

The way in which the data are presented and analysed (one-way analysis of variance – no error term or F-ratios tabled) makes it difficult to know how to evaluate these data. The authors went on to carry out further analyses (analysis of covariance) to remove unwanted variation introduced by client characteristics which did result in statistically significant results for each of the outcomes favouring family therapy. As presented, these data suggest that family therapy contributes to a better outcome when combined with methadone maintenance than does drug counselling, but the data remain difficult to interpret.

In a further analysis, the data from the four conditions were combined into two comparable groups – family therapy (paid and unpaid) and a control group (methadone maintenance control and family movie) – and then analysed according to whether subjects were found to have a poor, medium or good outcome. The allocation of poor, medium and good outcome categories was determined by combining all the outcome measures. Significant differences in favour of family therapy were found for legal opiates, illegal opiates, other illegal drugs and marijuana. No advantage for family therapy was found for alcohol consumption or employment. However, when the mortality rates for the two groups were examined, it was found that 10% of the control subjects had died in the period to follow-up compared with 2% of the family therapy subjects – a difference that was significant. Further follow-ups to five years after the completion of therapy were planned. A subsequent report (Todd, 1984) indicated that the positive effects for family therapy had persisted at two to three years after finishing treatment, but he presents no data to support this claim. We have been unable to find any other reports of further follow-ups for this study.

Taken overall, the Stanton *et al.* study was a well designed test of the use of family therapy in a methadone program. Patients who had the benefit of family therapy seem to have been able to reduce both their need for methadone and their use of illicit drugs. However, it has to be acknowledged that the eligibility criteria for the study meant that a defined subgroup of patients in the VA methadone program were compared with one another under a range of therapy conditions. Obviously, if a patient does not have contact with his or her family, or refuses to allow family members to become involved in the treatment process, then they are not suitable for family therapy. Further, structural family therapy is an intense and directive intervention that requires considerable interpersonal and observational skills of the therapist that can only be acquired through specialist training. It would seem then that if such a therapist was available and willing to go to the considerable effort of engaging a patient's family in treatment, and if the client was suitable for a family intervention, then family therapy may prove useful as an adjunct to traditional methadone maintenance treatment. It is impossible to say with any confidence on the basis of this single study, given the inadequate data presentation and analysis, whether such an intervention will or will not benefit a patient.

There has been one attempt to replicate the Stanton *et al.* study. Romijn *et al.* (1990) compared family therapy without methadone maintenance with low dose (20 mg) methadone maintenance plus drug counselling using two groups of subjects who were retrospectively matched on a range of client variables (age, sex, drug use, etc.). Using the same outcome criteria as in the original study, the two groups were compared on follow-up measures taken 18 months after the commencement of treatment. In addition to the outcomes used by Stanton *et al.*, crime and extent of drug culture involvement were assessed. The two groups differed significantly on only one measure – crime – and this favoured the methadone maintenance group.

This study differs obviously from the US study in a number of ways. First, it compares family therapy alone to methadone maintenance, whereas the original Stanton *et al.* study compared family therapy to drug counselling among methadone maintenance patients. Secondly, the USA study randomly allocated subjects to each of the conditions, an allocation procedure that is superior to matched controls, especially when it is taken into account that the family therapy and the methadone maintenance subjects in the Dutch study came from different geographical locations. Thirdly, a number of aspects of the study are not clear. No detail is given about the length of the family therapy, or about the average tenure of the patients in the methadone maintenance condition. No detail is given about the methadone maintenance program, making it difficult to assess the effectiveness of such a program. In this regard, doses of methadone as low as 20 mg have been consistently shown to be associated with treatment failure (see Chapter 9).

For all of the above reasons, it has to be concluded that the null result of the Dutch study does not overturn the promise for family therapy as part of a methadone maintenance program shown in the Philadelphia study. Of relevance also are two meta-analytic reviews of controlled studies of the effectiveness of family therapy for a range of disorders (which did not include drug dependence), both of which have independently found family therapy to be moderately effective when compared to no-treatment control groups (Hazelrigg *et al.*, 1987; Markus *et al.*, 1990). It is reasonable to assume that if family therapy is effective in other areas, (e.g., behaviour disorders in adolescents) then it may be effective in cases of drug dependence that are suitable for the intervention.

The extent to which this is desirable in methadone maintenance programs would have to be established: how many patients have sufficient contact with their family of origin and are willing to allow them to become involved in treatment? If there is a need, then further studies will need to establish whether such patients would benefit from family therapy if it was made available to them. The extent to which methadone maintenance program staff are willing to be trained in family therapy, or to which family therapists are willing to participate in methadone maintenance treatment, would also have to be established. Finally, the difficulties in getting methadone maintenance patients to attend family therapy sessions should not be underestimated. For example, Todd (1984) reports that paying patients did influence attendance at sessions in the Stanton *et al.* (1982) study. While all of the subjects and their families attended a minimum of four sessions in the paid family therapy condition, only 52% did so when they were not paid to attend.

Mandatory Psychotherapy?

Desmond and Maddux (1983) compared mandatory versus optional psychotherapy (described as supportive therapy and relationship therapy) over a one-year period and found no significant differences on a range of outcomes between the two groups. The pattern of results favoured the optional group, which is not surprising given that it is difficult to imagine how mandatory psychotherapy could be effective. Both groups received drug counselling as well as psychotherapy from the same counsellor, one for each group. It is unfortunate that the two groups were not compared to a third control group receiving drug counselling alone. The simple conclusion to be drawn from this study is that *mandatory* psychotherapy, if this needed to be demonstrated, should not be used as an adjunct to methadone maintenance. As others have remarked (Kaufman & Blaine, 1974), in methadone maintenance units where counselling or psychotherapy is mandatory, patients think of counselling sessions as a game they have to play to keep up their supply of methadone.

More recently, these investigators (Maddux *et al.*, 1995) have replicated their earlier result showing that mandatory counselling sessions were not superior to optional counselling on any of the measures reported. In fact, the results tended to favour the optional counselling patients who had better retention in treatment than the mandatory patients, even though they saw their counsellors only half as often. These results are suggestive that enforced attendance for counselling may be to the detriment of patients.

Therapist Effects

Do Therapists Differ in Their Impact on Patients?

An important finding arising out of the analysis of the results of the VA-Penn psychotherapy project was that there were significant differences in the effectiveness of different therapists within each of the types of therapy compared (Luborsky *et al.*, 1985). This finding confirms what is common knowledge among clinicians – that some therapists are better than others, no matter what style of therapy they subscribe to. This finding, which has since been replicated, has important implications for both treatment practices and future research on counselling, psychotherapy and (as will be seen) methadone maintenance treatment in general.

Most psychotherapy and counselling research has, until recently, compared the relative effectiveness of different types of interventions (for example, psychodynamic versus behavioural) and in doing so has assumed that one therapist is equivalent to another. Indeed, as Luborsky *et al.* (1986) point out, in the more than 500 studies that had been reported in the period to 1980 on psychotherapy, few examined whether there were differences between therapists within the various modalities that were being assessed. Luborsky *et al.* (1986) re-examined the data for four psychotherapy outcome studies (which included the seven-month follow-up data from the VA-Penn psychotherapy project) and found that differences between therapists were significantly related to patient outcome in all four. Importantly, therapist effects were found to be as, if not more, important as the contribution of therapy type to outcome. These findings have serious implications for the interpretation of research comparing different interventions that does not routinely control for therapist effects, that is, the therapist's as opposed to the therapy's influence on outcome.

Crits-Christoph and colleagues (1990) discuss in detail the implications of therapist effects for psychotherapy and counselling research. They argue that therapists are often treated in statistical analyses as if they were a fixed form of treatment, like a therapeutic drug, when they should be treated as if they were a random selection from the population of therapists who practise the particular form of therapy being investigated. In cases where the therapist is treated as a fixed form of treatment, the proper conclusion to be drawn is that the therapy concerned is effective as practised by the participating therapists. If there are no differences between therapists then this advice can be ignored. Crits-Christoph re-examined the data from eight psychotherapy studies to see how often this might occur. They found therapist effects in six out of eight of the studies. The largest therapist effect for any outcome measure in these studies meant that 55% of the variability in outcome seen in the patients was due to differences between therapists.

In order to determine the implications of therapist effects for study findings, Crits-Christoph *et al.* conducted a large series of simulated psychotherapy studies on computer using data generated randomly. Each of these 'studies' compared three treatment groups and varied both the number of therapists in each condition and the amount of variation in treatment effect contributed by differences between therapists. For each possible study, they then generated 2,000 analyses of variance using the randomly generated data. They found that neither the number of treatments, nor the number of therapists for each treatment would affect the results, but that the number of clients being treated by each therapist and the size of therapist effects would. In a study where there were 15 clients assigned to each therapist and where 25% of the variation seen in outcome was due to differences between therapists, one would expect a false positive result approximately 50% of the time. That is, one out of every two studies showing one intervention to be superior to another would be incorrect if differences between therapists were not investigated, and statistically controlled for if found.

The implications of this finding extend to studies of methadone maintenance treatment (Crits-Christoph *et al.*, 1990). Recent research (e.g., Ball and Ross, 1991) has found that methadone maintenance units differ in their effectiveness. This suggests that methadone maintenance units should be treated as random factors in treatment outcome studies that compare different modalities, unless it can be demonstrated that the variation in unit effect is zero. However, for the purposes of treatment practice, the most important implication of these findings is that an examination of therapist characteristics and their relationship to client improvement may lead to more effective therapies in general.

Characteristics of Effective Therapists

In addition to studies discussed in the previous section, there are two studies from the VA-Penn group, and findings from the alcohol treatment literature, which suggest that the therapist is an important factor in interventions with people with drug problems. In their investigation of the VA-Penn psychotherapy project data for therapist effects, Luborsky *et al.* (1985) found a number of aspects of both therapist and therapeutic style to be associated with improved outcomes when random samples of the therapy and counselling sessions were analysed. These findings can be summarised by four main points:

- therapists who were able to develop a warm, supportive relationship as a basis for working together (a therapeutic alliance) had better outcomes;
- components of sessions in all three modalities – supportive-expressive psychotherapy (SE), cognitive-behavioural psychotherapy (CB), and drug counselling (DC) – that were

coded as being part of SE or CB protocols from audio tapes of the sessions were associated with better outcomes, while DC techniques were not;

- the extent to which the psychotherapy sessions were consistent with the protocol for each of the therapies was related to better outcome, and this was true for comparisons between clients for individual therapists (i.e., those clients who received 'purer' SE or CB therapy did better);

- the extent to which therapists were judged to be well adjusted, skilled and interested in helping their patients was positively associated with a better outcome (although these were not statistically significant, perhaps as Luborsky *et al.* suggest, because of the small sample size of nine therapists).

Luborsky *et al.* (1985) interpreted these findings to mean that both personal characteristics of the therapist (adjustment, skill, interest in work, ability to establish a therapeutic alliance) and the psychotherapeutic techniques themselves (SE and CB) contributed to a better outcome. The latter point was highlighted by the finding that drug counsellors whose sessions were coded with more CB and SE components had clients who improved more. However, the data suggest that differences between therapists, rather than modalities, are the more powerful influence on client response. Luborsky *et al.* suggest that the most important characteristic in this regard is the ability to develop a therapeutic alliance.

In a further study from the VA-Penn group, McLellan (McLellan *et al.*, 1988) retrospectively examined the differences in outcome for four drug counsellors who were appointed to a large number of clients in a virtually random fashion after the sudden resignation of two counsellors on the VA methadone maintenance program in Philadelphia. They found consistent differences across a range of outcomes between the counsellors. While two counsellors were moderately effective, the third was very effective and the fourth was not effective at all. The most effective counsellor was able to bring his clients to a point over a six-month period where their drug use and unemployment were significantly reduced when compared with the six months prior to the change in counsellor, while at the same time reducing their use of both methadone and ancillary psychotropic prescriptions. By contrast, the clients of the least effective counsellor showed increased levels of unemployment, drug use and criminal activity, and needed more methadone and ancillary medication.

When the differences between counsellors were examined, it was found that the most effective counsellor had postgraduate qualifications in psychology, while the least effective counsellor was an ex-addict with no tertiary education; the two moderately effective counsellors also had tertiary education. The three more effective counsellors kept well organised case notes, saw their patients frequently, were consistent in the application of program rules, and often referred their patients to other members of staff within the methadone maintenance unit and to outside agencies for specialist help. The least effective counsellor did not keep adequate case management notes, saw clients relatively infrequently, was inconsistent in responding to rule infractions, and seemed not to refer clients for specialist help. McLellan *et al.* (1988) claimed that when the case notes were examined in detail for some indication of session content, it became clear that the most effective counsellor was able to help clients anticipate their problems and assist them in developing ways of dealing with them before they arose. This was the quality that most clearly distinguished this counsellor from the moderately effective ones who were similarly qualified. They went on to argue that the techniques reflected in the case notes were consistent with those features of psychotherapy that were found to be effective in comparison with DC in the psychotherapy project.

The findings discussed in this section suggest that two important qualities contribute to the effectiveness of a counsellor: the ability to establish a warm, supportive relationship with the client relatively quickly, and having specialist knowledge about how to manage that relationship once it has developed. The findings of the VA-Penn psychotherapy project overall suggest the latter is of most relevance when dealing with more disturbed clients. This also seems to be true of therapeutic relationships with 'difficult' methadone maintenance patients. Case management duties, which often involve dealing with rule infractions, conflict with the need to establish an alliance with clients. This is especially true of "difficult" patients who persistently break program rules. Zweben (1991) remarks that such rules are based on the notion that the behaviour of patients can be controlled through having rules and enforcing them. This, she argues, is in conflict with "the understanding on the part of most addiction treatment professionals that one person is essentially powerless to control the drug use of another" (p. 178). (See also Miller & Rollnick, 1991 for an extended discussion of this issue.) In dealing with ongoing illicit drug use, Zweben suggests that counsellors who use 'power tactics' when patients refuse to comply are merely demonstrating their lack of clinical skills. This point of view is consistent with that of others (Miller & Brown, 1991), who take the VA-Penn group's argument one step further and suggest that not only is establishing a therapeutic alliance important to a positive treatment response, but that confronting clients about their drug use contributes to a negative one.

The point has been made on a number of occasions that the importance of establishing supportive relationships when counselling clients with drug problems is simply a specific application of what has been found to be more generally true for counselling and psychotherapy (e.g., Luborsky *et al.*, 1985; Miller & Brown, 1991; Miller & Rollnick, 1991). Miller and his colleagues have been especially emphatic on this point, arguing that the traditional approach of confronting clients about their drug use in an attempt to get through to them works against everything that has been learned about how to change human behaviour. Miller and Brown (1991) interpret the Luborsky *et al.* (1985) findings as showing that counselling consisting solely of case management is ineffective. On this interpretation, this aspect of methadone maintenance treatment is conducive to a confrontational and directive style (see also Zweben, 1991). Forming an alliance with the counsellor has also been associated with less drug use and needle sharing (Tunis *et al.*, 1995), and is correlated with better outcomes in drug abuse treatment (Simpson *et al.*, 1995). In a study of clients with alcohol problems, it was found that the more therapists confronted clients, the less likely they were to reduce their drinking, and the more the therapist was empathic and supported the client, the more likely it was that they would reduce their drinking (Miller & Sovereign, 1989). Miller and Rollnick (1991) argue, on the basis of results like these, that the therapist is largely responsible for the extent to which the client resists therapy and, therefore, for the failure of therapy to the extent that it is the result of client resistance.

Conclusions

The evidence reviewed in this book suggests that methadone maintenance treatment is effective only with adequate doses of methadone and for the period that the person remains in treatment. The conclusion to be drawn from this evidence is that counselling is not a stand-alone treatment for opioid dependence, and that methadone maintenance treatment should not aspire to a goal of total abstinence in the belief that counselling makes such a goal possible.

However, it has to be acknowledged that the model of methadone maintenance treatment that the evidence supports as being effective is the Dole and Nyswander model – high-dose, maintenance-oriented treatment with high quality ancillary services to assist patients to recover (Chapter 2). The fears of the advocates of this model – that low intervention methadone maintenance is motivated by a desire to cut costs rather than the needs of the patient population – have some basis. The same motivation has been responsible for similar moves with other patient populations, such as the chronically mentally ill. However, this fear has to be tempered by the fact that it is unlikely all methadone maintenance patients need such a high level of intervention in their lives. The evidence we have reviewed shows that there are patients who need more assistance than others to get their lives in order, and counselling should be made available to them. On the other hand, it is hard to see why stabilised patients with no major life problems should need (or be required to routinely see) a counsellor at all. This is consistent with the main message of this book – that methadone maintenance patients are like any other treatment population. They have different needs and differ in their response to different components of treatment and therefore should have their treatment individualised for them.

Another issue arising from the literature reviewed in this chapter is that there is a clear need to develop protocols for counselling and training programs that are based on techniques shown to be useful elsewhere. Replacing confrontation with a client-centred style would be a step in this direction. Perhaps the most interesting findings reviewed in this chapter are those that suggest that not all counsellors are equally effective in bringing about change for their clients. Finding out more about the characteristics of effective counsellors is an obvious research need. As Luborsky *et al.* (1986) have remarked, it will be interesting to see to what extent these characteristics are teachable techniques, or are part of the effective counsellor's personality.

Summary

There is reasonable evidence to suggest that counselling does add to the effectiveness of methadone maintenance treatment for some patients. It has to be acknowledged that the model of methadone maintenance treatment that has been shown to be effective has usually included counselling as part of its service delivery. This remains the case even though methadone maintenance without counselling is not uncommon throughout the world. It is also the case that there is evidence that methadone alone does appear to reduce illicit opiate use. The role of counselling is important for those patients who want and need such assistance. The provision of mandatory counselling is not associated with better outcomes, the research showing, if anything, that such enforced attendance for counselling produces worse results in terms of retention.

There is limited evidence that methadone maintenance units with better quality counselling services have more success than units with lesser quality services. There is no evidence to suggest that ex-addict counsellors are more effective than other counsellors; if anything, the evidence suggests that they may be less effective. There is a need to define the word 'training' with regard to counselling in methadone maintenance programs. There is no evidence to suggest that an in-service trained person without formal counselling qualifications is any less effective than a person with formal counselling qualifications.

Studies of specific techniques, such as relaxation training, with methadone maintenance patients have failed to find any impact on the traditional outcomes of level of illicit drug use or criminal activity. The use of newer techniques (e.g., motivational interviewing) may prove to be useful in establishing a working relationship with patients and increasing their compliance with treatment, but require further research before they can be accepted as a necessary or integral part of treatment.

Psychotherapy (cognitive-behavioural or psychodynamic) might be a useful adjunct to methadone maintenance treatment for patients with psychiatric disorders that are amenable to such treatment (e.g., anxiety disorders, mood disorders). However, more research is needed to confirm this finding, which comes from one study. There is, however, no reason to believe that psychotherapy is a treatment for opioid dependence, or that it is indicated for methadone maintenance patients without psychiatric problems.

Patients with a diagnosis of ASPD do not appear to be amenable to psychotherapy unless they have a concurrent diagnosis of depression. Such patients are suitable for methadone maintenance treatment. Family therapy may be useful for methadone maintenance patients who qualify for family treatment and are willing to participate in it.

The limited evidence from one study for family therapy is positive. Further research is needed to establish its usefulness. Mandatory psychotherapy or counselling is unlikely to be of benefit to methadone maintenance patients and may have a negative impact on patient attitudes to treatment in general.

It has been established that some psychotherapists and counsellors are more effective than others. Differences between therapists (therapist effects) may be more important than differences between therapies, that is, differences in clients' responses to therapy may be more an effect of therapist characteristics than the relative effectiveness of particular therapies. The discovery that therapist effects exist has important implications for designing studies that compare different therapies.

The ability to establish a relationship with clients based on trust, known as a therapeutic alliance, is an important contributor to a positive outcome from therapy. As well, certain components of both psychodynamic and cognitive-behavioural therapy have been found to be associated with a better outcome, and the use of these components by therapists contributes in part to the differences seen in therapist effectiveness.

Evidence arising out of studies of differences between therapists suggests that counselling in methadone maintenance programs should be based on sound general counselling principles (reflective listening, establishing an empathic alliance, etc.) rather than confrontation.

REFERENCES

Abrahms, J. L. (1979). A cognitive-behavioral versus nondirective group treatment program for opioid-addicted persons: An adjunct to methadone maintenance. *International Journal of the Addictions, 14,* 503-511.

Aiken, L. S., LoSciuto, L. A., Ausetts, M. A., & Brown, B. S. (1984a). Paraprofessional versus professional drug counselors: Diverse routes to the same role. *International Journal of the Addictions, 19*(2), 153-173.

Aiken, L. S., LoSciuto, L. A., Ausetts, M. A., & Brown, B. S. (1984b). Paraprofessional versus professional drug counselors: The progress of clients in treatment. *International Journal of the Addictions, 19*(4), 383-401.

Anglin, M. D., Miller, M. L., Mantius, K., & Grella, C. (1993). Enhanced methadone maintenance treatment: Limiting the spread of HIV among high-risk Los Angeles narcotics addicts. In J.A.Inciardi, F. M. Tims, & B. W. Fletcher (Eds.), *Innovative approaches in the treatment of drug abuse: Program models and strategies* (pp. 3-19). London: Greenwood Press.

Australian Social Issues Research. (1991). *A descriptive study of New South Wales public methadone clinics* : Report prepared for the Drug & Alcohol Directorate, New South Wales Department of Health, Australia.

Baillie, A. J., Webster, P., & Mattick, R. P. (1992). An Australian survey of the procedures for the treatment of Opiate users. *Drug and Alcohol Review,* 11, 343-354.

Ball, J. C., & Ross, A. (1991). *The effectiveness of methadone maintenance treatment: Patients, programs, services, and outcome.* Vienna: Springer-Verlag.

Baranackie, K., & Crits-Christoph, P. K., (1992). Therapist techniques used during the cognitive therapy of opiate-dependent patients. *Journal of Substance Abuse Treatment,* 9, 221-228.

Borkovec, T. D. (1990). Control groups and comparison groups in psychotherapy outcome research. In L. S. Onken & J. D. Blaine (Eds.), *NIDA Research Monograph 104. Psychotherapy and Counseling in the Treatment of Drug Abuse.* (pp. 50-65). Rockville, MD: U.S. Department of Health and Human Services.

Brewington, V., Deren, S., Arella, L. R., & Randell, J. (1990). Obstacles to vocational rehabilitation: The clients' perspectives. *Journal of Applied Rehabilitation Counselling,* 21, 27-37.

Burgess, P. M., Gill, A. J., Pead, J., & Holman, C. P. (1990). Methadone: Old problems for new programs. *Drug and Alcohol Review,* 9, 61-66.

Calsyn, D. A., Saxon, A. J., Blaes, P., & Lee-Meyer, S. (1990). Staffing patterns of American methadone maintenance programs. *Journal of Substance Abuse Treatment,* 7, 255-259.

Carroll, K. M., Chang, K., Behr, H., & Clinton, B. (1995). Improving treatment-outcome in pregnant, methadone-maintained women: Results from a randomized clinical trial. *American Journal on Addictions,* 4, 56-59.

Childress, A. R., McLellan, A. T., Woody, G. E., & O'Brien, C. P. (1991). Are there minimum conditions necessary for methadone maintenance to reduce intravenous drug use and AIDS risk behaviors? In R. W. Pickens, C. G. Leukefeld, & C. R. Schuster (Eds.), *NIDA Research Monograph 106. Improving Drug Abuse Treatment.* (pp. 167-177). Rockville, MD: U.S. Department of Health and Human Services.

Coleman, S. B., & Davis, D. I. (1978). Family therapy and drug abuse: A national survey. *Family Process,* 17, 21-29.

Crits-Christoph, P., Beebe, K. L., & Connolly, M. B. (1990). Therapist effects in the treatment of drug dependence: Implications for conducting comparative treatment studies.

DeLeon, G., Staines, G. L., Perlis, T. E., Sacks, S., McKendrick, K., Hilton, R., & Brady, R. (1995). Therapeutic community methods in methadone maintenance (Passages): An open clinical trial. *Drug and Alcohol Dependence,* 37, 45-57.

Dennis, M. L., Karuntzos, G. T., McDougal, G. L., French, M. T., & Hubbard, R. L. (1993). Developing training and employment programs to meet the needs of methadone treatment clients. *Evaluation and Program Planning,* 16, 73-86.

Desmond, D. P., & Maddux, J. F. (1983). Optional versus mandatory psychotherapy in methadone maintenance. *International Journal of the Addictions,* 18, 281-290.

Dole, V. P., & Nyswander, M. (1967). Heroin addiction : A metabolic disease. *Archives of Internal Medicine,* 120, 19-24.

Dole, V. P., Robinson, J. W., Orraca, J., Towns, E., Searcy, P., & Caine, E. (1969). Methadone treatment of randomly selected criminal addicts. *New England Journal of Medicine,* 280, 1372-1375.

General Accounting Office. (1990). *Methadone maintenance: Some treatment programs are not effective; Greater federal oversight needed.* Washington, DC.: General Accounting Office.

Goldberg, R. J., Greenwood, J. C., & Taintor, Z. (1976). Alpha conditioning as an adjunct treatment for drug dependence. *International Journal of the Addictions,* 11, 1085-1089.

Grella, C. E., Anglin, M. D., Wugalter, S. E., Rawson, R. A., & Hasson, A. (1994). Reasons for discharge from methadone maintenance for addicts at high risk of HIV infection or transmission. *Journal of Psychoactive Drugs,* 26, 223-232.

Grönbladh, L., & Gunne, L.-M. (1989). Methadone-assisted rehabilitation of Swedish heroin addicts. *Drug and Alcohol Dependence,* 24, 31-37.

Gunne, L.-M., & Grönbladh, L. (1981). The Swedish methadone maintenance program: A controlled study. *Drug and Alcohol Dependence,* 7, 249-256.

Hagman, G. (1994). Methadone maintenance counselling: Definition, principles, components. *Journal of Substance Abuse Treatment,* 11, 405-413.

Hasson, A. L., Grella, C. E., Rawson, R., & Anglin, M. D. (1994). Case management within a methadone maitenance program: A research demonstration project for HIV risk reduction. *Journal of Case Management,* 3, 167-172.

Hazelrigg, M. D., Cooper, H. M., & Borduin, C. M. (1987). Evaluating the effectiveness of family therapies: An integrative review and analysis. *Psychological Bulletin,* 101, 428-442.

Houston, C. C., & Milby, J. (1983). Drug-seeking behaviour and its mediation: Effects of aversion therapy with narcotic addicts on methadone. *International Journal of the Addictions,* 18, 1171-1177.

Hubbard, R. L., Marsden, M. E., Rachal, J. V., Harwood, H. J., Cavanagh, E. R., & Ginzburg, H. M. (1989). *Drug abuse treatment: A national study of effectiveness.* Chapel Hill, NC: University of North Carolina Press.

Joe, G. W., Simpson, D. D., & Hubbard, R. L. (1991). Treatment predictors of tenure in methadone maintenance. *Journal of Substance Abuse, 3,* 73-84.

Kaufman, E., & Blaine, G. B. (1974). Full services in methadone treatment. *American Journal of Drug and Alcohol Abuse, 1,* 213-231.

Kleber, H. D. (1984). Is there a need for "professional psychotherapy" in methadone programs. *Journal of Substance Abuse Treatment, 1,* 73-76.

Kuna, D. J., Salkin, W., & Weinberger, K. (1976). Biofeedback, relaxation training, and methadone clients: An inquiry. *Contemporary Drug Problems, 5,* 565-572.

Longwell, B., Miller, J., & Nichols, A. W. (1978). Counselor effectiveness in a methadone maintenance program. *International Journal of the Addictions, 13,* 307-315.

LoSciuto, L., Aiken, L. S., Ausetts, M. A., & Brown, B. S. (1984). Paraprofessional versus professional drug abuse counselors: Attitudes and expectations of the counselors and their clients. *International Journal of the Addictions, 19,* 233-252.

Luborsky, L., Crits-Christoph, P., McLellan, A. T., Woody, G. E., Piper, W., Liberman, B., Imber, S., & Pilkonis, P. (1986). Do therapists vary much in their success? Findings from four outcome studies. *American Journal of Orthopsychiatry, 56,* 501-512.

Luborsky, L., McLellan, A. T., Woody, G. E., O'Brien, C. P., & Auerbach, A. (1985). Therapist success and its determinants. *Archives of General Psychiatry, 42,* 602-611.

Maddux, J. F., Desmond, D. P., & Vogtsberger, K. N. (1995). Patient-regulated methadone dose and optional counseling in methadone maintenance. *American Journal on Addictions, 4,* 18-32.

Markus, E., Lange, A., & Pettigrew, T. F. (1990). Effectiveness of family therapy: A meta-analysis. *Journal of Family Therapy, 12,* 205-221.

McLellan, A. T., Arndt, I. O., Metzger, D. S., Woody, G. E., & O'Brien, C. P. (1993). The effects of psychosocial services in substance abuse treatment. *Journal of the American Medical Association, 269,* 1953-1959.

McLellan, A. T., Childress, A. R., Ehrman, R., O'Brien, C. P., & Pashko, S. (1986). Extin-guishing conditioned responses during opiate dependence treatment: Turning laboratory findings into clinical procedures. *Journal of Substance Abuse Treatment, 3,* 33-40.

McLellan, A. T., Woody, G. E., Luborsky, L., & Goehl, L. (1988). Is the counselor an "active ingredient" in substance abuse rehabilitation? An examination of treatment success among four counselors. *Journal of Nervous and Mental Disease, 176,* 423-430.

Miller, W. R., & Brown, J. M. (1991). Self-regulation as a conceptual basis for the prevention and treatment of addictive behaviours. In N. Heather, W. R. Miller, & J. Greeley (Eds.), *Self-control in the addictive behaviours* (pp. 3-79). Melbourne: Maxwell Macmillan.

Miller, W. R., & Rollnick, S. (1991). *Motivational interviewing: Preparing people to change addictive behavior.* New York: Guilford.

Miller, W. R., & Sovereign, R. G. (1989). The check-up: A model for early intervention in addictive behaviors. In T. L. Berg, W. R. Miller, P. E. Nathan, & G. A. Marlatt (Eds.), *Addictive behaviors: Prevention and early intervention* (pp. 219-231). Amsterdam: Swets & Zeitlinger.

Newman, R. (1974). The role of ancillary services in methadone maintenance treatment. *American Journal of Drug and Alcohol Abuse,* 1, 207-212.

Newman, R. G., & Peyser, N. (1991). Methadone treatment: Experiment and experience. *Journal of Psychoactive Drugs,* 23, 115-121.

Newman, R. G., & Whitehill, W. B. (1979). Double-blind comparison of methadone and placebo maintenance treatments of narcotic addicts in Hong Kong. *Lancet, 8 September,* 485-488.

Platt, J. J., Husband, S. D., Hermalin, J., & Cater, J. (1993). A cognitive problem-solving employment readiness intervention for methadone clients. *Journal of Cognitive Psychotherapy,* 7, 21-33.

Ramer, B. S., Zaslove, M. O., & Langan, J. (1971). Is methadone enough? The use of ancillary treatment during methadone maintenance. *American Journal of Psychiatry,* 127, 80-84.

Renner, J. A. (1984). Methadone maintenance: Past, present, and future. *Addictive Behaviours,* 3, 75-90.

Rogers, C. R. (1957). The necessary and sufficient conditions of therapeutic personality change. *Journal of Consulting Psychology,* 21, 95-103.

Romijn, C. M., Platt, J. J., & Schippers, G. M. (1990). Family therapy for Dutch drug abusers: Replication of an American study. *International Journal of the Addictions,* 25, 1127-1149.

Rounsaville, B. J., Glazer, W., Wilber, C. H., Weissman, M. M., & Kleber, H. D. (1983). Short-term interpersonal psychotherapy in methadone-maintained opiate addicts. *Archives of General Psychiatry,* 40, 629-636.

Rounsaville, B. J., Kosten, T. R., Weissman, M. M., & Kleber, H. D. (1986). A 2.5-year follow-up of short-term interpersonal psychotherapy in methadone-maintained opiate addicts. *Comprehensive Psychiatry,* 27, 201-210.

Saunders, B., & Wilkinson, C. (1990). Motivation and addiction behaviour: A psychological perspective. *Drug and Alcohol Review,* 9, 133-142.

Saunders, B., Wilkinson, C., & Phillips, M. (1995). The impact of a brief motivational intervention with opiate users attending a methadone programme. *Addiction,* 90, 415-424.

Saxon, A. J., Wells, E. A., Fleming, C., Jackson, T. R., & Calsyn, D. A.

(1996). Pre-treatment characteristics, program philosophy and level of ancillary services as predictors of methadone maintenance treatment outcome. *Addiction,* **91**(8), 1197-1209.

Siassi, I., Angle, B. P., & Alston, D. C. (1977). Who should be counselors in methadone maintenance programs: Ex-addicts or nonaddicts. *Community Mental Health Journal,* **13**, 125-132.

Simpson, D. D., Joe, G. W., Rowan-Szal, G., & Greener, J. (1995). Client engagement and change during drug abuse treatment. *Journal of Substance Abuse,* 7, 117-134.

Snowden, L. R. (1978). Personality tailored covert sensitization of heroin abuse. *Addictive Behaviors,* **3**, 43-49.

Stanton, M. D., Todd, T. C., & Associates (Eds.). (1982). *The family therapy of drug abuse and addiction.* New York: Guilford.

Stark, M. J., & Campbell, B. K. (1991). A psychoeducational approach to methadone maintenance treatment: A survey of client reactions. *Journal of Substance Abuse Treatment,* **8**, 125-131.

Todd, T. C. (1984). A contingency analysis of family treatment and drug abuse. In J. Grabowski, M. L. Stitzer, & J. E. Henningfield (Eds.), *NIDA Research Monograph 46. Behavioural intervention techniques in drug abuse treatment.* (pp. 104-114). Rockville, MD: U.S. Department of Health and Human Services.

Tunis, S. L., Delucchi, K. L., Schwartz, K., Banys, P., & Sees, K. L. (1995). The relationship of counsellor and peer alliance to drug use and HIV risk behaviors in a six-month methadone detoxification program. *Addictive Behaviors,* **20**, 395-405.

Willet, E. A. (1973). Group therapy in a methadone treatment program: An evaluation of changes in interpersonal behaviour. *International Journal of the Addictions,* **8**, 33-39.

Woody, G. E., Luborsky, L., McLellan, A. T., & O'Brien, C. P. (1986). Psychotherapy as an adjunct to methadone treatment. In R. E. Meyer (Ed.), *Psychopathology and Addictive Disorders* (pp. 9-25). New York: Guilford Press.

Woody, G. E., Luborsky, L., McLellan, A. T., O'Brien, C. P., Beck, A. T., Blaine, J., Herman, I., & Hole, A. (1983). Psychotherapy for opiate addicts. Does it help. *Archives of General Psychiatry,* **40**, 639-645.

Woody, G. E., McLellan, A. T., Luborsky, L., & O'Brien, C. P. (1985). Sociopathy and psychotherapy outcome. *Archives of General Psychiatry,* **42**, 1081-1086.

Woody, G. E., McLellan, A. T., Luborsky, L., & O'Brien, C. P. (1987). Twelve-month follow-up of psychotherapy for opiate dependence. *American Journal of Psychiatry,* **144**, 590-596.

Woody, G. E., McLellan, A. T., Luborsky, L., & O'Brien, C. P. (1990). Psychotherapy and counseling for methadone-maintained opiate addicts: Results of research studies. In L. S. Onken & J. D. Blaine (Eds.), *NIDA*

Research Monograph 104. Psychotherapy and Counseling in the Treatment of Drug Abuse. (pp. 9-23). Rockville, MD: U.S. Department of Health and Human Services.

Woody, G. E., McLellan, A. T., Luborsky, L., & O'Brien, C. P. (1995). Psychotherapy in community methadone programs: A validation study. *American Journal of Psychiatry,* 152, 1302-1308.

Woody, G. E., McLellan, A. T., Luborsky, L., O'Brien, C. P., Blaine, J., Fox, S., Herman, I., & Beck, A. T. (1984). Severity of psychiatric symptoms as a predictor of benefits from psychotherapy: The Veterans Administration-Penn study. *American Journal of Psychiatry,* 141, 1172-1177.

Yancovitz, S. R., Des Jarlais, D. C., Peyser, N. P., Drew, E., Freidmann, P., Trigg, H. L., & Robinson, J. W. (1991). A randomised trial of an interim methadone maintenance clinic. *American Journal of Public Health,* 81, 1185-1191.

Zweben, J. E. (1991). Counseling issues in methadone maintenance treatment. *Journal of Psychoactive Drugs,* 23, 177-190.

12

HOW LONG IS LONG ENOUGH? ANSWERS TO QUESTIONS ABOUT THE DURATION OF METHADONE MAINTENANCE TREATMENT

JEFF WARD, RICHARD P. MATTICK
AND WAYNE HALL

INTRODUCTION

During the 1970s, the expansion of methadone maintenance programs in the United States and in other countries around the world was accomplished in an atmosphere of controversy about what the appropriate goal and optimal duration of treatment should be. The treatment philosophy developed by the originators of this form of opioid replacement therapy had been based on the idea that opioid dependence was a chronic, metabolic disease not unlike diabetes mellitus (Dole & Nyswander, 1967). It followed from this conception of opioid dependence that the appropriate goal of treatment was indefinite maintenance on methadone. Critics of this treatment philosophy, who came from both within and outside the methadone treatment system, argued that abstinence from all drugs including methadone was an attainable goal of treatment for many patients and that this goal could be achieved in a relatively short period of time (e.g., 2 years). As a result, an alternative treatment philosophy developed based on a model of opioid dependence which emphasised its psychological and social antecedents. These two methadone treatment philosophies have been identified and described by a number of authors (Cole & James, 1975; Graff & Ball, 1976; Hubbard *et al.,* 1989; Rosenbaum, 1985). Focusing on the duration of treatment considered to be desirable according to the two models, they can be conveniently referred to for the purposes of this discussion of the duration of treatment as long-term maintenance and short-term maintenance. Broadly speaking the long-term maintenance philosophy advocates successful maintenance on methadone as an appropriate goal of treatment, and the short-term maintenance philosophy advocates abstinence from all drugs including methadone after a relatively short period of treatment.

As we have argued previously (Hall, 1993; Mattick & Hall, 1993; Ward *et al.,* 1992) and in the other chapters in this volume, we believe that the only valid way in which to evaluate such controversies as the one outlined above is by reference to what the best available research has to tell us. In this chapter, therefore, we examine the extent to which these two treatment philosophies are supported by the research evidence, and, in doing so, we provide answers to the following commonly asked questions: (a) Is abstinence a viable goal of methadone maintenance treatment? (b) What is the optimum duration for methadone maintenance treatment? (c) What factors predict premature exit from methadone maintenance treatment? and (d) Does methadone maintenance prolong opioid dependence?

The answers to these questions have implications for any consideration of the appropriate duration of methadone maintenance treatment. For example, the methadone program in Australia has been rapidly expanded over the past decade and there are currently approximately 18,000 people in treatment. The cost of this program and the limited number of free, public treatment places has given rise to familiar debates about how much treatment is enough and to what extent long-term treatment recipients are blocking access for younger heroin users who would like to enter treatment. The evidence reviewed in this chapter is complex and, at times, difficult to interpret. Keeping this in mind, we believe that a coherent, evidence-based position on what is an appropriate goal and duration for methadone treatment has to be built from a number of different sources of evidence. In the following sections, we review this evidence and develop our argument along the way. After differentiating between outcome during and after treatment, we move on to review the evidence on the relationship between length of stay and these two outcomes. We then examine the evidence on the relationship between reason for leaving treatment and post-treatment outcome. This includes follow-up studies of patients who have left treatment and a small number of studies that have investigated the fate of patients whose treatment was abruptly terminated. This is followed by a section that reviews the evidence on patient and program characteristics associated with retention in treatment. In the final part of the chapter we use the evidence that has been reviewed to evaluate the two treatment philosophies.

WHEN TO MEASURE OUTCOME?

The two different treatment philosophies described above, the long-term and short-term maintenance philosophies, have differing views on when outcome from methadone maintenance treatment should be measured. These views are a direct consequence of the differing views that each of the proponents hold on the aetiology of opioid dependence. The advocates of the long-term maintenance philosophy view opioid dependence as primarily a biological phenomenon, which is usually hypothesised as being an inherited or acquired opioid receptor disorder (e.g., Dole, 1988; Goldstein, 1991; Kreek, 1992; Newman, 1991). By contrast, the advocates of the short-term maintenance philosophy see opioid dependence as a secondary manifestation of more fundamental psychological and social problems (e.g., Alexander, 1990). The latter view is shared by cognitive-behavioural, psychodynamic and sociological theorists (Alexander, 1990).

As Alexander (1990) has pointed out, what the various psychosocial schools of thought have in common is that they differ from biological theories in two important ways. Whereas biological theorists suggest that opioid dependence is the cause of the many problems observed among opioid users, psychosocial theorists suggest that the use of opioids and other drugs is a result of, and a way of dealing with, these problems. Secondly, while biological theorists view addiction to be a direct consequence of exposure to opioids, psychosocial theorists see pre-existing problems as being important in making drug exposure significant. It follows from these two views of opioid dependence that biological theorists who are advocates of the long-term maintenance treatment philosophy will see methadone as the central component of treatment, and that psychosocial theorists who advocate the short-term maintenance philosophy will see methadone as a short-term adjunct to psychological and social interventions that will ameliorate and redress the causes of opioid dependence. In terms of measuring outcome, the long-term maintenance philosophy clearly suggests that maintenance on methadone is the goal of treatment and that outcome should be measured during treatment, whereas the short-term maintenance philosophy suggests that outcome should be measured after the patient has been treated for the underlying causes of their opioid dependence and after the administration of methadone has ceased.

We agree with Sisk and colleagues (1990) that both the biological and the psychosocial theorists are right in some respects. Furthermore, we would suggest that there is no necessary connection between these two classes of theories of opioid dependence and the two treatment philosophies that have been connected with them. For example, even if one accepts that there are psychosocial factors that contribute to the genesis and maintenance of opioid dependence, it does not necessarily follow that the amelioration or elimination of these factors is within the power or the ability of clinicians. For the purposes of this chapter, we accept that measuring outcome both during and after treatment are equally valid.

DOES LONGER DURATION PREDICT BETTER OUTCOME?

In this section, we examine research that has investigated the relationship between length of time spent in methadone maintenance and treatment outcome. This literature has been reviewed previously by Hargreaves (1983). For practical and ethical reasons, the use of experimental designs to assess the impact of shorter and longer durations of methadone maintenance treatment is not feasible. Therefore, in the absence of rigorous experimental evidence, the effect of treatment duration on outcome has to be assessed on the basis of a range of observational outcome studies, most of which use non-equivalent control group or pre-post designs. Some of these studies use statistical techniques to control for the influence of extraneous variables and can therefore be interpreted with more confidence than those that do not. Others, however, merely report correlations between duration and outcome and, in such cases, it is unclear whether it is the duration of treatment that is related to outcome or whether this apparent relationship could be explained by some other factor. The most likely alternative explanation for such a correlation is selective attrition, that is, the biased loss of a proportion of the original study sample (Hall, 1983). Bias is introduced because, as we shall see in the section below on patient characteristics as predictors of retention, patients who have more serious problems are more likely to respond poorly and leave treatment early. As these poorer functioning patients leave treatment, the performance of the diminishing remainder appears to improve, when in actual fact the reported averages (e.g., for heroin use) are diminishing due to changes in the composition of the group rather than to the accumulating impact of treatment. Where such predictors have been measured and adjusted for in the statistical analysis, we can more confidently rule out selective attrition as the explanation for any observed relationship between time spent in treatment and treatment outcome.

The finding that the longer a patient spends in methadone maintenance the more likely they are to benefit, has been reported from a number of studies (Cushman, 1981; Dole & Joseph, 1978; Hubbard *et al.,* 1989; Kang & De Leon, 1993; McGlothlin & Anglin, 1981a; Simpson, 1979, 1981; Simpson & Sells, 1982; Stimmel *et al.,* 1978; White *et al.,* 1994). In one of the first large-scale studies to investigate this issue, Dole and Joseph (1978) examined the long-term outcomes of 1,544 patients admitted to methadone maintenance in the period 1966 to 1967 and in 1970 in New York. They found that for the 846 patients who had been discharged or had left methadone maintenance, a favourable outcome in terms of relapse to heroin use and criminal activity was associated with having spent a longer time in methadone maintenance. Cushman (1981), in another follow-up study conducted in New York, also found a relationship between time spent in methadone maintenance and post-treatment outcome, with patients staying longer than three years doing significantly better than those who stayed for less than three years. In a further study conducted in New York, Stimmel *et al.* (1978) followed up patients admitted to methadone maintenance during the period March 1969 to February 1976 who had left by May 1977. They found a positive association between time spent in methadone maintenance and illicit opioid use at follow-up. Eighty-six percent of patients who had spent less than 12 months in methadone maintenance had relapsed compared with 79% who had one to two years of maintenance, 67%

who had two to three years of maintenance, and 60% of those who had more than three years of maintenance. However, as will be shown below, once reason for leaving treatment was adjusted for this relationship between time in treatment and outcome disappeared, suggesting that the relationship between treatment duration and outcome after treatment may be more complex than appears at first glance.

In a study conducted in California in the 1970s, McGlothlin and Anglin (1981a) compared the outcome of patients from three methadone programs at an average of 6.6 years after entry to methadone maintenance. Two of the programs followed a high dose, long retention policy (i.e., long-term maintenance), while the third program used low dose methadone, imposed a two-year maximum duration and adopted a strict policy of expulsion for program rule violations (i.e., short-term maintenance). Overall, the patients in the two high dose, long retention programs were doing better at follow-up. Of special interest was the difference in treatment duration among those who did and did not become dependent again after leaving treatment. Of the patients who had left methadone maintenance, those who had not become dependent averaged 32 months of maintenance compared to 18 months for those who became dependent.

Some of the most widely cited results supporting the relationship between length of time spent in methadone maintenance and positive treatment outcome are those arising out of the Drug Abuse Reporting Program (DARP) study discussed in detail in Chapter 2 (Simpson, 1979, 1981; Simpson & Sells, 1982). For the three major treatment modalities concerned – methadone maintenance, therapeutic community and outpatient drug-free treatment – a positive outcome was correlated with a longer time spent in treatment. This relationship was evident after three-months' stay and was linear (Simpson & Sells, 1982). The association between time in treatment and outcome was consistently found among various sub-samples of the follow-up group, whether single or composite outcome measures were used, whether different post-methadone maintenance time periods were examined, after statistical procedures were employed to control for background and baseline differences between clients, and when post-DARP treatment was examined in the same way (Simpson, 1979, 1981; Simpson & Sells, 1982). However, as Hargreaves (1983) has pointed out, it is difficult to know what these findings mean in clinical terms, when it is acknowledged that the correlation between time spent in treatment and outcome reported by Simpson (1981) accounts for only 4% of the variation seen in outcome.

The Treatment Outcome Prospective Study (TOPS) study was a second large-scale, multi-site treatment outcome study carried out in the USA (Hubbard *et al.,* 1989; see Chapter 2 for a detailed discussion of this study.) The analysis of the data in the TOPS study made use of statistical procedures to test various hypotheses about the relationship between a wide range of variables and the outcomes observed. Outcome for patients at follow-up was compared with a comparison group of patients who had left treatment within the first week. These analyses revealed that overall for the three modalities that showed an effect of treatment in the study (methadone maintenance, therapeutic communities, outpatient drug-free), one of the best predictors of a positive outcome was the length of time spent in treatment. This finding remained consistent for each of the modalities examined separately, for each of the three annual cohorts followed, for different groups of patients, and for different programs participating in the study. However, an examination of the findings for time in treatment by outcome in the TOPS study (see Table 2.3, Chapter 2) reveals that for methadone maintenance a statistically significant reduction in heroin use was only observed after spending more than a year in maintenance, and significant reductions in criminality were only observed in those patients who had remained continuously in methadone maintenance during the follow-up period (i.e., they were still in methadone maintenance at the time of their follow-up interview). This suggests that for heroin use at least one year of treatment was necessary for reductions to persist after leaving treatment. There was no post-treatment effect of treatment duration for crime. Rather, there was a reduction of crime as a result of being in treatment compared with not being in treatment.

In a further study from the U.S., Ball and Ross (1991) in their report on the Three Cities Study (discussed in detail in Chapter 2) found that heroin use and crime were both related to length of stay when examined individually. However, once other relevant characteristics were statistically controlled for, time spent in treatment was not related to levels of heroin use or crime reported at one-year follow-up. These findings suggest that the relationship between reductions in heroin use and crime and length of time spent in treatment may well have been due to selective attrition.

An Australian study of the impact of methadone maintenance on rate of recorded convictions in Western Sydney, found that increasing duration of maintenance was associated with a decreasing risk of being convicted for property or drug offences (Bell *et al.,* 1992). Unlike the Three Cities Study, this relationship persisted after adjusting for important predictor variables. In a more recent Australian study carried in Adelaide, White *et al.* (1994) found the incidence of recent injecting among methadone clients to be related to time in treatment. However, no adjustments were made for key predictor variables, so it is unclear whether this relationship could be accounted for by selective attrition. Nevertheless, in a similar study carried out in New York, Kang and De Leon (1993) found time spent in treatment to be the strongest predictor of recent injecting, after adjusting for other likely predictors of this outcome.

The studies reviewed in this section suggest that there is a relationship between longer stays in methadone maintenance treatment and improved outcome after leaving treatment. Given the consistency with which this relationship has been observed across a number of studies that have employed statistical adjustment to control for selective attrition, it is unlikely that the findings are solely due to this form of bias. There are fewer studies that have examined length of stay and outcome during treatment, but the weight of the evidence suggests that outcome improves over time. Again some studies have shown that this relationship remains after statistical adjustment, but the finding that this was not the case in the Three Cities Study suggests that selective attrition may be more likely to influence this relationship for outcomes during treatment.

REASON FOR LEAVING TREATMENT AND POST-TREATMENT OUTCOME

In this section, we examine to what extent the reason for leaving treatment might be related to outcome after treatment. Patients leave methadone maintenance treatment for a variety of reasons. Common reasons are: (a) *treatment completion* where a patient detoxifies with staff assent; (b) *premature detoxification* where a patient detoxifies against the advice of staff; (c) *expulsion* where a patient infringes a program rule and is expelled; (d) *absconding* where a patient fails to appear for treatment; and, (e) *imprisonment* for cases where a patient is imprisoned. A number of studies have found reason for leaving treatment to be an important predictor of post-treatment outcome and, in general, these studies suggest that patients who complete methadone treatment are more likely to have a successful outcome than those who leave for other reasons (Cushman, 1978, 1981; Des Jarlais *et al.*, 1981; Dole & Joseph, 1978; Simpson & Sells, 1982; Stimmel *et al.*, 1978). Teasing out the relative contributions of length of time spent in treatment and reason for leaving to outcome after treatment is a difficult task. In this section, we review the few studies that have examined the relative contributions of length of time spent in treatment and reason for leaving treatment, and then we review a series of studies that have examined the fate of those who leave treatment for reasons other than treatment completion. The latter studies are of special interest, because they are pertinent to the question of whether long-term maintenance should be the goal of treatment for individuals who have not shown clinically significant recovery during their treatment tenure.

Patients Who Complete Treatment

In this section, we examine three studies that have attempted to disentangle the contribution of length of time spent in treatment to post-treatment outcome independent of reason for leaving.

In the first of these studies, Stimmel *et al.* (1978) estimated the risk of relapse to opioid use for patients who had different reasons for leaving treatment. They studied a cohort of patients who were detoxified from methadone maintenance between 1969 and 1976 in New York. Patients who completed treatment were found to have spent a longer time in treatment compared with patients who left for other reasons and, having spent a longer time in treatment, were associated with lower rates of relapse to opioid use. The risk of relapse for patients who did not complete treatment was estimated to be almost five times (relative risk = 4.7) that of those who had completed treatment. However, after statistical adjustment (using proportional hazards regression modelling) for reason for leaving treatment, a longer time spent in treatment was no longer associated with lowered rates of relapse. In fact, the reverse relationship was observed, with the risk of relapse increasing by 20% for each additional year spent in treatment. It is not clear, however, what would have occurred if time in treatment had been entered into the model first and the risk of relapse then estimated for treatment completion versus other reasons for leaving treatment (Hargreaves, 1983). It may be the case that reason for leaving treatment is best seen as an intervening variable in the path that begins with a longer time in treatment leading to treatment completion which in turn leads to a lowered likelihood of relapse.

The only other published report that has specifically attempted to disentangle the relative contributions of reason for leaving treatment and length of time spent is an analysis of the DARP data set published by Simpson in 1981. This study used a global score that comprised measures of criminality, opioid use, non-opioid drug use, alcohol use and employment as the outcome. Simpson found an effect on outcome of time in treatment but there was no effect for reason for leaving treatment. In comparing this finding with that of Stimmel and colleagues (1978), we have to take into account the different outcome measures employed and the different statistical procedures used (hierarchical Cox regression versus ANOVA). It remains difficult, however, on the basis of these two studies which report contradictory findings to draw any definite conclusions about reason for leaving treatment and post-treatment outcome. In order to do so we need to examine other related evidence.

The conclusion that treatment completion is related to a more positive post-treatment outcome is indirectly supported by the findings of a number of other studies that have reported an association between positive behaviour change during methadone maintenance and success after leaving treatment (Ball & Ross, 1991; Dole & Joseph, 1978; McGlothlin & Anglin, 1981a). It is further supported by the findings of Cushman (1978) who reported that for a group of patients who had completed methadone maintenance (i.e., detoxified with the assent of staff) the average time spent in maintenance for successful patients (defined as not relapsing to heroin use) was not significantly different from the average stay for those patients who had relapsed to heroin use. The most plausible interpretation of the evidence reviewed in this section as a whole is that a longer rather than a shorter stay in treatment is usually necessary for treatment completion, as is by definition behaviour change during treatment. It is the combination of treatment duration and behaviour change leading to treatment completion that predicts a positive post-treatment outcome rather than any of these factors operating independently.

Patients Who Do Not Complete Treatment

In a series of articles published in the late seventies and early eighties, Dole and his colleagues presented data in support of the long-term maintenance model, arguing that because of the high rates of relapse to illicit opioid use that were observed among patients after methadone maintenance treatment, it was advisable to adopt long-term maintenance as the most viable goal of treatment (Des Jarlais *et al.*, 1981; Dole & Joseph, 1977, 1978). In response to various government agencies that sought to place a limit on the length of methadone maintenance, they conducted a series of follow-up studies of patients who completed, left or were discharged from methadone maintenance. In this section, we examine in detail the two larger of these studies (Des Jarlais *et al.*, 1981; Dole & Joseph, 1978), as well as evidence from the Three Cities Study (Ball & Ross, 1991).

As already described above, in 1978 Dole and Joseph reported on a comparison of patients in New York who remained in methadone maintenance with those who did not. The subjects consisted of two cohorts: the first cohort comprised all the patients admitted to methadone maintenance during 1966 to 1967; the second consisted of a stratified random sample drawn from the approximately 17,000 first-admission patients that entered methadone maintenance during 1972. This amounted to 1,544 subjects, 92% (1,413) of whom were followed up. Of these, 567 had remained in treatment continuously and 846 had left or been expelled one or more times. The results of this study generally support the conclusion that being in methadone maintenance effectively suppresses illicit opioid use (10%), while most of the patients who had left treatment had relapsed (70%). Of those who had left treatment, only 20% could be said to have completed treatment. When the general outcome for this group was compared to those who left prematurely or were expelled, it was found that while 34% of the treatment completers could be said to be doing well, only 2% of those who dropped out and 1% of those who were expelled could be said to be doing so. These findings suggest that the prognosis for patients who leave treatment or who are expelled before completion is very poor.

In a second study reported from Dole's group, Des Jarlais *et al.* (1981) presented data from a sample of 956 patients who entered methadone maintenance during 1965 to 1966 and 1972 and who subsequently left or were discharged at least once. Information was acquired through interviews (528 people) and agency records (357 people). Ninety-three per cent of the original sample was followed up in this way. Seventy-two per cent of the group relapsed to opioid use after discharge: 56% of the treatment completers, 76% of those who left prematurely, and 84% of those who were expelled.

As part of the analysis of the data collected for the Three Cities Study Ball and Ross (1991) reported on the fate of 105 patients who had left treatment during the one-year follow-up period and were able to be found. Because patients left the programs at different times during the follow-up period Ball and Ross examined rates for relapse to injecting drug use as a function of time out of treatment. These rates are summarised in Table 12.1

Table 12.1
Three Cities Study: Per cent relapsed to injecting drug use by time out of treatment

Months out of treatment	n	Percent relapsed
1-3	12	46
4-6	34	58
7-9	31	73
10-12 or more	28	82
Total	105	68

Source: Ball & Ross (1991)

As Table 12.1 shows, 68% of the whole group had relapsed by the time of their follow-up interview. When examined by the time spent out of treatment, the relapse rate was observed to increase as time out of treatment increased. While 46% of those who had been out of treatment for 1 to 3 months had relapsed at the time of their follow-up interview, this increased to 82% for those who had been out of treatment for 10 months or more. While the results are not analysed separately according to reason for leaving treatment, Ball and Ross (1991) report on the fate of the 23 (22%) individuals who had completed treatment. Of these, only 7 (30%) had not relapsed by the time of their follow-up interview.

Studies of Time-Limited Methadone Treatment

Three studies have been published that have looked at the effect on patients of removing methadone treatment either through program closure or by instituting an arbitrary maximum time limit for methadone maintenance (Anglin *et al.*, 1989; McGlothlin & Anglin, 1981b; Rosenbaum *et al.*, 1988). McGlothlin and Anglin (1981b; see Chapter 3 for a more detailed account of this study) examined the effect of the closure of a methadone maintenance program on its patients and compared outcome at two-year follow-up with patients from a similar program that continued operating during the follow-up period. In comparison to the patients who remained in methadone maintenance, the patients who had to leave treatment were substantially worse off. Anglin *et al.* (1989) report a similar study conducted after the closure of the San Diego County methadone program in 1978. In this case, they found few overall differences between the San Diego patients and a comparison group, because the majority of the San Diego patients entered private methadone maintenance programs. However, when the fate of those patients who did not enter another treatment program was examined it was found that they had poorer outcomes in terms of their greater involvement in crime, drug dealing and daily drug use.

In a similar study, Rosenbaum and colleagues (1988) examined the impact on patients of the adoption of a two-year limit for public methadone maintenance in Alemada County, California. After two years of publicly-funded methadone maintenance, patients had to detoxify or begin paying US$200 a month if they wanted to stay on methadone. The sample (N = 143) consisted of nearly half the patients on public methadone maintenance in Alemada who were affected by the new policy at the time of its introduction. Each of the patients was interviewed at this time and at six-month intervals thereafter for two-and-a-half years.

Rosenbaum *et al.* found that the patients they interviewed fell into three broad groups and that each of these groups responded to the two-year limit in different ways. They described these three groups of patients as being 'model', 'stabilised' and 'marginal'. Model patients (6% of sample) tended to have some history of employment, a minimal involvement in crime, did not use illicit drugs during treatment and had found work while on methadone maintenance. These patients used the advent of the two-year limit to successfully get off methadone maintenance. At the other end of the spectrum, marginal patients (25% of sample) were described as having long histories of opioid dependence and criminal activity, having little or no past employment, being poorly educated, being poly-drug using, and as having entered methadone maintenance as a last resort rather than out of a desire to rehabilitate. While in methadone maintenance they used heroin and other illicit drugs, regularly missed appointments, and tended to be abusive to program staff. Because these patients had not really abandoned their pre-methadone maintenance lifestyle, the imposition of the two-year limit meant for them simply an intensification of their illicit drug use and the lifestyle associated with it.

The majority of the patients (69%) were in the stabilised group. These patients responded to methadone maintenance and became stabilised, although their backgrounds were similar to the marginal patients. Many of this group had mental health problems. They continued to use heroin occasionally after entry to methadone maintenance, but this had tapered off over time. Methadone maintenance stabilised their lives and they responded in a positive fashion as their drug use and criminal activity diminished. The introduction of the two-year limit was catastrophic for this group as a whole with many becoming dependent on heroin again. The results of this study, as the authors point out, expose the irony involved in arbitrarily limiting the duration of methadone maintenance. The population that methadone maintenance is most suitable for – the stabilised group – was the one most disadvantaged by the policy.

Overall, the findings from studies of time-limited methadone maintenance suggest that imposing arbitrary time limits on the availability of methadone, either for financial purposes or in the belief that a limit will foster rehabilitation, does not contribute to a positive treatment outcome for the patients most in need of it. They also, in combination with the findings concerning reason for leaving treatment, suggest that until such time as the patient can be said to be ready to detoxify, methadone treatment should be a *maintenance* intervention.

DURATION, REASON FOR LEAVING AND TREATMENT OUTCOME: CONCLUSIONS

Overall, the evidence reviewed above suggests that the longer a patient remains in methadone maintenance treatment the more likely they are to evince the behavioural and lifestyle changes necessary to be able to complete treatment and have a reasonable chance of not returning to opioid use after detoxifying from methadone. If treatment is interrupted, for whatever reason, the above evidence suggests that most patients will relapse within the first year of leaving treatment.

When taken as a whole this research supports the long-term maintenance treatment philosophy. While a small proportion of patients remain abstinent after a relatively short period of methadone maintenance, these patients tend to be relatively stable individuals with short histories of opioid dependence and crime (Dole & Joseph, 1978; Rosenbaum *et al.*, 1988). Furthermore, as Dole and Joseph (1978) point out, there is no published large-scale study which has shown that a relatively short period of methadone maintenance produces any significant or enduring period of abstinence in a chronically opioid-dependent and criminally active population. The combined weight of the evidence concerning the high risk of relapse among methadone patients who leave treatment prematurely has led a number of other authors besides ourselves to conclude that detoxification from methadone maintenance and a drug-free life is not a realistic goal for many patients (e.g., Ball & Ross, 1991; Cushman, 1981; Hubbard *et al.*, 1989; Institute of Medicine, 1995; McGlothlin & Anglin, 1981b; McLellan, 1983; Rosenbaum *et al.*, 1988; Sisk *et al.*, 1990; Stimmel *et al.*, 1978). Rather than encouraging patients to leave treatment, the evidence, on the contrary, suggests that efforts should made to maximise retention. In the section that follows, we review the evidence that has been published concerning patient and program characteristics associated with premature exit from treatment.

PREDICTORS OF RETENTION IN METHADONE MAINTENANCE

The evidence reviewed in the preceding sections suggests that most patients who leave treatment before completion do poorly. In this section, we survey the research on patient and treatment characteristics that have been found to be associated with retention in methadone maintenance. First, we review the evidence concerning patient characteristics that predict both retention and post-treatment outcome, in order to characterise those patients who are more or less likely to remain in treatment and those who are more or less likely to do well after leaving treatment. Second, we review the clinical and research literature on treatment characteristics and retention, in order to ascertain if there are some treatment practices that might be employed to increase retention.

Patient Characteristics and Retention

As Payte and Khuri (1993) have pointed out, the length of time a given patient will stay in treatment is influenced by a number of factors, including their ability and willingness to keep attending for treatment. As will be shown below, the background and resources that a given patient brings to treatment predict how long he or she will remain in treatment and what will happen after leaving treatment. This literature has been comprehensively reviewed in the past by Szapocznik and Ladner (1977) and McLellan (1983). Rather than go over the early literature again, where applicable we report the conclusions of these two reviews and provide an update for studies published since that time.

Age

Although age is predictive of retention in methadone maintenance, with older patients tending to stay longer, it does not seem to be simply related to post-treatment outcome (McLellan, 1983). A number of recent studies have confirmed the association between being older and staying longer in treatment (Grella *et al.*, 1994; Maddux *et al.*, 1995a; Torrens *et al.*, 1996).

Gender

At the time of McLellan's (1983) review, he reported that there had been no studies that had reported on gender as a predictor of outcome or retention. Subsequent studies have been contradictory, with some failing to find an association between gender and retention (e.g., Torrens *et al.*, 1996), and others finding that males are more likely to leave treatment than females (Grella *et al.*, 1994).

Criminal History

One of the most consistent predictors of retention and subsequent post-treatment behaviour reported in the literature is the extent of pre-treatment criminal involvement (McLellan, 1983). The findings of earlier studies have been confirmed in recently published reports (Bell *et al.*, 1992; Caplehorn & Bell, 1991; Hubbard *et al.*, 1989; Maddux *et al.*, 1995a). This evidence suggests that patients who have an extensive criminal history have problems remaining in treatment and do not do well when they leave.

Opioid Use History

In 1983, McLellan concluded that severity of opioid dependence was only weakly related to outcome during and after leaving treatment. However, a number of studies have since found that the duration and intensity of pre-treatment opioid use is associated with an increased probability of relapse to opioid use after leaving treatment (Ball & Ross, 1991; Dole & Joseph, 1978; Hubbard *et al.*, 1989; Simpson & Sells, 1982). The evidence suggests that patients who have a long history of heavy opioid use will not do well if they leave methadone maintenance.

Psychological Adjustment

McLellan (1983) concluded that descriptive measures of personality variables or psychopathological symptoms had not been predictive of retention or post-treatment outcome, but that studies which had used quantitative measures of psychopathology were suggestive of a relationship between more severe symptomatology and lower retention rates. Subsequent studies have tended to confirm this finding (e.g., Joe *et al.*, 1991).

Employment

In 1983, McLellan concluded that employment history and status at entry to treatment were associated with longer stays in treatment and better outcomes after leaving treatment. More specifically, the best predictor of post-treatment employment in both the DARP and TOPS studies was having been employed before entry to methadone maintenance (Hubbard *et al.*, 1989; Simpson & Sells, 1982).

Living with Family/Partner

Stimmel *et al.* (1978) found that patients completing treatment were more likely to be living with family than patients who left methadone maintenance for other reasons. More recently, Torrens *et al.* (1996) have found living with family members to be associated with longer stays in treatment. Turning more specifically to marital status, McLellan (1983) concluded that being married or living with a partner was associated with longer retention in treatment and this conclusion is supported by subsequent research. For example, Hubbard *et al.* (1989) also report a relationship between length of stay in methadone maintenance and being married. These results are consistent with common sense in suggesting that those patients with more social support do better in methadone maintenance (McLellan, 1983).

Alcohol Use

High levels of alcohol use have been found to be negatively associated with retention (Szapocznik & Ladner, 1977; Torrens *et al.,* 1996) and overall treatment outcome (Judson & Goldstein, 1982), and predict post-treatment level of alcohol use (Hubbard *et al.,* 1989).

Poly-Drug Use

Poly-drug use is predictive of shorter stays in treatment (McLellan, 1983; Joe *et al.,* 1991; Szapocznik & Ladner, 1977). The TOPS study subsequently confirmed that patients who use only opioids tend to stay in methadone maintenance longer (Hubbard *et al.,* 1989).

Motivation and Expectations Regarding Treatment

In 1983, McLellan mentioned that a number of authors had hypothesised that motivation to change is an important variable in predicting treatment outcome. He noted, however, that while this is plausible, there were no measures of motivation available to test this hypothesis. One recent study has since found stronger motivation and a greater desire for help to be associated with retention in the early stages of methadone maintenance (Simpson & Joe, 1993). This study also found that realistic, as opposed to unrealistic, expectations regarding treatment were also associated with remaining in treatment.

The evidence reviewed in this section suggests that patients who have a long history of opioid dependence and criminal activity will do poorly if they leave methadone maintenance prematurely. This should be seen in the light of the more general point that patients who leave methadone maintenance for reasons other than completing treatment with staff assent have a high risk of relapsing. As common sense would dictate, patients who have less severe drug and legal problems, who have some form of social support, who have few or no psychological problems, and who find work, are more likely to reach a point after a relatively short period of methadone maintenance where they have a reasonable chance of capitalising on the positive behaviour changes they have made while in treatment. In the next section we consider ways in which methadone maintenance programs might maximise retention rates for patients with more serious problems who need longer periods of methadone maintenance.

Treatment Characteristics and Retention

It is clear from the evidence reviewed in the previous sections that a substantial proportion of patients leave methadone maintenance before they have any likelihood of even short-term success in recovering from their dependence. Ironically, these are the patients most in need of methadone maintenance in that they have more severe drug and drug-related problems. This section examines ways in which characteristics of the treatment delivered affect patient retention in order to identify ways in which retention rates might be improved.

Methadone Dose

For a full discussion of the importance of methadone dose see Chapter 9. For the purposes of this chapter, it can be noted that methadone dose is an important predictor of retention in methadone maintenance (e.g., Ling *et al.,* 1996; Strain *et al.,* 1993). Patients who are maintained on higher doses of methadone stay in treatment longer. Patients who are maintained on low doses of methadone as a consequence of the clinic following a low dose policy, rather than dose being determined on an individual basis, tend to drop out of treatment.

Treatment Philosophy

Clinics that follow a short-term maintenance philosophy have poorer retention rates than those who follow a long-term maintenance philosophy (Caplehorn *et al.,* 1993; McGlothlin & Anglin, 1981a). While at first glance this might seem obvious given that short-term treatment is what the short-term maintenance philosophy espouses, an examination of the two studies that have investigated this issue suggest that the short-term maintenance philosophy is associated with poorer retention independent of treatment goal. For example, in the study conducted by McGlothlin and Anglin (1981a) described above, an examination of the numbers of patients who completed treatment, absconded or were expelled is revealing (Hargreaves, 1983). While 12% and 18% of the patients completed treatment in the two long-term maintenance programs, only 2% did so in the short-term maintenance program. Furthermore, while 10% and 16% absconded from the long-term maintenance programs, 29% did so from the short-term maintenance program. Finally, while 18% and 22% of patients were expelled from the long-term maintenance programs, 44% were expelled from the short-term maintenance program. These figures suggest that the short-term maintenance program was associated with less success in terms of patients completing treatment, more failure in terms of keeping their patients in methadone maintenance, and less capacity to change patients' behaviour without expelling them. Similarly, Caplehorn *et al.,* (1993) found that the short-term maintenance philosophy of treatment was associated with poorer retention when compared with the long-term philosophy and that this relationship persisted after methadone dose and the maximum allowable treatment period had been adjusted for.

Ancillary Services

The term 'ancillary services' refers to services provided by methadone maintenance programs other than the dispensing of methadone. These services may include such things as medical treatment, counselling (see Chapter 11) and job training. While there has been considerable speculation about the possible role of ancillary services in increasing treatment retention, there are few well-conducted studies and their results are inconsistent. In an extensive analysis of the data collected for the TOPS study, which examined treatment characteristics associated with retention, Joe *et al.* (1991) found exposure to medical, psychological and financial services during treatment to be associated with increased retention. Similarly, in another analysis of this data set, Condelli (1993) found increased retention to be associated with a higher patient rating of the quality of social services available in the clinic. This suggests that it may not be the provision of services *per se,* but their quality that is important. A recent study reported by Maddux *et al.,* (1995b) also suggests that the level of service provision may need to be appropriate to client needs. They compared mandatory to optional counselling and found that patients in the optional counselling condition attended half as many counselling sessions as the mandatory counselling group, yet were retained longer in treatment. These findings suggest that the level of service provision within methadone clinics has to be tailored to the needs of patients and has to also take account of the extent to which they want and will make use of them.

Clinic Accessibility

The extent to which the clinic is accessible has been found to be associated with retention in the TOPS study (Condelli, 1993; Joe *et al.,* 1991). Although no research has been reported on the issue, Payte and Khuri (1993) suggest plausibly that the accessibility of treatment (e.g., convenient clinic hours) is likely to influence retention.

Treatment Fees

The provision of methadone treatment, like many other aspects of medicine, has undergone considerable privatisation in recent years (Bell *et al.,* 1995; Britton, 1994). Maddux and colleagues (1994) recently compared fee-for-service methadone maintenance with free treatment and found that the patients in the fee-for-service condition had poorer retention rates than those who did not have to pay.

Take-Home Methadone Doses

The provision of take-home methadone doses has been found to be related to retention in two studies. Grabowski *et al.* (1993) compared the effects of providing five versus two take-home methadone doses to two groups of patients who were maintained on either a high (80 mg per day) or low (50 mg per day) dose of methadone. In both groups the provision of more take-home methadone doses was associated with increased retention. In another study that examined the clinical impact of a nation-wide prohibition on take-home methadone that was implemented in Italy in January 1991, Pani *et al.* (1996) found that the restriction of take-home methadone was associated with a lowered retention rate.

Rapid Assessment

Having a rapid as opposed to a slow assessment process has been found to be associated with better subsequent retention in treatment in two studies (Bell *et al.,* 1994; Woody *et al.,* 1975). In a recent study employing a randomised design, Maddux *et al.* (1995a) failed to find a statistically significant difference between a rapid and a more protracted assessment process, but more patients initiated treatment in the rapid assessment group and although not statistically significant there was a trend towards increased retention in this group.

Contingency Contracting

As noted in Chapter 10, the use of negative consequences such as reductions in methadone doses as a response to illicit drug use has been associated with losing patients from treatment in a number of studies (Stitzer *et al.,* 1993).

The studies reviewed in this section suggest a number of strategies that could be employed to maximise retention in methadone maintenance treatment. These strategies can be summarised as the provision of accessible and effective treatment in a form that is appropriate to the target population. The relationship between providing *effective* treatment and the willingness of patients to remain in treatment has not often been emphasised. Given that the main "need" that patients present with is to be helped with their opioid dependence, it is highly likely that one important determinant of retention is the extent to which they quickly receive the help they are seeking in a form that they find acceptable. Rapid assessment, adequate methadone dosing and a treatment philosophy that allows for long-term treatment seem to be important ingredients in providing this help in an appropriate manner.

PHILOSOPHIES OF TREATMENT AND DURATION OF METHADONE MAINTENANCE

In this section, we consider the two treatment philosophies identified at the beginning of the chapter in the light of the evidence we have reviewed. This evidence clearly supports the long-term maintenance treatment philosophy. An orientation towards long-term maintenance is associated with effective treatment and superior retention rates and is consistent with what is likely to be achieved in the short term with the target population. The evidence concerning the high rate of relapse to heroin use among patients who leave treatment suggests long-term maintenance is a pragmatic response to a chronic condition that reappears once treatment is removed.

While the research evidence favours the long-term maintenance philosophy, it does not mean that one has to accept the theory that opioid dependence is a metabolic disease. Newman (1991), for example, has argued that the only plausible explanation for the success of methadone maintenance is that opioid dependence is a metabolic disease. There is, however, no necessary connection between the long-term maintenance philosophy and the metabolic disease hypothesis. In fact, we see no reason at this time to make any assumptions about the aetiology of opioid dependence in order to explain the success of dispensing methadone in reducing opioid use and drug-related crime. The most parsimonious explanation is that methadone maintenance works because it provides, in a controlled fashion, an opioid substance that is acceptable to patients as an alternative to illegally obtained opioids such as heroin.

While the disease model may have advantages in the U.S., it may be disadvantageous in other countries for the long-term maintenance philosophy to depend so heavily on disease theories of dependence which not all disciplines and drug treatment workers accept. Another major disadvantage of employing these notions is that by telling patients they have a disease for which they will need to take methadone indefinitely, patients may develop the belief that they will never be able to recover from their dependence, thereby creating a self-fulfilling prophecy (D'Amanda, 1983).

We would also emphasise that it is wise to avoid creating unrealistic expectations about early recovery. Rosenbaum (1985) found patients who attended short-term maintenance clinics were often told by treatment staff that they should be able to overcome their problems and lead a drug-free life. To this end they were encouraged to detoxify after relatively short periods of methadone maintenance. They would then relapse and return to treatment only to repeat the cycle time and time again. Rosenbaum (1985) suggests this cycle of detoxification, failure and return to methadone maintenance, which the short-term maintenance approach induces, erodes the patient's already fragile sense of self-worth and self-efficacy. The short-term maintenance treatment philosophy may, therefore, not only be ineffective but harmful in the long run to the best interest of the patients.

DOES METHADONE TREATMENT PROLONG DEPENDENCE?

Over the past three decades, critics of the long-term maintenance approach have argued that there is a substantial risk of prolonging the opioid dependence of patients attending for long-term opioid replacement therapy. This view has had a substantial influence on the widespread acceptance of the short-term maintenance treatment philosophy and regulations governing methadone treatment. For example, a two-year review became part of federal regulations in the USA in the early 1970s. It arose not out of research or clinical practice, but out of political pressure that was brought to bear as a result of a concern that methadone maintenance patients were being sentenced to a life of methadone dependence – a view that was shared by proponents of the short-term maintenance model and social critics who saw methadone treatment as a form of social control (Attewell & Gerstein, 1979; Newman, 1977).

In considering the risk that methadone maintenance might prolong dependence, it has to be remembered that nearly every pharmacotherapy employed in modern medicine poses risks to the patient that have to be weighed against the benefits derived from administering the drug concerned. The decision to use or not use a given therapy has to be made in the light of knowledge about what will happen if the therapy is not employed. As Nies (1990) has succinctly summarised the issues involved in such decision making:

> The utility of a regimen can be defined as the benefit it produces plus the dangers of not treating the disease minus the sum of the adverse effects of therapy. (p. 74).

The benefits of methadone maintenance treatment have been demonstrated in terms of reductions in heroin use, crime, premature mortality and rates of HIV infection (see Chapters 2 & 3). The dangers of not treating opioid-dependent individuals can be stated in terms of the ongoing risks posed by continued heroin use and the lifestyle associated with it. The adverse effects of therapy have been discussed in detail by Mattick and Hall (1993). For the purposes of the current chapter, the key adverse effect would be the prolongation of opioid dependence for longer than would otherwise occur if an alternative treatment were employed or even, as argued by some, if no treatment were employed. Follow-up studies of dependent opioid users suggest that the rates of long-term recovery are equivalent among untreated individuals, individuals who have been receiving methadone maintenance (Goldstein & Herrera, 1995; Hser *et al.,* 1993) and individuals who have been treated in the major alternative modality, the therapeutic community (Maddux & Desmond, 1992). This evidence suggests that the benefits of long-term methadone maintenance are not provided at the expense of a prolonged opioid dependence.

CONCLUSION

In general terms the question we have tried to answer in this chapter is one that is often asked by patients, their family members, the community and policy makers: For opioid replacement therapies such as methadone maintenance treatment, how long is long enough? We have attempted, on the basis of the accumulated research evidence and clinical literature concerning methadone treatment to answer this and other subsidiary questions. In brief, the evidence clearly suggests that only a minority of individuals will require relatively short periods of methadone maintenance. Such individuals are a minority who come to treatment with a short history of opioid dependence and significant social and psychological resources at their disposal which can be deployed in the recovery process. For the majority of entrants to methadone programs, it is more appropriate to have maintenance as a goal and to maximise retention rates so that the benefits of treatment are realised for both the individual and the community. There is therefore no specifiable, optimal duration for methadone maintenance treatment.

SUMMARY

There are two broad treatment philosophies of methadone maintenance. One philosophy, which is primarily medically based, views opioid dependence as a metabolic disease and the goal of treatment as successful maintenance on methadone; the other philosophy, which is non-medical, views opioid dependence as the manifestation of underlying social and psychological problems and the goal of treatment as abstinence from all drugs including methadone. According to the latter philosophy, a relatively brief period of methadone maintenance is seen as a useful period within which the patient can be rehabilitated and then detoxified and able to lead a drug-free life. This chapter examines these treatment philosophies from the perspective of their viability as indicated by research findings. Research findings pertinent to an evaluation of these two philosophies comes from a variety of sources. They include studies that have examined aspects of treatment duration and its relationship to post-treatment outcome; the relationship between reason for leaving treatment and post-treatment outcome; the outcome of individuals who have had their treatment removed for reasons unrelated to their clinical management; and predictors of treatment tenure.

The research suggests that there is an association between longer stays in methadone maintenance and a positive post-treatment outcome as measured by reduced illicit opioid use and criminal activity. This evidence suggests that periods of at least two to three years of continuous methadone maintenance are more likely to benefit a majority of patients than are briefer periods. However, the evidence does not allow the specification of an optimum duration for methadone maintenance which would be applicable to all individuals. That is, in general terms, the evidence indicates that longer stays are better than shorter stays, and that being in methadone maintenance is better than not being in methadone maintenance. Studies of the fate of individuals who have had their treatment removed for financial reasons indicates that limiting the duration of methadone maintenance, whether for financial or philosophical reasons, has serious negative consequences for a majority of patients.

Studies that have examined the relationship between patient characteristics and post-treatment outcome suggest that patients with the following characteristics will relapse to drug use and/or criminal activity if they leave treatment:

- a longer and heavier history of opioid use;
- a longer and more extensive criminal history;
- leaving methadone maintenance against staff advice;
- exhibiting little behaviour change during treatment;
- not living with family or partner;
- not finding employment before, during or after methadone maintenance.

On the other hand, patients with less severe drug problems, who have little history of criminal activity, who have reasonable social support, and who become employed have a better chance of success if they complete methadone maintenance. Overall, the evidence on patient characteristics suggests that patients should not be encouraged to leave methadone maintenance before they show these signs of rehabilitation (i.e., employment, stable social adjustment, no illicit drug use, etc.). On the contrary efforts should be made, where possible, to retain such patients in treatment.

Recent research on the relationship between treatment program characteristics and retention suggests that some forms of methadone maintenance are more successful at retaining their patients than others. Programs that are affordable, provide rapid access to treatment, prescribe higher methadone doses, have a flexible policy regarding dosage, a non-punitive approach to illicit drug use and are oriented toward maintenance rather than abstinence are more likely to meet the needs of their patients than programs that do not. Similarly, programs that are accessible, that have convenient hours, and employ staff with positive attitudes towards methadone treatment and their patients are more likely to retain their patients.

Even though there is very little research to support it, until recently, the short-term philosophy of methadone maintenance had a strong influence on government policy and treatment practice. The original program devised by Dole and Nyswander (1967) for methadone maintenance was a maintenance regimen. A return to this basic philosophy is suggested by the evidence reviewed above. The optimum duration for methadone maintenance is, therefore, for as long as the patient benefits from taking a daily dose of methadone, and given the chronic, relapsing nature of opioid dependence, there is no reason to believe that this would be for a short period of time while heroin remains relatively freely available in our society.

REFERENCES

Alexander, B. K. (1990). The empirical and theoretical bases for an adaptive model of addiction. *Journal of Drug Issues,* **20**, 37-65.

Anglin, M. D., Speckart, G. R., Booth, M. W., & Ryan, T. M. (1989). Consequences and costs of shutting off methadone. *Addictive Behaviors,* **14**, 307-326.

Attewell, P., & Gerstein, D. R. (1979). Government policy and local practice. *American Sociological Review,* **44**, 311-327.

Ball, J. C., & Ross, A. (1991). *The effectiveness of methadone maintenance treatment: Patients, programs, services, and outcome.* New York: Springer-Verlag.

Bell, J., Caplehorn, J. R. M., & McNeil, D. R. (1994). The effect of intake procedures on performance in methadone maintenance. *Addiction,* **89**, 463-471.

Bell, J., Hall, W., & Byth, K. (1992). Changes in criminal activity after entering methadone maintenance. *British Journal of Addiction,* **87**, 251-258.

Bell, J., Ward, J., Mattick, R.P., Hay, A., Chan, J., & Hall, W. (1995). *An evaluation of private methadone clinics* (National Drug Strategy Report Series No. 4). Canberrra, Australia: Australian Government Publishing Service.

Britton, B. M. (1994). The privatization of methadone maintenance; changes in risk behavior associated with cost related detoxification. *Addiction Research,* **2**, 171-181.

Caplehorn, J. R. M., & Bell, J. (1991). Methadone dosage and retention of patients in maintenance treatment. *Medical Journal of Australia,* **154**, 195-199.

Caplehorn, J. R. M., McNeil, D. R., & Kleinbaum, D. G. (1993). Clinic policy and retention in methadone maintenance. *International Journal of the Addictions,* **28**, 73-89.

Cole, S. G., & James, L. R. (1975). A revised treatment typology based on the DARP. *American Journal of Drug and Alcohol Abuse,* **2**, 37-49.

Condelli, W. S. (1993). Strategies for increasing retention in methadone programs. *Journal of Psychoactive Drugs,* **25**, 143-147.

Cushman, P. (1978). Abstinence following detoxification and methadone maintenance treatment. *American Journal of Medicine,* **65**, 46-52.

Cushman, P. (1981). Detoxification after methadone treatment. In J. H. Lowinson & P. Ruiz (Eds.), *Substance abuse: Clinical problems and perspectives* (pp. 389-395). USA: Williams Wilkins.

D'Amanda, C. (1983). Program policies and procedures associated with treatment outcome. In J. R. Cooper, F. Altman, B. S. Brown, & D. Czechowicz (Eds.), *Research on the treatment of narcotic addiction: State of the art* (pp. 637-679). Rockville, MD: National Insitute on Drug Abuse.

Des Jarlais, D. C., Joseph, H., & Dole, V. P. (1981). Long-term outcomes after termination from methadone maintenance treatment. *Annals of the New York Academy of Sciences,* 362, 231-238.

Dole, V. P. (1988). Implications of methadone maintenance for theories of narcotic addiction. *Journal of the American Medical Association,* 260, 3025-3029.

Dole, V. P., & Joseph, H. J. (1977). Methadone maintenance: Outcome after termination. *New York State Journal of Medicine,* 77, 1409-1412.

Dole, V. P., & Joseph, H. J. (1978). Long-term outcome of patients treated with methadone maintenance. *Annals of the New York Academy of Sciences,* 311, 181-189.

Dole, V. P., & Nyswander, M. (1967). Heroin addiction: A metabolic disease. *Archives of Internal Medicine,* 120, 19-24.

Goldstein, A. (1991). Heroin addiction: Neurobiology, pharmacology, and policy. *Journal of Psychoactive Drugs,* 23, 123-133.

Goldstein, A., & Herrera, J. (1995). Heroin addicts and methadone treatment in Albuquerque: A 22-year follow-up. *Drug and Alcohol Dependence,* 40, 139-150.

Grabowski, J., Rhoades, H., Elk, R., Schmitz, J., & Creson, D. (1993). Clinicwide and individualized behavioral interventions in drug dependence treatment. In L. S. Onken, J. D. Blaine, & J. J. Boren (Eds.), *Behavioral treatments for drug abuse and dependence* (NIDA Research Monograph 137, pp. 37-71). Rockville, MD: National Insitute on Drug Abuse.

Graff, H., & Ball, J. C. (1976). The methadone clinic: Function and philosophy. *International Journal of Social Psychiatry,* 22, 140-146.

Grella, C. E., Anglin, M. D., Wugalter, S. E., Rawson, R., & Hasson, A. (1994). Reasons for discharge from methadone maintenance for addicts at high risk of HIV infection or transmission. *Journal of Psychoactive Drugs,* 26, 223-232.

Hall, S. M. (1983). Methadone treatment: A review of the research findings. In J. R. Cooper, F. Altman, B. S. Brown, & D. Czechowicz (Eds.), *Research on the treatment of narcotic addiction: State of the art* (pp. 575-632). Rockville, MD: National Institute on Drug Abuse.

Hall, W. (1993). Perfectionism in the therapeutic appraisal of methadone maintenance. *Addiction,* 88, 1173-1175.

Hargreaves, W.A. (1983). Methadone dosage and duration for maintenance treatment. In J.R. Cooper, F. Altman, B.S. Brown, & D. Czechowicz (Eds.), *Research on the treatment of narcotic addiction: State of the art* (pp. 19-79). Rockville, MD: National Institute on Drug Abuse.

Hser, Y., Anglin, M. D., & Powers, K. (1993). A 24-year follow-up of California narcotics addicts. *Archives of General Psychiatry,* 50, 577-584.

Hubbard, R.L., Marsden, M.E., Rachal, J.V., Harwood, H.J., Cavanaugh, E.R., & Ginzburg, H.M. (1989). *Drug abuse treatment: a national study of effectiveness.* Chapel Hill, NC: University of North Carolina Press.

Institute of Medicine. (1995). *Federal regulation of methadone treatment.* Washington, DC: National Academy Press.

Joe, G. W., Simpson, D. D., & Hubbard, R. L. (1991). Treatment predictors of tenure in methadone maintenance. *Journal of Substance Abuse, 3,* 73-84.

Judson, B. A., & Goldstein, A. (1982). Prediction of long-term outcome for heroin addicts admitted to a methadone maintenance program. *Drug and Alcohol Dependence, 10,* 383-393.

Kang, S., & De Leon, G. (1993). Correlates of drug injection behaviors among methadone outpatients. *American Journal of Drug and Alcohol Abuse, 19,* 107-118.

Kreek, M. J. (1992). Rationale for maintenance pharmacotherapy of opiate dependence. In C. P. O'Brien & J. H. Jaffe (Eds.), *Addictive states* (Research publications: Association for Research in Nervous and Mental Disease Vol. 70, pp. 205-230). New York: Raven Press.

Ling, W., Wesson, D. R., Charuvastra, C., & Klett, J. (1996). A controlled trial comparing buprenorphine and methadone maintenance in opioid dependence. *Archives of General Psychiatry, 53,* 401-407.

Maddux, J. F., & Desmond, D. P. (1992). Methadone maintenance and recovery from opioid dependence. *American Journal of Drug and Alcohol Abuse, 18,* 63-74.

Maddux, J. F., Desmond, D. P., & Esquivel, M. (1995). Rapid admission and retention on methadone. *American Journal of Drug and Alcohol Abuse, 21,* 533-547.

Maddux, J. F., Desmond, D. P., & Vogtsberger, K. N. (1995). Patient-regulated methadone dose and optional counseling in methadone maintenance. *American Journal on Addictions, 4,* 18-32.

Maddux, J. F., Prihoda, T. J., & Desmond, D. P. (1994). Treatment fees and retention on methadone maintenance. *Journal of Drug Issues, 24,* 429-443.

Mattick, R. P., & Hall, W. (Eds.). (1993). *A treatment outline for approaches to opioid dependence.* Canberra, Australia: Australian Government Publishing Service.

McGlothlin, W. H., & Anglin, M. D. (1981a). Long-term follow-up of clients of high- and low-dose methadone programs. *Archives of General Psychiatry, 38,* 1055-1063.

McGlothlin, W. H., & Anglin, M. D. (1981b). Shutting off methadone: Costs and benefits. *Archives of General Psychiatry, 38,* 885-892.

McLellan, A. T. (1983). Patient characteristics associated with outcome. In J. R. Cooper, F. Altman, B. S. Brown, & D. Czechowicz (Eds.), *Research on the treatment of narcotic addiction: State of the art* (pp. 500-529). Rockville, MD: National Insitute on Drug Abuse.

Newman, R. G. (1977). *Methadone treatment in narcotic addiction: Program management, findings and prospects for the future.* New York: Academic Press.

Newman, R. G. (1991). What's so special about methadone maintenance? *Drug and Alcohol Review,* **10,** 225-232.

Nies, A. S. (1990). Principles of therapeutics. In A. G. Gilman, T. W. Rall, A. S. Nies, & P. Taylor (Eds.), *The pharmacological basis of therapeutics* (7th Edition ed., pp. 62-83). USA: Pergamon.

Pani, P. P., Pirastu, R., Ricci, A., & Gessa, G. L. (1996). Prohibition of take-home dosages: Negative consequences on methadone maintenance treatment. *Drug and Alcohol Dependence,* **41,** 81-84.

Payte, J. T., & Khuri, E. T. (1993). Treatment duration and patient retention. In M. W. Parrino (Ed.), *State methadone treatment guidelines* (pp. 119-124). Rockville, MD: Center for Substance Abuse Treatment, U.S. Department of Health and Human Services.

Rosenbaum, M. (1985). A matter of style: Variation among methadone clinics in the control of clients. *Contemporary Drug Problems,* **12,** 375-400.

Rosenbaum, M., Irwin, J., & Murphy, S. (1988). De facto destabilization as policy: The impact of short-term methadone maintenance. *Contemporary Drug Problems,* **15,** 491-517.

Simpson, D. D. (1979). The relation of time spent in drug abuse treatment to posttreatment outcome. *American Journal of Psychiatry,* **136,** 1449 1453.

Simpson, D. D. (1981). Treatment for drug abuse: Follow-up outcomes and length of time spent. *Archives of General Psychiatry,* **38,** 875-880.

Simpson, D. D., & Joe, G. W. (1993). Motivation as a predictor of early dropout from drug abuse treatment. *Psychotherapy,* **30,** 357-368.

Simpson, D. D., & Sells, S. B. (1982). Effectiveness of treatment for drug abuse: An overview of the DARP research program. *Advances in Alcohol and Substance Abuse,* **2,** 7-29.

Sisk, J. E., Hatziandreu, E. J., & Hughes, R. (1990). *The effectiveness of drug abuse treatment: Implications for controlling AIDS/HIV infection.* Washington, DC: Congress of the United States, Office of Technology Assessment.

Stimmel, B., Goldberg, J., Cohen, M., & Rotkopf, E. (1978). Detoxification from methadone maintenance: Risk factors associated with relapse to narcotic use. *Annals of the New York Academy of Sciences,* **311,** 173-180.

Stitzer, M. L., Iguchi, M. Y., Kidorf, M., & Bigelow, G. E. (1993). Contingency management in methadone treatment: The case for positive incentives. In L. S. Onken, J. D. Blaine, & J. J. Boren (Eds.), *Behavioral treatments for drug abuse and dependence* (NIDA Research Monograph 137, pp. 19-35). Rockville, MD: National Institute on Drug Abuse.

Strain, E. C., Stitzer, M. L., Liebson, I. A., & Bigelow, G. E. (1993). Dose-response effects of methadone in the treatment of opioid dependence. *Annals of Internal Medicine,* 119, 23-27.

Szapocznik, J., & Ladner, R. (1977). Factors related to successful retention in methadone maintenance: A review. *International Journal of the Addictions,* 12, 1067-1085.

Torrens, M., Castillo, C., & Pérez-Solá , V. (1996). Retention in a low-threshold methadone maintenance program. *Drug and Alcohol Dependence,* 41, 55-59.

Ward, J., Mattick, R. P., & Hall, W. (1992). *Key issues in methadone maintenance treatment.* Sydney, Australia: New South Wales University Press.

White, J. M., Dyer, K. R., Ali, R. L., Gaughwin, M. D., & Cormack, S. (1994). Injecting behaviour and risky needle use amongst methadone maintenance clients. *Drug and Alcohol Dependence,* 34, 113-119.

Woody, G., O'Hare, K., Mintz, J., & O'Brien, C. (1975). Rapid intake: A method for increasing retention rate of heroin addicts seeking methadone treatment. *Comprehensive Psychiatry,* 16, 165-169.

13

MAKING THE TRANSITION FROM MAINTENANCE TO ABSTINENCE: DETOXIFICATION FROM METHADONE MAINTENANCE TREATMENT

JEFF WARD, RICHARD P. MATTICK
AND WAYNE HALL

INTRODUCTION

In Chapter 12 in this volume, two conclusions were drawn from the accumulated research evidence about the optimum duration of methadone maintenance treatment. The first was that a majority of patients soon relapse to heroin use if they cease taking methadone. The second was that the reason for leaving treatment was a reasonable predictor of whether a given patient would relapse. Patients who had made significant changes during their tenure in treatment were more likely to succeed than those who left before such changes had taken place.

Moolchan and Hoffman (1994) have suggested that for most patients who have made significant changes in their lifestyle and functioning, there is a point when they begin to contemplate leaving treatment. The task for treatment staff at this point is to assist the patient to make a reasoned decision based on his or her likelihood of success and the advantages and disadvantages of the options of remaining in or leaving treatment. The important focus for such discussions is the extent to which the patient is able to lead a rewarding and fulfilling life, not simply whether it is desirable to continue taking methadone or not.

For some patients, long-term methadone maintenance may be the best option, because withdrawing from methadone may be destabilising. However, such patients no longer require a highly structured treatment program and one option for continuing treatment is "medical" maintenance (Novick & Joseph, 1991) – the term "medical" indicating that their medication can be managed as it is with other patients with chronic conditions such as diabetes or epilepsy. Other patients may be ready to leave treatment and this chapter discusses issues related to the most humane and effective way of facilitating their exit from treatment. The discussion is also applicable to patients who exercise their free will and leave treatment, even though staff may think that this is not their best option at that particular time. One important hurdle that patients leaving treatment must negotiate is the inevitable withdrawal syndrome that occurs when the use of opioids is ceased. The following sections consider the withdrawal syndrome consequent upon the cessation of methadone ingestions and the procedures that have been developed to reduce the suffering associated with the transition from maintenance to abstinence.

THE METHADONE WITHDRAWAL SYNDROME

As with other opioids, when people who are dependent on methadone abruptly cease taking the drug, they exhibit a set of signs and symptoms that are collectively referred to as a withdrawal or abstinence syndrome. While the details of the physiological processes involved in the manifestation of this syndrome are not fully known, it is thought that regular exposure to exogenous opioids causes changes in neuronal functioning in the brain. When exposure suddenly stops or the dose being taken is sharply reduced, a rebound-like effect occurs resulting in hyper-excitability. In short, it is thought that certain endogenous systems in the central nervous system adapt to chronic opioid use and that when this use ceases it takes some time for the body to readjust.

According to Jaffe (1990):

> The abrupt withdrawal of methadone produces a syndrome that is qualitatively similar to that of morphine, but it develops more slowly and is more prolonged, although usually less intense. The addict has few or no symptoms until 24 to 48 hours after the last dose, and then complains of weakness, anxiety, anorexia, insomnia, abdominal discomfort, headaches, sweating, pain in muscles and bones, and hot and cold flashes. As with morphine withdrawal, there is nausea, vomiting, and an increase in body temperature, blood pressure, pulse, respiratory rate, and pupillary size. In general, after abrupt withdrawal, the primary or early abstinence syndrome reaches its maximal intensity by about the third day and may not begin to decrease until the third week; apparent recovery may not occur until the sixth or seventh week (p. 534).

This first or primary phase of withdrawal is succeeded by a secondary and more prolonged abstinence syndrome in which both subjective symptoms of distress and physiological signs of abnormal functioning may be observed (Martin *et al.,* 1973).

The existence of a withdrawal syndrome, unpleasant as it may be, is not sufficient to explain the very high rates of relapse observed among opioid users after detoxification. Opioid-dependent individuals are capable of fully or partially detoxifying themselves and use a variety of methods to achieve this goal without professional assistance (Gossop *et al.,* 1991). This is also the experience of detoxification programs that are quite successful as long as the goal of detoxification is seen as completing the withdrawal process. Such programs would, however, have to be seen as unsuccessful, if there is the unrealistic expectation that the people who briefly pass through them will go on to lead a drug-free life (Mattick & Hall, 1996; Newman, 1983).

DETOXIFICATION FEAR

The distress associated with withdrawing from opioids is better tolerated by some individuals than others. A number of factors are thought to be associated with this. Andrews and Himmelsbach (1944) demonstrated that the greater the amount of opioid required to prevent withdrawal, the more intense the syndrome will be when withdrawal occurs. Similarly, it is widely believed that the longer the person has been dependent, the more intense the withdrawal syndrome will be (Kleber, 1981). However, contrary to these beliefs, Phillips and colleagues (1986) found that neither the dose of methadone required to stabilise patients at the beginning of a detoxification program, nor the length of opioid dependence were associated with the level of withdrawal distress. Instead, they found stronger associations between withdrawal symptoms and neuroticism (as assessed by the Eysenck Personality Questionnaire) and expectations about withdrawal distress.

The role of expectations about how distressing withdrawal might be has led some authors to describe what has been referred to as an abstinence "phobia" or pathological detoxification fear. Hall (1979) characterised abstinence phobia in methadone maintenance patients who are attempting to slowly withdraw from methadone as an exaggerated anxious reaction to comparatively mild withdrawal symptoms. She notes that anxiety is a common symptom of the opioid withdrawal syndrome, but that in the cases she is referring to extreme levels of anxiety are observed which evoke a phobic-like response (i.e., a refusal to attempt or to proceed with the detoxification). Hall suggests that this reaction is probably the result of previous experiences of traumatic, sudden and involuntary withdrawal such as may occur in detention, experiences of observing others suffer severe withdrawal symptoms, or the result of inaccurate information about the severity of methadone withdrawal that circulates within the heroin-using subculture.

Hall (1979) proposed that abstinence phobia might, like other phobias, be amenable to treatment. Hall *et al.* (1984) tested this proposition by examining whether the addition of a cognitive-behavioural intervention (relaxation training tied to anxiety as cue plus cognitive restructuring of withdrawal symptoms) assisted patients who wished to detoxify from methadone. When they compared two stratified random samples of methadone maintenance patients, they found no discernible influence for the intervention on reductions in methadone dose, detoxification rate or detoxification anxiety. However, the findings of the study did support the existence and importance of a phenomenon of detoxification anxiety. Patients who were assessed as being anxious about detoxifying at the beginning of the study showed only minimal changes in their maintenance dosage, and assessed levels of detoxification anxiety were found to increase as dose decreased.

Milby and his colleagues have developed an instrument for assessing detoxification fear (Gentile & Milby, 1992; Milby *et al.*, 1987; Milby *et al.*, 1986; Milby *et al.*, 1994; Raczynski *et al.*, 1988). Milby *et al.* (1986, 1994) make a distinction between mild anxiety in anticipation of an unpleasant experience and unrealistic fear which is out of proportion to the symptoms experienced in a dose reduction withdrawal procedure. They agree with Hall (1979) and suggest that such apparently unrealistic fear may have a realistic component if it is based on experiences that have been very traumatic, such as unassisted detoxification in a prison or police station.

Milby *et al.* (1986) surveyed methadone maintenance patients from three cities in the USA and found 28% to be suffering from high levels of detoxification fear. They also found that significantly more women than men suffered from this fear. This finding is consistent with the observation of Rosenbaum and Murphy (1984) that women may experience the emotional dimensions of withdrawal more intensely than men do and evidence that women are more likely to experience anxiety disorders than men (Robins *et al.*, 1991). In a further study, Milby *et al.* (1994) also found that patients suffering from high levels of detoxification fear were more likely to also be suffering from a depressive or anxiety disorder, suggesting that detoxification fear may be a manifestation of a more general neurotic personality.

The clinical usefulness of identifying patients with detoxification fear has been established in two studies (Milby *et al.*, 1994; Schumacher *et al.*, 1992). Both of these studies found that patients assessed as having high levels of detoxification fear stayed in methadone treatment longer and made fewer attempts to withdraw from methadone than did patients assessed as having little or no detoxification fear. Milby *et al.* (1994) further reported that patients with high levels of detoxification fear who sought psychotherapy to assist them to detoxify were more likely to succeed than similar patients who did not seek additional therapy. This finding is in contradiction to those of Hall *et al.* (1984) reported above and suggests that there may be some benefit to providing additional psychological help and support to patients with high levels of detoxification fear.

In summary, sufficient evidence exists to suggest that there is a subgroup of methadone maintenance patients who are fearful of detoxifying from methadone for this to be an impediment to completing withdrawal. The contradictory findings reported above for attempts to overcome this impediment, suggest that further research is warranted into the nature of this anxiety and the application of existing therapies to alleviate it. One simple intervention that has shown some success in alleviating anxiety in withdrawing opioid users is reported by Green and Gossop (1988). They based their procedure on the assumption that clear, accurate information may reduce the distress involved in withdrawal, as has been found in other areas of medicine where unpleasant interventions have to be employed. Green and Gossop compared the responses of opioid-dependent individuals randomly assigned to an information and no-information condition for a 21-day methadone detoxification program. The subjects who received the information were more likely to complete detoxification and experienced less subjective withdrawal distress during the period immediately after their methadone dose reached zero. The implications of this study are that accurate information may also be useful in alleviating anxiety among withdrawing methadone maintenance patients. The extent to which this would also be true for patients with severe detoxification anxiety is unclear.

WITHDRAWAL METHODS AND REGIMENS

In this section, different methods and regimens for detoxifying opioid-dependent individuals are considered. In order to make detoxification a more humane process, there has been a constant search for medications and procedures that alleviate the suffering involved, and a startling array have been tried over the years (see Kleber, 1981). The treatment of choice for detoxification regimens has for some time been a course of diminishing doses of methadone, so that individuals detoxifying could do so with as little distress as possible. This has also been the procedure of choice for methadone maintenance patients when they are leaving treatment. Recent experimentation with other medications (e.g., clonidine) has shown promise, but when the disadvantages associated with the use of these medications are taken into account, tapering off from methadone still remains the most effective and humane method for withdrawing opioid-dependent individuals, including methadone maintenance patients.

Methadone-Assisted Withdrawal

There have been few studies that have examined the relative

effectiveness of different methadone withdrawal regimens in detoxifying methadone maintenance patients. Mintz *et al.* (1975) randomly assigned patients to a withdrawal regimen (reduction in dose by 10% per week over two days for 14 weeks) or to continued methadone maintenance under double-blind conditions. Although the study was thwarted by nearly all the patients leaving the experiment by the end of the study period, one finding did emerge: under double-blind conditions, methadone maintenance patients whose dose was being reduced by 10% per week reported withdrawal symptoms, which because of the double-blind design were unlikely to be the result of patient expectation.

In a more successful study, Senay and colleagues (1977) found that under double-blind conditions a slow (3% per week) dose reduction withdrawal regimen was better than a faster (10%) regimen which was associated with higher drop-out rates, more heroin use and greater subjective distress. The inclusion of both blind and open methadone maintenance conditions in the study allowed the authors to estimate the influence of expectation on withdrawal symptoms. They found that in the blind methadone maintenance condition and the slow withdrawal condition (remembering that subjects did not know what conditions they were in) more withdrawal symptoms were observed than in the methadone maintenance condition in which patients knew their dose, suggesting that the uncertainty about whether their dose was being reduced or not induced withdrawal symptoms in the blind methadone maintenance condition. By contrast, both the blind methadone maintenance condition and the slow withdrawal condition exhibited less withdrawal symptoms than the fast withdrawal condition, demonstrating that rate of detoxification also played a part. This study is consistent with the result of Mintz *et al.* in demonstrating that withdrawal phenomena are related to both rate of methadone reduction and to patient expectations about withdrawal symptoms.

Given that patient expectations appear to play a role in the withdrawal process, it may be possible to devise conditions in which these expectations assist in achieving detoxification from methadone. Panepinto *et al.* (1977) report on a procedure used in a methadone maintenance program for pregnant women and their partners in which the patients knew their doses and had some control over their detoxification schedule. Using this procedure, they found that 63% of a group of patients successfully completed the detoxification process. An important part of the regimen was regular attendance at a group held for detoxifying methadone maintenance patients, in which issues of relevance to the patients were discussed. The arguments put forward for both the open schedule and the importance of detoxification groups are plausible, but the unusual characteristics of the study participants make it difficult to accept that the findings can be generalised to the population of all methadone maintenance patients. Pregnant women were over-represented in the sample (74%), which means presumably that at the time of detoxification all would have had young babies to take care of. The small number of men in the sample, in comparison to the usual methadone maintenance patient population where men usually outnumber women, were all partners of these women. The significance of the influence children may have on methadone maintenance patients may be considerable. Rosenbaum (1981, 1991) has found in two surveys that both opioid addicts out of treatment and methadone maintenance patients report that having children spurs them on to make an extra effort to deal with their opioid dependence.

The three studies discussed above (Mintz *et al.,* 1975; Panepinto *et al.,* 1977; Senay *et al.,* 1977) raise the main issues that need to be addressed in a withdrawal regimen: (a) the rate at which the methadone dose should be reduced and whether this relates to maintenance dose level; (b) whether the reductions in dose should be blind or open; and (c) whether group or individual counselling is an important part of the process.

The clinical consensus concerning the rate of withdrawal is that withdrawing patients from methadone maintenance should be done in a slow, gradual fashion (Kleber, 1977). For example, Lowinson and colleagues (1976) recommend dose reductions of 10 mg per fortnight until a daily dose of 40 mg is reached; thereafter the patient should be split-dosed and further reductions made at 5 mg per fortnight until the daily dose reaches 10 mg. When 10 mg is reached, they recommend reductions of 2-3 mg per week which are introduced according to individual response. Cushman (1981) suggests reductions of 5 mg per week until the daily dose reaches 20 mg, when the reduction rate should be halved to 2.5 mg per week.

Two conclusions emerge from these recommendations: that the process should be gradual and that there is a point where the tapering of the dose is slowed down. In this regard, it is widely believed that many patients begin to experience difficulties with the withdrawal procedure when the dose reaches around 20 mg (Goldstein, 1971;

Lowinson *et al.*, 1976). If a patient begins to experience withdrawal symptoms, it is preferable to readjust the methadone dose rather than offer ancillary medications, such as the benzodiazepines, which are often abused by methadone maintenance patients.

With regard to whether dose reductions should be known to the patient or not, there is no evidence to suggest that either blind or open dose reduction schedules are more effective. As Kleber (1977) points out, when patients know their dose reduction schedule they are encouraged to participate in the procedure, and to take some responsibility for each dose reduction decision, but their knowledge may lead to anxiety when the dose gets close to zero. Blind withdrawal lessens this anxiety, and for this reason is preferred by some patients. Letting patients know that both options are available, and the relative advantages and disadvantages of each, is probably the best way of maximising participation, while allowing for individual differences in anxiety before and during the detoxification process.

There is probably no optimum method for tapering methadone dosage that is applicable to all patients. Cushman and Dole (1973) conducted a prospective study with 48 methadone maintenance patients who were detoxifying from methadone with the assent of program staff because they were considered to have been rehabilitated. All patients were blind to the dose reduction schedule. It was found that the patients could be categorised into four distinct groups according to their response to being detoxified:

- a small number of patients who, even though they did not experience withdrawal symptoms, became anxious about their dose before it reached 30 mg and asked for methadone maintenance to be reinstated;

- a small number of patients whose dose went below 30 mg and asked for methadone maintenance to be reinstated because they could not tolerate the withdrawal symptoms;

- about one-half of the overall majority of patients who successfully detoxified but who re-entered methadone maintenance because of relapse to drug use or an inability to tolerate the protracted withdrawal syndrome they were experiencing;

- the other half of the detoxified group who were successful in getting off methadone maintenance and leading an opioid-free life.

Cushman and Dole (1973) note that 93% of the patients overall experienced a withdrawal syndrome, and that secondary withdrawal was sufficiently intense to make 25% of the study group return to methadone maintenance after being detoxified. According to the authors, the implication of these findings is that both program staff and patients have to realise that a withdrawal syndrome of some sort is inevitable when a patient leaves methadone maintenance, regardless of the degree of rehabilitation achieved during treatment.

Clonidine

Clonidine is a non-opioid medication (alpha adrenergic blocking agent) that has been mainly used in the treatment of hypertension. In the mid-seventies, it was discovered that clonidine reduced the signs of withdrawal in rats and it was then trialed towards the end of the decade for the detoxification of opioid-dependent humans. In a series of experiments it was found to effectively suppress the opioid withdrawal syndrome. With methadone maintenance patients, it was found that administration of clonidine for the duration of the primary withdrawal period (first 10 days) reduced both the observable signs and subjective distress of the study participants (see Ginzburg, 1983).

When clonidine has been compared with tapered methadone withdrawal, it has usually been found to be equally effective in reducing the signs and symptoms of the abstinence syndrome. However, the two regimens differ in the times during withdrawal when patients experience difficulty. For clonidine, the first few days seem to be difficult, while for methadone tapering, the end of the tapering regimen as the dose nears zero seems to be the time at which many patients suffered the most (Ginzburg, 1983; Gossop, 1988). Given that the methadone withdrawal regimen is the preferred treatment for detoxifying opioid-dependent individuals, the apparent equal efficacy of clonidine is an important finding (Gossop, 1988). For methadone maintenance patients, there would also appear to be an advantage in the use of clonidine. Using a methadone tapering regimen, it may take many months before the patient becomes completely detoxified from methadone. According to its advocates, using clonidine can shorten this period to 10 days. In a number of studies, it has been found that when clonidine was used in combination with the narcotic antagonist naltrexone, the detoxification period can be shortened to a few days (Stine & Kosten, 1992). The usual purpose in achieving this rapid detoxification is to initiate maintenance with an opioid antagonist like naltrexone, a treatment that would effectively block the effects of any opioids taken by the patient.

Marked problems have, however, been found to be associated with the outpatient use of clonidine. These have been serious enough for the two authors who have reviewed the literature on the use of clonidine in opioid detoxification to conclude that there are serious disadvantages with the procedure when it is compared to a tapered methadone regimen (Ginzburg, 1983; Gossop, 1988). Clonidine has a number of undesirable effects when used at the dose levels necessary to suppress withdrawal symptoms. The most unpleasant of these effects are sedation and a lowering of blood pressure. These untoward effects are serious enough to require the close medical supervision of patients who are being administered clonidine at levels necessary for opioid detoxification. Most of the trials of clonidine have accordingly been conducted with hospitalised subjects. When outpatient trials have been conducted, the delicate balance between administering an adequate dose to suppress withdrawal and one which will not result in too great a lowering of blood pressure and sedation has not easily been achieved. Patients also often have difficulty sleeping when taking clonidine during withdrawal and, in some early studies, the procedure induced psychosis in a small number of patients (although this outcome is less likely if patients are screened for a history of psychiatric disorder).

Clonidine, as well as having the disadvantage of serious side-effects, appears to be no more effective than methadone in alleviating the opioid withdrawal syndrome. As Gossop (1988) has pointed out in his comprehensive review of the literature, although clonidine advocates claim that it is more effective than methadone tapering, the evidence does not really indicate this. More recent results confirm Gossop's view. In a randomised controlled trial comparing clonidine to methadone tapering, San *et al.* (1990) found methadone to be more effective at eliminating withdrawal signs and symptoms than clonidine. Similarly, Ghodse and colleagues (1994) found no advantage over a placebo for the addition of clonidine to an in-patient methadone tapering regimen for detoxifying methadone patients in reducing either the symptoms or signs of withdrawal.

There would seem to be little reason to recommend the use of clonidine for detoxifying methadone maintenance patients. Although becoming detoxified from methadone is required in order to complete the recovery process, it does not mean that it is a desirable goal in its own right. Many patients now in methadone maintenance would probably successfully detoxify rapidly using clonidine if this was done in a hospitalised setting. However, we know from the evidence reviewed in Chapter 12 on the duration of methadone maintenance that most patients would quickly relapse to heroin use after leaving hospital. This was confirmed by Rawson *et al.,* (1984) who compared the outcome of methadone maintenance patients detoxified over 10 days using clonidine, who either did or did not then go on to naltrexone maintenance. They found that most of the clonidine-only subjects relapsed because of urges to use heroin rather than because they experienced withdrawal symptoms. This finding emphasises that, just as in the case of illicit opioids, successful detoxification from methadone is a relatively easy goal to achieve under controlled conditions, but that this has very little meaning in terms of recovery from opioid dependence in the long term. This result is fully consistent with what we know from other substance dependence disorders (Mattick & Baillie, 1992; Mattick *et al.,* 1993).

Adjunctive Counselling

There is a clinical consensus that withdrawal from methadone maintenance is a difficult time for most patients and that additional support is needed (Cushman, 1981; Kleber, 1977; Lowinson *et al.,* 1976; Resnick, 1983). Milby (1988), who has reviewed this literature, concluded that some form of psychotherapy or counselling, as distinct from merely providing information, probably assists the withdrawal process, but, given the paucity of studies in this area, was unable to state that the research strongly indicated the importance of counselling for successful withdrawal. Similarly, there was no research evidence available to assess whether group or individual counselling is superior in this regard (Kleber, 1977). As already mentioned earlier in this chapter, some methadone maintenance programs do form 'detox' groups for patients who are ready to leave treatment (Kleber, 1977; Panepinto *et al.,* 1977). Such groups allow individuals going through the same experience to get together and encourage and support one another.

In a survey of staff and patient attitudes to withdrawing from methadone maintenance, Gold and colleagues (1988) found that three-quarters of the patients and nearly of all of the staff members surveyed thought that counselling and psychotherapy would contribute to successfully leaving methadone maintenance. Besides anxiety about withdrawal and difficulties due to withdrawal symptoms, many patients experience a sense of loss about leaving treatment, especially if they have been in methadone maintenance for a long period of time. The patients in the Gold *et al.* survey indicated that they would miss contact with clinic staff and the counselling provided within the program more than coming to the clinic itself or the contact this made possible with the other patients. There is also the loss associated with giving up opioids which have been at the centre of the patient's life for many years (Rosenbaum & Murphy, 1984).

Although there is little research evidence on which to base such a conclusion, it is likely from the observations set out in the clinical literature that supportive counselling during the detoxification process does contribute to a more successful weaning from methadone maintenance for most patients. However, before resources were allocated to such counselling, it would be prudent to ensure that the benefits were demonstrable in independently evaluated research projects and of a sufficient magnitude to warrant the cost. In the next section, we look at the importance of paying attention to patients' motivation for wanting to leave methadone maintenance and the further role that counselling and self-help groups can play once the patient has passed through withdrawal and moved into the post-treatment phase.

REASONS FOR LEAVING METHADONE TREATMENT

A number of factors have been identified as influencing a patient's readiness to attempt withdrawal from methadone maintenance. These include staff attitudes to methadone maintenance and withdrawal, the influence of significant others in the patient's life, and the gains that the patient has made during his or her time in treatment. A patient who has improved during methadone maintenance and who leaves with the blessing of program staff has a reasonable chance of success in leading an opioid-free life (Milby, 1988).

As we have noted previously (see Chapter 12), patients withdraw from methadone for a variety of reasons. These reasons can be broadly classified into three categories:

(a)   patients who have made significant life changes and will be able to leave without these gains being destabilised or relapsing to heroin use;

(b)   patients who leave against the advice of program staff; and

(c)   patients who leave involuntarily because they have been sentenced to prison or have broken program rules and are being mandatorily detoxified.

In the first and last categories the precursors to exit from the program are reasonably clear. In the first case, a long period of not heavily or regularly using the more serious illicit drugs in combination with other signs of change will be evident to program staff. In the case of involuntary withdrawal from methadone maintenance, serious infraction of program rules or being sentenced by a court are usually the immediate precursors.

With the second category – leaving contrary to advice – a number of factors might precipitate a premature exit from treatment. Initially, patients who enter methadone maintenance may have unrealistic expectations about what is possible for them. Often they think that after many years of opioid dependence they will be able to get themselves together and get off methadone within a few months (Caplehorn & Bell, 1991; Stimmel *et al.*, 1977). A patient who wishes to leave methadone maintenance after a short period should be offered the opportunity to discuss their reasons for wanting to detoxify with program staff. Other pressures that methadone maintenance patients feel are the stigma associated with being a methadone maintenance patient (Murphy & Irwin, 1992) and the burden of having to come into the clinic regularly. In other cases, patients are coerced into leaving treatment by family or friends who do not understand the treatment or its goals. In all of the instances discussed in this paragraph, staff can clarify with the patient the reasons why they feel they have to leave treatment at that particular point and assist, if necessary, in ensuring the patient is treated fairly (e.g., at other sites within the health care system) or in educating family and friends about methadone maintenance treatment and the rationale for its use (Kleber, 1977; Lowinson *et al.*, 1976).

The attitudes of staff may also affect a patient's decision to leave treatment. Lowinson *et al.* (1976) suggest that the best course to take is to develop an attitude that is at the same time neutral (in the sense of not subscribing to any given duration of methadone maintenance as being the best) and patient-centred. If staff members appear either eager or pessimistic about leaving treatment they may thwart any attempts in the latter case, or they may make the patient feel that they cannot live up to staff expectations in the former. The issue of the way in which staff attitudes to the optimum duration of treatment may unduly influence patients is discussed in more detail in Chapter 12. Being patient-centred also means that if a patient decides after consultation that he or she wants to leave treatment at a time that staff feel is inappropriate, then the decision should be respected and full encouragement and support offered as would occur in other cases.

AFTERCARE

It is widely acknowledged that individuals who have left methadone maintenance need assistance and support for some time afterwards with the aim of minimising lapses and relapses to opioid use (e.g., Gold *et al.,* 1988; Goldstein, 1972; Lowinson *et al.,* 1976). Former methadone maintenance patients may experience a protracted withdrawal syndrome and may also have to contend with a renewed desire to use heroin in response to environmental cues and emotional states that arise. Relapse to heroin use is associated with an inability to remove oneself from drug using networks, family problems, social isolation, and negative emotional states (Hawkins & Catalano, 1985). Aftercare is designed to assist patients to deal with these problems and may involve a range of services and activities such as regular individual counselling sessions, relapse prevention training and attendance at self-help groups.

As Kleber (1977) has noted, however, although aftercare is often recommended and offered to many former methadone maintenance patients, it is unusual for them to remain in contact with the program once they have detoxified. Providing aftercare that former methadone maintenance patients will take advantage of is an important aspect of methadone maintenance treatment that has not been adequately developed in most countries which offer opioid replacement therapy. In this section, we examine the types of aftercare that have been proposed and the results of the few studies that have investigated their effectiveness.

One suggestion for assisting in the transition from methadone maintenance to abstinence has been for the tapering process to take place while the patient resides in a therapeutic community (Sorensen *et al.*, 1984a). Results of research examining this mode of getting off methadone maintenance suggest that it may be a useful form of aftercare, but that, as is true of the therapeutic community treatment generally, it is acceptable to very few patients (Sorensen *et al.*, 1984b). Wermuth and colleagues (1987) describe an aftercare service that can be delivered by methadone maintenance units on an outpatient basis that involves individual counselling, group meetings, relapse prevention training and referral to Narcotics Anonymous. Wermuth *et al.* suggest that at least six months of aftercare is necessary to help patients get over what they refer to as the post-methadone syndrome. Other suggestions for aftercare have included opioid antagonist maintenance and the integration of 12-step style programs into methadone maintenance programs (Weddington, 1990–91).

The best available evidence for the effectiveness of aftercare in enabling opioid-dependent individuals to make a new life for themselves is provided by a randomised controlled trial conducted in Hong Kong and the USA. This study compared a structured aftercare program with assistance on request which was provided by both study and former treatment personnel (McAuliffe, 1990; McAuliffe & Ch'ien, 1986). The aftercare program, which was trialed in this study, consisted of a combined recovery training and self-help group approach. Subjects had been treated in a range of treatment modalities (methadone maintenance, therapeutic communities, detoxification programs). Each recovery group met for three hours each week for a period of six months, or for longer if participants wished to continue. Half the time the group was led by a trained counsellor who conducted relapse prevention sessions, while the rest of the time was devoted to an unstructured self-help meeting led by one of the group participants. Group members were encouraged to attend extra-curricular social activities and to use the 'buddy' system if they felt themselves at risk of relapsing. The study found that, in comparison with the control condition, the intervention reduced the risk of relapse, self-reported crime and helped unemployed subjects find work. All of the subjects participating in the study were highly motivated individuals who wanted to lead a drug-free life. It remains unclear, however, what proportion of methadone maintenance treatment populations would fall into this category.

Although methadone maintenance patients rarely return to their former programs for assistance, it may be that patients would be more likely to return if specialised aftercare services were made available and presented as part of the treatment process. One possible impediment to providing aftercare services is their cost. However, two things should be kept in mind when the costs of such services are considered. The first is that every patient who is successful is one less patient who will return for another course of treatment (McAuliffe, 1990). The second is that it may be possible to offer such services within existing programs. Wermuth *et al.* (1987), for example, suggest appointing one member of staff as the aftercare specialist who will organise the aftercare program and keep up with developments in the area.

CONCLUSION

Withdrawing from methadone is only one part of the process of leaving methadone maintenance. However, it is important to recognise that the withdrawal process is difficult and that many patients are fearful of the process itself and its consequences. A slow tapering of the patient's methadone dose, in combination with an individualised approach to the rate of reduction and matters such as blinding of dose decreases, is indicated by both research and clinical experience. During the detoxification process, patients are also likely to benefit from accurate information about what they are experiencing, as well as supportive counselling to help them to deal with any difficulties that arise during their transition from maintenance to abstinence. Even when conducted under ideal conditions, it is important to recognise that the success rate of achieving successful abstinence is likely to be low. In the light of this information, it is important to remember that abstinence is only one option available to the patient and that an otherwise fulfilling life while attending for methadone maintenance is another.

SUMMARY

Methadone maintenance patients, like other people who are dependent on opioids, will experience a characteristic withdrawal syndrome if the administration of methadone is ceased abruptly. Because of the relatively long elimination half-life of methadone and the fact that it accumulates in body tissue during maintenance treatment, the methadone withdrawal syndrome is more protracted than that of shorter acting opioids like morphine and heroin, but is also said to be less intense.

As is probably the case with any incipient unpleasant experience, most methadone maintenance patients experience a mild anticipatory anxiety when faced with the prospect of withdrawing from methadone. Providing clear, accurate information about what is about to happen may be helpful in alleviating some of this anxiety. In some patients, however, this mild anxiety becomes a fear of phobic proportions and may make the prospect of leaving treatment difficult. At present, there is no intervention known to be effective in ameliorating this detoxification fear.

The most effective and humane procedure for withdrawing methadone maintenance patients from methadone at the end of treatment has been a slow course of diminishing doses of methadone. The limited research available suggests that the slower the course the better, although clinically the pace is best set individually in consultation with the patient. Tapering can occur in an open fashion in which the patient knows the details of the dose reduction schedule, or in a blind manner in which the patient does not know these details. Some patients prefer to be blind to dose reductions in order to reduce anxiety and prevent expectancy effects. Informing patients about what is possible when withdrawing from methadone maintenance and allowing them to decide what is the best for them is the optimum method for allowing for differences between patients, and of maximising their participation in decision-making process. Supportive counselling is also thought to be an important part of withdrawing from methadone maintenance. There is a clinical consensus that this is a particularly difficult time for patients and that the disengagement process should be seen as part of the treatment process, not the end of it.

The decision to leave methadone maintenance may have complex features associated with it. New patients often have unrealistic notions about detoxifying from methadone quickly and then leading a problem-free life. Some patients are pressured by family and friends who do not understand that recovery from opioid dependence takes time. Patients may also feel that there is a stigma associated with being on methadone. And finally, staff may, through their beliefs and attitudes about the desirability of either abstinence or maintenance, influence patients to either attempt or abandon withdrawal from methadone maintenance no matter what their state of readiness. A patient-centred approach to these issues is one where staff orient their attitudes about treatment to the patient rather than to their own beliefs about the desirability of this or that practice.

Most ex-methadone maintenance patients suffer what has been referred to as a post-methadone syndrome. This consists of the mild symptoms of the protracted phase of the withdrawal syndrome and the issues involved in leading an opioid-free life without the regular counselling and contact with clinic staff that is part of methadone maintenance treatment. There has long been a clinical consensus that supportive counselling should be continued after the administration of methadone has ceased, but few patients take up this option. Recent developments in research on relapse prevention have led to the development of aftercare services, which involve a mix of education, skills training and features derived from self-help groups like Narcotics Anonymous. The research available suggests that well-motivated patients leaving treatment are more likely to be successful if they participate in an aftercare program.

REFERENCES

Andrews, H. L., & Himmelsbach, C. K. (1944). Relation of the intensity of the morphine abstinence syndrome to dosage. *Journal of Pharmacology and Experimental Therapeutics,* **81**, 288-293.

Caplehorn, J. R. M., & Bell, J. (1991). Methadone dosage and retention of patients in maintenance treatment. *Medical Journal of Australia,* **154**, 195-199.

Cushman, P. (1981). Detoxification after methadone treatment. In J. H. Lowinson & P. Ruiz (Eds.), *Substance abuse: Clinical problems and perspectives* (pp. 389-395). USA: Williams Wilkins.

Cushman, P., & Dole, V. P. (1973). Detoxification of rehabilitated methadone-maintained patients. *Journal of the American Medical Association,* **226**, 747-752.

Gentile, M. A., & Milby, J. B. (1992). Methadone maintenance detoxification fear: A study of its components. *Journal of Clinical Psychology,* **48**, 797-807.

Ghodse, H., Myles, J., & Smith, S. E. (1994). Clonidine is not a useful adjunct to methadone gradual detoxification in opioid addiction. *British Journal of Psychiatry,* **165**, 370-374.

Ginzburg, H. M. (1983). Use of clonidine or lofexidine to detoxify from methadone maintenance or other opioid dependencies. In J. R. Cooper, F. Altman, B. S. Brown, & D. Czechowicz (Eds.), *Research on the treatment of narcotic addiction: State of the art* (pp. 174-211). Rockville, MD: National Institute of Drug Abuse.

Gold, M. L., Sorensen, J. L., McCanlies, N., Trier, M., & Dlugosch, G. (1988). Tapering from methadone maintenance: Attitudes of clients and staff. *Journal of Substance Abuse Treatment,* **5**, 37-44.

Goldstein, A. (1971). Blind dosage comparisons and other studies in a large methadone program. *Journal of Psychedelic Drugs*, 4, 177-181.

Goldstein, A. (1972). Heroin addiction and the role of methadone in its treatment. *Archives of General Psychiatry*, 26, 291-297.

Gossop, M. (1988). Clonidine and the treatment of the opiate withdrawal syndrome. *Drug and Alcohol Dependence*, 21, 253-259.

Gossop, M., Battersby, M., & Strang, J. (1991). Self-detoxification by opiate addicts: A preliminary investigation. *British Journal of Psychiatry*, 159, 208-212.

Green, L., & Gossop, M. (1988). Effects of information on the opiate withdrawal syndrome. *British Journal of Addiction*, 83, 305-309.

Hall, S. M. (1979). The abstinence phobia. In N. A. Krasnegor (Ed.), *Behavioral analysis of substance abuse* (NIDA Research Monograph 25, pp. 55-67). Rockville, MD: National Institute on Drug Abuse.

Hall, S. M., Loeb, P. C., & Kushner, M. (1984). Methadone dose decreases and anxiety reduction. *Addictive Behaviors*, 9, 11-19.

Hawkins, J. D., & Catalano, R. F. (1985). Aftercare in drug abuse treatment. *International Journal of the Addictions*, 20, 917-945.

Jaffe, J. H. (1990). Drug addiction and drug abuse. In A. G. Gilman, T. W. Rall, A. S. Nies, & P. Taylor (Eds.), *The pharmacological basis of therapeutics* (7th Edition ed., pp. 522-573). USA: Pergamon.

Kleber, H. D. (1977). Detoxification from methadone maintenance: The state of the art. *International Journal of the Addictions*, 12, 807-820.

Kleber, H. D. (1981). Detoxification from narcotics. In J. H. Lowinson & P. Ruiz (Eds.), *Substance abuse: Clinical problems and perspectives* (pp. 317-338). U.S.A.: Williams & Wilkins.

Lowinson, J., Berle, B., & Langrod, J. (1976). Detoxification of long-term methadone patients: Problems and prospects. *International Journal of the Addictions*, 11, 1009-1018.

Martin, W. R., Jasinski, D. R., Haertzen, C. A., Kay, D. C., Jones, B. E., Mansky, P. A., & Carpenter, R. W. (1973). Methadone: A re-evaluation. *Archives of General Psychiatry*, 28, 286-295.

Mattick, R. P., & Baillie, A. (Eds.). (1992). *An outline for approaches to smoking cessation: Quality assurance project.* Canberra, Australia: Australian Government Publishing Service.

Mattick, R. P., Baillie, A., Grenyer, B., Hall, W., Jarvis, T., & Webster, P. (Eds.). (1993). *An outline for the management of alcohol problems: Quality assurance project.* Canberra, Australia: Australian Government Publishing Service.

Mattick, R. P., & Hall, W. (1996). Are detoxification programmes effective? *Lancet*, 347, 97-100.

McAuliffe, W. E. (1990). A randomized controlled trial of recovery training and self-help for opioid addicts in New England and Hong Kong. *Journal of Psychoactive Drugs*, 22, 197-209.

McAuliffe, W. E., & Ch'ien, J. M. N. (1986). Recovery training and self help: A relapse-prevention program for treated opiate addicts. *Journal of Substance Abuse Treatment, 3,* 9-20.

Milby, J.B. (1988). Methadone maintenance to abstinence: How many make it. *Journal of Nervous and Mental Disease, 176,* 409-422.

Milby, J. B., Gurwitch, R. H., Hohmann, A. A., Wiebe, D. J., Ling, W., McLellan, A. T., & Woody, G. E. (1987). Assessing pathological detoxification fear among methadone maintenance patients: The DFSS. *Journal of Clinical Psychology, 43,* 528-538.

Milby, J. B., Gurwitch, R. H., Wiebe, D. J., Ling, W., McLellan, A. T., & Woody, G. E. (1986). Prevalence and diagnostic reliability of methadone maintenance detoxification fear. *American Journal of Psychiatry, 143,* 739-743.

Milby, J. B., Hohmann, A. A., Gentile, M., Huggins, N., Sims, M. K., McLellan, A. T., Woody, G., & Haas, N. (1994). Methadone maintenance outcome as a function of detoxification phobia. *American Journal of Psychiatry, 151,* 1031-1037.

Mintz, J., O'Brien, C. P., O'Hare, K., & Goldschmidt, J. (1975). Double-blind detoxification of methadone maintenance patients. *International Journal of the Addictions, 10,* 815-824.

Moolchan, E. T., & Hoffman, J. A. (1994). Phases of treatment: A practical approach to methadone maintenance treatment. *International Journal of the Addictions, 29,* 135-160.

Murphy, S., & Irwin, J. (1992). "Living with the dirty secret": Problems of disclosure for methadone maintenance clients. *Journal of Psychoactive Drugs, 24,* 257-264.

Newman, R. G. (1983). Critique [of R. Resnick, Methadone detoxification from illicit opiates and methadone maintenance]. In J. R. Cooper, F. Altman, B. S. Brown, & D. Czechowicz (Eds.), *Research on the treatment of narcotic addiction: State of the art* (pp. 168-171). Rockville, MD: National Institute on Drug Abuse.

Novick, D. M., & Joseph, H. (1991). Medical maintenance: The treatment of chronic opiate dependence in general medical practice. *Journal of Substance Abuse Treatment, 8,* 233-239.

Panepinto, W., Arnon, D., Silver, F., Orbe, M., & Kissin, B. (1977). Detoxification from methadone maintenance in a family-oriented program. *British Journal of Addiction, 72,* 255-259.

Phillips, G. T., Gossop, M., & Bradley, B. (1986). The influence of psychological factors on the opiate withdrawal syndrome. *British Journal of Psychiatry, 149,* 235-238.

Raczynski, J. M., Wiebe, D. J., Milby, J. B., & Gurwitch, R. H. (1988). Behavioral assessment of narcotic detoxification fear. *Addictive Behaviors, 13,* 165-169.

Rawson, R. A., Washton, A. M., Resnick, R. B., & Tennant, F. S. (1984).

Clonidine hydrochloride detoxification from methadone treatment: The value of naltrexone aftercare. *Advances in Alcohol and Substance Abuse,* **3,** 41-49.

Resnick, R. (1983). Methadone detoxification from illicit opiates and methadone maintenance. In J. R. Cooper, F. Altman, B. S. Brown, & D. Czechowicz (Eds.), *Research on the treatment of narcotic addiction: State of the art* (pp. 160-167). Rockville, MD: National Institute on Drug Abuse.

Robins, L. N., Locke, B. Z., & Regier, D. A. (1991). An overview of psychiatric disorders in America. In L. N. Robins & D. A. Regier (Eds.), *Psychiatric disorders in America: The epidemiologic catchment area study* (pp. 328-366). New York: The Free Press.

Rosenbaum, M. (1981). *Women on heroin.* U.S.A.: Rutgers University Press.

Rosenbaum, M. (1991). Staying off methadone. *Journal of Psychoactive Drugs,* **23,** 251-260.

Rosenbaum, M., & Murphy, S. (1984). Always a junkie? The arduous task of getting off methadone maintenance. *Journal of Drug Issues,* **14,** 527-552.

San, L., Camí, J., Peri, J. M., Mata, R., & Porta, M. (1990). Efficacy of clonidine, guanifacine and methadone in the rapid detoxification of heroin addicts: A controlled clinical trial. *British Journal of Addiction,* **85,** 141-147.

Schumacher, J. E., Milby, J. B., Fishman, B. E., & Huggins, N. (1992). Relation of detoxification fear to methadone maintenance outcome: 5-year follow-up. *Psychology of Addictive Behaviors,* **6,** 41-46.

Senay, E. C., Dorus, W., Goldberg, F., & Thornton, W. (1977). Withdrawal from methadone maintenance: Rate of withdrawal and expectation. *Archives of General Psychiatry,* **34,** 361-367.

Sorensen, J. L., Acampora, A. P., & Deitch, D. A. (1984a). From maintenance to abstinence in a therapeutic community: Preliminary results. *Journal of Psychoactive Drugs,* **16,** 73-77.

Sorensen, J. L., Acampora, A. P., & Iscoff, D. (1984b). From maintenance to abstinence in a therapeutic community: Clinical treatment methods. *Journal of Psychoactive Drugs,* **16,** 229-239.

Stimmel, B., Goldberg, J., Rotkopf, E., & Cohen, M. (1977). Ability to remain abstinent after methadone detoxification: A six year study. *Journal of the American Medical Association,* **237,** 1216-1220.

Stine, S. M., & Kosten, T. R. (1992). Use of drug combinations in treatment of opioid withdrawal. *Journal of Clinical Psychopharmacology,* **12,** 203-209.

Weddington, W.W. (1990-91). Towards a rehabilitation of methadone maintenance: Integrations of relapse prevention and after care. *International Journal of the Addictions,* **25,** 1201-1224.

Wermuth, L., Brummett, S., & Sorensen, J. L. (1987). Bridges and barriers to recovery: Clinical observations from an opiate recovery project. *Journal of Substance Abuse Treatment,* **4,** 189-196.

III SPECIAL ISSUES

14

TRAINING HEALTH PROFESSIONALS TO DELIVER METHADONE TREATMENT

JAMES BELL

INTRODUCTION

Considerable emphasis has been placed on the role of education in responding to social problems in the contemporary world. In relation to the problems of drug abuse and drug dependence, three broad educational approaches have been employed: The largest effort – and the one with perhaps the most disappointing results (Schaps *et al.,* 1981) – has been in the development of education programs aimed at young people, designed to prevent drug abuse. Efforts to produce more sophisticated, integrated approaches to informing people about the risks of drug abuse continue (Wragg, 1992), but there remains little firm evidence that educational programs reduce drug abuse by young people. The second approach has been the role of education within treatment programs. The increasing influence of cognitive-behavioural treatment has been reflected in an emphasis on "psycho-educational" components of treatment for dependency problems. The role of patient education and information in methadone treatment has not been extensively investigated, although prima facie it seems likely that education of clients (particularly in the broadest sense, addressing not just information but skills and attitudes) has an important role in improving treatment outcomes. The third area in which education is being proposed to have an important role is in the training of staff treating people with dependency problems. It is this aspect of education and training which is the subject of this chapter.

In the last decade, issues of training the work-force have acquired a new significance. In most areas of employment, including the health care industry, changing technology has thrown open the need for flexibility, new skills, constant upgrading of skills, and a greater degree of specialisation. Continuing education programs and recertification of health care professionals have become an established feature of the health industry.

There are particularly cogent reasons for offering training and continuing education programs for clinicians involved in delivering methadone maintenance treatment. There is clear evidence that the outcomes of treatment vary according to how it is delivered, and it appears that the role of staff is important in influencing treatment outcomes (Ball & Ross, 1991). Furthermore, treatment philosophy, attitudes and beliefs can influence outcome of treatment (Szapocznik & Ladner, 1979; Bell *et al.,* 1995a). Thus, specific training for medical, dispensing and counselling staff is potentially one avenue towards improving the outcomes of methadone maintenance treatment.

There is another, more pragmatic reason for offering health professionals training in the skills and knowledge required to deliver methadone maintenance treatment. One feature of the published literature of continuing medical education is that areas of medicine often avoided or neglected by practitioners receive special attention. For example, training programs for medical practitioners in smoking cessation (Montner *et al.,* 1994), preventive medicine (Cohen *et al.,* 1994) and HIV medicine (Irvine *et al.,* 1993) have been described in the last few years. The role of such courses is not merely to provide doctors with knowledge and skills, but to attract their interest and involvement in valuable activities often neglected by doctors. Such considerations pertain to methadone treatment, and it is no coincidence that training programs for medical practitioners have been reported in jurisdictions where local policy is to encourage involvement of medical practitioners in delivering methadone treatment (Greenwood, 1992; Bell, 1995). In Australia, the need to recruit primary care practitioners to provide methadone maintenance has led to considerable emphasis on training, particularly for doctors and pharmacists. This paper sets out how training programs have developed in Australia, and examines the lessons learnt. The concluding section discusses what can realistically be expected of professional training in improving the treatment system.

TRAINING IN METHADONE MAINTENANCE TREATMENT

Apart from these recent reports on training primary care practitioners, the topic of training has received little attention in the literature on methadone. Most published research related to training addresses the question of whether ex-addicts or professionally trained counsellors achieve better results. These studies have generally been interpreted as showing little difference between professional and ex-addict counsellors, as concluded in the review by Hall (1983). However, a series of studies from a group in Philadelphia suggest clear benefits from structured psychotherapy, delivered according to detailed manuals by well-organised therapists (Luborsky *et al.*, 1985; McLellan *et al.*, 1988). These studies provide evidence that, even if the nature of professional qualifications is not directly relevant, training in delivery of treatment is an important aspect of therapist effectiveness. Although the findings from this group have not been replicated by other researchers within methadone treatment, they are consistent with the literature on psychotherapy and provide a strong argument that training staff to deliver planned and structured treatment has the potential to improve treatment outcomes.

There are several possible explanations for the lack of attention to training in methadone treatment, but they may all be traced back to the central problem which has bedevilled methadone treatment since its inception – scepticism over whether opioid replacement is a bona fide basis for treatment. Such scepticism has had a corrosive effect on the evolution of methadone treatment. Empirical findings about treatment effectiveness have been ignored as irrelevant. Worse, community and political doubt about the validity of methadone maintenance has been most constricting and damaging, through the imposition of regulations covering most aspects of treatment. Rather than evolving as a professional treatment, methadone treatment has been stifled by regulations which stipulate most of what takes place in treatment (Molinari *et al.*, 1994). In an atmosphere dominated by morality rather than science, and regulations rather than professional practice, it is no surprise that there has been relatively little emphasis on professional training, skills and knowledge.

Methadone Treatment in Australia

In order to understand the development of training programs in Australia, it is helpful to understand the evolution of methadone treatment in Australia. There has been a dramatic expansion of methadone treatment in the last decade. In 1985, when the decision to expand treatment was taken, there were 2,000 people receiving methadone maintenance treatment. In 1995, there 15,000 people in treatment, and the number is continuing to rise by about 15% per annum.

The expansion of treatment, and evolution into its present form, has been shaped by the nature of funding which has been available. Initially, Federal Government funding to establish methadone clinics was made available in 1985. This was used to establish methadone clinics offering free treatment including counselling and medical services. Subsequent continuing demand for treatment, without further increases in specific funding, have been based on the Australian system of universal health insurance, Medicare. Medicare allows medical practitioners to directly charge the government for consultations, providing patients with treatment at no cost. This remuneration available to medical practitioners has permitted the continued expansion of availability of treatment, and has resulted in the appearance of two further models of methadone service delivery.

The first is through private methadone clinics, usually treating large numbers of patients, in which prescribers derive their income from regular consultations charged to Medicare, while the running costs of the clinics are met by charging dispensing fees which are paid by patients. Most of the expansion of treatment in recent years has taken place in private methadone clinics. The other form of private treatment involves primary care practitioners prescribing methadone for small numbers of patients (usually less than 25) who are dispensed their methadone from a retail pharmacy, paying the pharmacist a dispensing fee. This latter model of treatment involves no specialist clinics, minimal infrastructure, and a decentralised system of methadone distribution making use of existing medical practitioners and retail pharmacies. The availability of universal health care has thus shaped a treatment system in which most care other than dispensing is delivered by medical practitioners.

The expansion of treatment has not been without problems. Most medical practitioners and retail pharmacists have been reluctant to become involved in delivering methadone treatment. More seriously, concerns over treatment delivered by inexperienced and untrained doctors began to be voiced in the state of Victoria in 1990, following a report that there had been a number of methadone overdose deaths among patients during the first week of treatment (Drummer *et al.,* 1990). The State Coroner recommended that doctors proposing to use methadone in the treatment of addiction be given training. This inauspicious circumstance led to the development of training programs for medical practitioners, and there are now active training programs in most Australian states.

CONTENT OF TRAINING PROGRAMS

Several hundred medical practitioners and pharmacists have now completed training courses around Australia. The course in New South Wales, the largest of the 6 Australian states, has been extensively evaluated and modified (Bell, 1995). However, all clinicians involved in training shared concerns over the validity of what was being taught.

Among clinicians working in methadone maintenance treatment, there has been persisting dissension over the nature of addiction, the principles upon which treatment should be based, and the goals of treatment. Such lack of agreement on fundamental issues has had many deleterious consequences. Treatment practices are often idiosyncratic, reflecting the assumptions and beliefs of staff rather than being based on research evidence as to how treatment is most effectively delivered (D'Aunno & Vaughn, 1992). Within methadone clinics, different staff members often hold contradictory views about addiction (Ball & Ross, 1991). Given the confusion of values and priorities, apparent in the literature on methadone maintenance, it seemed a crucial challenge to undertake a process to validate the basis of training. To this end, a national committee was convened, comprising experienced prescribers working in a range of settings. The aim of this committee was to systematically identify the work involved in managing patients on methadone. The committee divided the activities of treatment, of necessity somewhat arbitrarily, into a series of headings. Under each heading, treatment practices were described and skills identified. The learning objectives identified are summarised in the next sections.

1. Assessment

Assessment was seen by the committee as covering two distinct processes. The first of these was the task of *determining suitability for treatment,* while the second aspect of assessment is a more comprehensive exploration of *health, welfare and psychological* issues relevant to treatment. The reason for separating out initial and ongoing assessment was the perception of the committee that it was important not to overload the initial interview with material experienced by the patient as tangential to their main concern – whether and when they could receive their first dose of methadone. Taking a detailed history at this time was seen as less likely to yield useful information than performing such detailed assessment once the patient was stabilised on methadone, and no longer felt they had to prove something to be accepted into treatment.

The tasks involved in *establishing suitability for methadone* were (1) assessing the presence and severity of opioid dependence, and (2) obtaining informed consent for treatment. There was agreement that naloxone testing has a very limited role in the assessment of opioid dependence, which is diagnosed on the basis of history – of drug use, attendant problems, and of features of dependency. The important learning objective was that trainees demonstrated the ability to interview a patient, document a drug-use history and identify the features and assess the severity of opioid dependence. Included in the assessment of dependence is documentation of focused physical examination (for signs of vein damage, intoxication and withdrawal from opioids and other psychoactive drugs).

Theoretical knowledge which trainees are expected to demonstrate includes the role of methadone in pregnancy, and drug interactions with methadone which need to be anticipated prior to commencing treatment.

To demonstrate that they could gain *informed consent* to treatment, trainees need to demonstrate that they can explain to patients what is involved in methadone treatment, the rationale for treatment, what is expected of clients, and where they can get information about methadone. Trainees were expected to demonstrate a knowledge of other treatment modalities for opioid dependence, so that options could be discussed with patients. Finally, trainees need to demonstrate that they could perform a mental state examination, documenting cognition, affect and orientation, as part of ensuring patients can give valid informed consent to treatment.

Comprehensive assessment was seen as an ongoing process throughout treatment – the basis of a doctor-patient relationship in which the doctor documents the major psychological, social and medical issues in the patient's life. Usually, such assessment begins early in treatment, once the patient has been stabilised on methadone. The first learning objective relating to comprehensive assessment is for trainees to document an assessment adequately covering (1) drug use history (2) medical and psychiatric history (3) personal history – family and other relationships, significant life events, education and employment (4) current circumstances and functioning. This objective is assessed either through a written case history, or in an observed clinical interview.

The other objectives relating to comprehensive assessment are generic skills in interviewing, observed either in a clinical interview or role play. Trainees are expected to demonstrate sensitivity and appropriateness in relating to patients and making them feel comfortable. It is also expected that trainees will demonstrate specific interviewing skills – reflective listening and asking open-ended questions.

2. Prescribe Methadone Safely and Effectively

The committee agreed that adequate theoretical knowledge, such as could be tested in a written examination, was the first learning objective within this area of competence. Two broad areas of knowledge were identified. Firstly, trainees need to demonstrate knowledge of methadone pharmacology, including effects and side-effects, pharmacokinetics, and drug interactions. Trainees need to describe safe initial dose levels and safe rates of incremental increase of methadone dose, and management of methadone overdose. The second topic area is a knowledge of the research findings regarding factors which contribute to better treatment outcomes – adequate dose, longer duration of treatment, good therapeutic relationship, and identification and treatment of coexisting medical and psychiatric problems.

The second major learning objective was identified as being able to respond appropriately to continuing illicit drug use by those in treatment. Committee members agreed that this was often a major source of concern and conflict within methadone treatment, and that the challenge for clinicians was to find ways of responding which avoid punitive and controlling responses. It was agreed that training needed to cover two issues – theoretical knowledge and treatment philosophy.

Theoretical knowledge needed to respond to continuing heroin use was identified as knowledge of patterns of drug use within methadone treatment, the role of adequate methadone dose in reducing heroin use, and the prognosis for people prematurely discharged from treatment. Regarding abuse of drugs other than heroin, trainees should be able to identify the risks associated with abuse of alcohol, benzodiazepines, cannabis and stimulants by patients on methadone, and to be aware of the treatment options for these problems, such as antidepressants, selective detoxification, and supervised disulfiram.

The committee agreed that more important than basic knowledge was for training to provide clinicians with the opportunity to scrutinise their own attitudes and assumptions about drug abuse and dependence. Such scrutiny includes clarifying assumptions about the goals of methadone maintenance treatment. The first specific learning objective on this topic was to define a range of potential objectives of treatment, ranging from retaining people in maintenance through to achieving abstinence from all drugs. It was agreed that an important aspect of training was to introduce the philosophy of harm minimisation. Application of this philosophy involves tailoring the goals of treatment to the specific problems and disabilities of the individual patient. The specific learning objectives incorporating these considerations were for trainees to (1) describe policies to respond to continuing drug use in treatment, and (2) develop a treatment plan for an individual patient with continuing dependence on multiple drugs.

The third aspect of competence to prescribe methadone effectively was identified as the management of withdrawal from methadone. Specific learning objectives were identified as being (1) indications for and alternatives to involuntary discharge from treatment (2) how to advise patients seeking voluntary withdrawal, and (3) rate of reduction, symptoms associated with gradual withdrawal, and the role of supportive care in voluntary withdrawal from methadone.

3. Deliver Appropriately Structured Methadone Treatment

Methadone maintenance treatment is a highly structured form of treatment. Structure is in part an important behavioural component of treatment, but it also reflects the level of regulations surrounding the prescribing and dispensing of methadone. Such regulations are frequently irksome, particularly to medical practitioners accustomed to making their own decisions about patient care and unused to bureaucratic regulation. It was therefore considered desirable in training to emphasise that all treatment must comply with national and local jurisdictional requirements. Therefore, the first learning objective is for trainees to list the major legal requirements to prescribe methadone.

The second area of structure relates to the use of urine tests, and the availability of take-home doses. This represents one of the contentious areas of methadone practice, and the committee felt that the task in training programs should be to ensure trainees were able to summarise usefulness and limitations of urine testing, and the benefits, risks, and jurisdictional policy concerning the availability of take-home medication.

The third learning objective under this heading relates to the perception of the committee that more effective treatment was usually well organised and coherent, with good communication between clinicians involved in treatment. This has been documented in methadone clinics (Bell *et al.*, 1995b), but is also probably important in the primary care setting, where communication between the prescribing doctor and the dispensing pharmacist are desirable. For example, it is important that there are agreed policies and procedures for patients who miss consecutive doses, and for patients who present intoxicated for treatment. This was expressed in the learning objective that trainees describe policies for delivering treatment which reflect the need for agreed goals of treatment and clear communication among clinicians involved in delivering methadone treatment.

The fourth learning objective is for trainees to demonstrate knowledge of how to handle disruptive incidents and conflict. This involves two components. First, trainees are expected to understand the importance of containing anger and acting out behaviour, and to demonstrate clinical skills in handling aggressive, upset and impulsive patients. They should demonstrate tolerance and patience in their interaction with drug users. The second component is a matter of policy and procedures. Trainees should understand the importance of setting reasonable limits (e.g., regarding dosing times, keeping appointments, standards of behaviour in the waiting room or retail pharmacy) which are fairly but flexibly enforced. They should describe the value of having a grievance system for dealing with patient complaints.

The fifth learning objective relates to record keeping and review of treatment. Trainees should be able to list the features of treatment review, be able to develop a treatment plan, and demonstrate that they can adequately document a clinical interview.

Finally, the committee agreed that part of appropriately structured treatment is a knowledge of other services relevant to the potential needs of patients on methadone. The importance of this is that clinicians need to recognise their own limitations in managing patients, and be aware of when it is desirable to refer them for further management. Two examples of services are specialist obstetric services for addicted pregnant women, and HIV treatment services.

4. Address the Individual Health Care Needs of Patients on Methadone

The committee identified knowledge of HIV, HCV, HBV, and consequences of non-sterile injection as important medical information which should be familiar to doctors working in methadone treatment. In addition, such doctors should be familiar with intoxication and withdrawal states from commonly used drugs, including alcohol. Knowledge of psychiatric illness – including personality disorders, anxiety, and depression — was also considered desirable. The committee also agreed that prescribers needed some knowledge about the management of acute pain in patients with concomitant opioid dependence, and the role of methadone in chronic pain management. Prescribers should know the role of methadone in pregnancy, and the risks to the foetus of opioid intoxication and withdrawal. Finally, it was considered essential that methadone prescribers be able to identify the risks commonly associated with opioid dependence – including HIV risk taking, overdose risks, and potentially dangerous drug interactions.

The final learning objective involved translating this knowledge into practice, by the trainee demonstrating that he/she could develop a management plan for an individual patient.

5. Maintain Professional Conduct in Delivering Methadone Treatment

The committee identified several potential difficulties in working with dependent patients. At one extreme, some health professionals are at risk of becoming over-involved and enmeshed in trying to assist their patients. At the other, some professionals adopt adversarial, voyeuristic, and censorious ways of relating to addicted patients. These concerns were addressed in the learning objective that trainees demonstrate that they could relate to patients in a respectful and appropriate manner. A related objective was for trainees to maintain patient privacy and confidentiality.

The other important aspect of professionalism in delivering methadone treatment was expressed in the learning objective that practitioners maintain involvement in professional development – through participation in relevant courses, conferences, and meetings.

DELIVERING TRAINING

In New South Wales, a state with just over 9,000 people in methadone maintenance treatment, training for medical practitioners has comprised a written manual, an interactive workshop, and a supervised clinical placement. The training has been evaluated and progressively modified in the light of feedback from participants and observers.

Feedback from trainees has revealed that participants liked the training, and valued all aspects of it, particularly the use of clinical vignettes and case studies. The most often expressed problem was that a one-day interactive workshop was too short to cover all the material. Surveyed 6 to 18 months after undertaking the training program, most trainees indicated that they were prescribing methadone, and expressed a strong interest in continuing education and peer support (Bell, 1995).

The most valuable feedback on the training process came from observers who attended the first four workshops. Observers and facilitators met after each workshop to identify difficulties which had arisen. It was quickly apparent that the key challenge in training did not relate to lack of knowledge, but to the assumptions and attitudes with which medical practitioners approached methadone treatment.

The attitudes to addicts and addiction which were most problematic were those which polarised at two extremes. At one extreme were the medical practitioners who expressed negative views of drug users, and who saw the goal of treatment as being to achieve abstinence from all drugs. For these doctors, the justification for methadone treatment was that it serves as a way of controlling deviant behaviour. Their understanding was that methadone is offered to patients in return for compliance with the expectations of the prescriber. This contractual basis of treatment essentially sees methadone as a system of rewards and punishments designed to encourage patients to abstinence and to behave in less antisocial ways.

At the other extreme, there was a group of trainees who expressed more positive views of drug addicts, seeing them not as individuals with problems but as people making particular lifestyle choices – choices which were discriminated against by social policy. For these "progressives" there is little that is inherently problematic about dependence on heroin; rather, the problems associated with heroin addiction arise because the drug is illegal, and supplies are therefore expensive and impure. Such views have been developed in the literature in recent years (see, e.g., Gerlach & Schneider, 1990). To this group, it seemed it would be more rational to prescribe heroin than methadone, but as a matter of political compromise methadone is given instead.

Both these perspectives conceptualise methadone maintenance as a system of controlled drug distribution designed to reduce the harmful consequences of heroin addiction (a view expressed occasionally in the literature – see, for example, Berridge, 1993). For both groups, and for many politicians and administrators, methadone maintenance is a matter of social policy, a pragmatic solution to a social problem, rather than a treatment of individuals. In this frame of reference, regulations about how methadone should be prescribed and dispensed are more relevant than principles of treatment.

To the committee organising the training program, this frame of reference was problematic. It identifies methadone treatment as a different activity from "mainstream" medical practice, not part of the duty of care owed to individual patients seeking treatment. Within the regulatory framework, usual assumptions about patient care are often not seen as applying; rather, any practices which fit within the regulations are acceptable. In contrast, "treatment" involves assumptions about individual patient care and professionalism which are a better defence against poor practice than regulations.

A related problem identified in the workshops relates to the nature of treatment of drug dependence. Many medical practitioners had difficulties coming to terms with the motivational and interactive nature of treatment of dependence. Trainees expected clear guidelines for how to respond to clinical problems. For example, many asked how to respond to the problem of benzodiazepine abuse among patients on methadone. However, instead of clear directions on how to proceed, they would receive responses suggesting that what to do depended on what the patient was willing or able to do, and that even when a plan was negotiated, they should not be surprised when it was not adhered to. They found difficulty with the suggestion that sometimes the most helpful response is to advise, wait and observe, and avoid being provoked into fruitless attempts to control patients' behaviour. Treatment as something passive, something which at best permits change to occur, is an unfamiliar and challenging concept to people trained in a biomedical framework. The frustration of working in this way is another obstacle to perceiving methadone maintenance as a "real" form of treatment.

Addressing the Problems Identified in Training

In the light of these identified problems, the manual and workshop were progressively modified. The first session of the workshop was devoted to exercises aimed at exploring trainees' attitudes to addicts and addiction. Most doctors share community antipathy towards heroin users, and for many doctors, this attitude is exacerbated by the occasional experience of treating difficult, hostile, drug-seeking patients. Such experiences often give rise to an adversarial approach to treating heroin users. An exercise to address these difficulties was adopted to place methadone treatment in the context of medical practice, identifying the types of patients whom doctors find difficult. Heroin users presented as examples of patients embodying many of the traits which doctors find difficult. The skills needed to respond appropriately were emphasised as generic skills of value in all areas of medical practice.

A similar approach was adopted to deal with trainees' beliefs about heroin addiction. Here too, medical practitioners tend to reflect community assumptions about addiction to heroin, and a crucial aspect of training was to avoid either exaggerating or trivialising the problems of dependence on heroin. This was addressed by considering problems of dependence on a variety of drugs – benzodiazepines, alcohol, tobacco – and to the biopsychosocial factors promoting vulnerability to dependence.

In dealing with the frustration of patients who continue to abuse drugs while in treatment, the manual and workshop were modified to clarify that treatment of dependence is permissive, not causing people to change but allowing them to do so. The goal of treatment is to allow patients a greater degree of control over their own lives: treatment with methadone can reduce the level of behavioural dependence on opioids, allowing patients the opportunity – depending on their circumstances – to lead more normal and productive lives. The fact that some patients are unable to take advantage of this respite is something clinicians – and policy makers – must acknowledge.

The final and perhaps most important lesson from the training program was to recognise the limitations of a single training session, particularly in dealing with attitudinal issues. A system of continuing education, based around case discussions and clinical problems, has now been developed.

WHAT CAN EDUCATION AND TRAINING ACHIEVE?

Reading the research reviews in this book, it is possible to gain an image of methadone treatment as a well-validated, empirically-based treatment extensively practised around the world. The sad reality is that methadone treatment in many countries – perhaps all – continues to be marginalised, a subject of continual controversy over the basic question of whether it is a valid modality of treatment. If there are brief periods when methadone maintenance is supported, it is predictable that in time the support will wane. As a politically unpopular modality of treatment, limited resources are devoted to methadone treatment, and demand for treatment almost always exceeds availability. Most clinics are shabby, reflecting the grudging level of support and the marginalised status of the clientele. Most health professionals are reluctant to become involved in this treatment, a problem exacerbated by the fact that budgetary constraints limit the extent to which well-qualified staff can be employed.

Training of staff cannot compensate for a lack of resources devoted to treatment. While training can serve as a valuable way to recruit professionals by raising their interest in methadone treatment, it will only succeed in doing so if people work in reasonably satisfactory conditions in delivering treatment. The Australian experience of expanding treatment in the primary care setting, and remunerating methadone maintenance as a medical procedure, has been moderately successful, as have similar approaches in Germany.

However, methadone treatment in Australia is still well short of being a "mainstream" medical treatment. Most health professionals share community attitudes, and tend to be reluctant to become involved in treatment of addicts. Staff who share the prevalent fear and intolerance probably contribute to less effective treatment. The assumption that methadone maintenance is essentially a legitimised form of drug distribution is widespread in the community, and is shared by many heroin users. It constitutes a significant problem for the methadone treatment system and is a barrier to health professionals being involved in this form of treatment, a barrier to patients entering treatment, a barrier to good treatment, and a justification for maintaining high levels of bureaucratic regulation.

In summary, the major difficulty confronting methadone treatment is that prevailing attitudes to addiction entrench the alienation of heroin users, and make treatment more difficult. Most staff working in clinics find that their views tend to be out of step with community attitudes, an uncomfortable situation for many professionals. Initial and ongoing training, with an emphasis on value clarification, informed by empirical findings in relation to addiction treatment, is an appropriate response to this problem. Although there are no data to indicate whether specific training programs can improve the effectiveness of treatment, the Australian experience indicates that training can help recruit people to deliver methadone maintenance treatment, and is also valued by staff already working in this modality of treatment.

REFERENCES

Ball, J.C., & Ross, A (1991). *The effectiveness of methadone maintenance treatment: Patients, programs, services and outcome.* New York: Springer-

Verlag.

Bell, J. (1995). Lessons from a training program for methadone prescribers. *Medical Journal of Australia,* **162,** 143-144.

Bell, J., Chan, J., & Kuk, A. (1995a). Investigating the effect of treatment philosophy on outcome of methadone maintenance. *Addiction,* **90,** 823-830.

Bell, J., Ward, J., Mattick, R.P., Hay, A., Chan, J., & Hall, W. (1995b). *An evaluation of private methadone clinics* (National Drug Strategy Report Series No. 4). Canberra, Australia: Australian Government Publishing Service.

Berridge, V. (1993). Harm minimisation and public health: an historical perspective. In Heather, N., Wodak, A., Nadelmann, E., & O Hare, P. (Eds.), *Psychoactive drugs and harm reduction: From faith to science* (pp. 55-64). London: Whurr.

Cohen, S.J., Halvorson, H.W., & Gosselink, C.A. (1994). Changing physician behavior to improve disease prevention. *Preventive Medicine,* **23(3),** 284-91.

D'Aunno, T., & Vaughn, T.E. (1992). Variations in methadone treatment practices: Results from a national study. *Journal of the American Medical Association,* **267,** 253-258.

Drummer, O.H., Syrjanen, M., Opeskin, K., & Cordner, S. (1990). Deaths of heroin addicts starting on a methadone maintenance programme. *Lancet,* **335,** 108.

Gerlach, R., & Schneider, W. (1990). Abstinence and acceptance? The problematic relationship between the German abstinence paradigm, low-threshold oriented drug work, and methadone. *Drug and Alcohol Review,* **10,** 417-421

Greenwood, J. (1992). Persuading general practitioners to prescribe - good husbandry or a recipe for chaos? *British Journal of Addiction,* **87,** 567-575.

Hall, S.M. (1983). Methadone maintenance: An overview of research findings. In J. R. Cooper, F. Altman, B. S. Brown, & D. Czechowicz (Eds.), *Research on the treatment of narcotic addiction: State of the art* (pp. 575-632). Rockville, MD: National Institute on Drug Abuse.

Irvine, S., Penny, R., & Anns, M. (1993). Developing quality primary care services in HIV/AIDS care: The educational imperative. *Journal of Acquired Immune Deficiency Syndromes Suppl* 1, *6,* S72-6.

Luborsky, L., McLellan, A.T., Woody, G., O Brien, C.P., & Auerbach, A. (1985). Therapist success and its determinants. *Archives of General Psychiatry,* **42,** 602-611

McLellan, A.T., Woody, G., Luborsky, L., & Goelh, L (1988). Is the counselor an "active ingredient" in substance abuse rehabilitation? An examination of treatment success among four counsellors. *Journal of Nervous and Mental Disease,* **176,** 423-430.

Molinari, S.P., Cooper, J.R., & Czechowicz, D.J. (1994). Federal Regulation of clinical practice in narcotic addiction treatment: Purpose, status, and alternatives. *Journal of Law, Medicine and Ethics,* **22(3)**, 231-239.

Montner, P., Bennett, G., & Brown, C. (1994). An evaluation of a smoking cessation training program for medical residents in an inner-city hospital. *Journal of the National Medical Association,* **86(9)**, 671-5.

Schaps, E., di Bartolo, R., Moskowitz, J., Palley C.S., & Churgin, S. (1981). A review of 127 drug abuse prevention evaluations. *Journal of Drug Issues,* **11**, 17-43.

Szapocznik, J., & Ladner, R. (1979). Factors related to successful retention in methadone maintenance: A review. *International Journal of the Addictions,* **12**, 1067-1085

Wragg, J. (1992). *An evaluation of a model of drug education.* Canberra, Australia: Australian Government Publishing Service.

15

THE PROVISION OF METHADONE WITHIN PRISON SETTINGS

KATE DOLAN, WAYNE HALL AND ALEX WODAK

INTRODUCTION

The use of illicit drugs is associated with risk of serious health, social and legal consequences. Methadone maintenance treatment has been shown to reduce these complications including HIV transmission (Metzger *et al.*, 1993), mortality (Grönbladh *et al.*, 1990) and criminal involvement (Dole *et al.*, 1969). While illicit drug use is known to continue in prison, albeit at lower levels than in the community (Dolan, 1993), the role of methadone treatment in reducing any of these consequences among prisoners remains to be determined.

This chapter examines the rationale, implementation and likely benefits of providing methadone programs to prisoners. The arguments against prison methadone programs are examined and the limited published research into prison-based methadone programs is reviewed. Alternative drug treatment for inmates (National Institute on Drug Abuse, 1992) and service delivery in prison (Anonymous, 1992) have been reviewed elsewhere.

Injecting drug users (IDUs) have an increased risk of imprisonment, primarily because of the illegal activities they engage in to generate funds for the purchase of drugs. A review of 15 studies in the US found the proportion of IDUs among prison populations ranged from 20 to 50 percent (Gaughwin *et al.,* 1991). Similar proportions of IDUs among prison populations have been reported in Australia (Crofts *et al.,* 1996) and slightly lower levels in the UK (Gore *et al.,* 1995; Maden *et al.,* 1992). Likewise, a high proportion of IDUs report having been imprisoned. In a 12 city study of IDUs, the proportion reporting a history of imprisonment ranged from 60 to 95 percent (WHO, 1994).

Multiple episodes of imprisonment are more common for IDU inmates than for non-injecting inmates. Gore *et al.* (1995) reported the difference in periods of imprisonment for general inmates and for IDU inmates in a Glasgow prison. The differences in the number of imprisonments for IDU inmates and non-IDU inmates (general inmates minus IDU inmates) is shown in Table 15.1.

Table 15.1
Number of imprisonments for IDUs and non-IDU inmates

Times in prison	IDUs %(n=75)	Non-IDUs* %(n=209)
once	12	39
twice	4	13
3-5	27	22
5 or more	57	26

* Calculated from Gore *et al.,* 1995.

IDU prisoners in Gore's study were significantly more likely to have been in prison on five or more occasions than non-IDU prisoners (p<0.0001). Non-IDU inmates were significantly more likely to have experienced only one period of incarceration than IDUs inmates (p<0.0001). One study estimated that the cumulative time IDUs spend in prison can amount to one-tenth of their drug-using careers, (Wodak, 1991). Moreover, IDUs in the US are more likely to have contact with correctional facilities than drug treatment agencies (Brewer *et al.,* 1988). The concentration of IDUs among inmate populations suggests that provision of drug treatment within prison might be more cost-effective than in the community.

The prison environment is a dynamic one. For example, in the US, the annual turnover is approximately 800 percent in jails (which accommodates short term inmates) and 50 percent in prisons. The daily national prison census now exceeds one million inmates in the US (Glaser & Greifinger, 1993). There are a remarkable 10 million entries and exits in US correctional facilities each year (Glaser & Greifinger, 1993). In New South Wales, the most populous state in Australia, the daily prison census is about 6,000 (Walker *et al.,* 1992), with 14,000 entrants and 20,000 internal transfers between prisons (Department of Corrective Services, 1994) annually. This dynamic nature of prison populations creates an efficient mechanism for transmission of infections such as HIV and tuberculosis. This rapid turnover of prison populations also creates opportunities (and challenges) for the provision of treatment and prevention to vast numbers of individuals who are generally disadvantaged. Prison health services are usually grossly under-funded and occupy a low position in the health care hierarchy. These two factors predict poor quality health care for a population whose health status is already very marginal (General Accounting Office, 1994). Furthermore, prison populations have substantially increased in many countries, suggesting that the health care service may deteriorate further unless additional funding is provided (Mauer, 1995).

ARE METHADONE PROGRAMS NECESSARY FOR PRISONERS?

The introduction or expansion of methadone programs in prison has been recommended by a number of prominent organisations (World Health Organization, 1993; UK's Advisory Council on the Misuse of Drugs, 1993; Scottish Affairs Committee, 1994). The large proportion of IDUs among prison entrants means heroin withdrawal is common in prison (Jeanmonod *et al.,* 1991). The increasing numbers of IDUs in community-based methadone programs means that methadone withdrawal, which is more protracted than heroin withdrawal, will also become common among prison entrants. The provision of methadone on a detoxification basis alleviates withdrawal symptoms and reduces anxiety in the stressful environment of a prison. For detoxification, methadone provision is required for approximately 10 to 20 days (Ward *et al.,* 1992). Other detoxification agents are available, such as clonidine, and may have advantages such as a shorter half-life and cause less conflict over dose levels (Mattick & Hall, 1996).

The provision of methadone to prisoners who are nearing release can be justified on two grounds. Newly released IDUs often resume drug injecting (Turnbull *et al.*, 1991; Dolan *et al.*, 1990) but with little or no tolerance to heroin. Under these circumstances, they are at increased risk of suffering either a fatal (Zador *et al.*, 1995) or non-fatal overdose (Darke *et al.*, 1994). Stabilising IDU inmates on methadone prior to prison release increases tolerance and reduces the risk of overdose. The second factor is that as drug injectors resume injecting, they also often resume illegal activities and risk being arrested and incarcerated. As methadone maintenance treatment reduces illegal activities among newly released IDUs (Dole *et al.*, 1969), enrolling IDUs into methadone treatment prior to prison release also reduces the likelihood of being reincarcerated (Dole *et al.*, 1969). In order to control these problems, methadone provision in prison would only be required for the brief period prior to release. The justification of extended periods of methadone provision in prison, especially on a maintenance basis, depends upon other considerations.

Prison methadone maintenance programs may seem inappropriate because heroin injecting is infrequent (and therefore heroin dependence is rare) among prisoners (Dolan *et al.*, 1996d; Turnbull *et al.*, 1991). Among inmates who inject, which is about one in every four or five prisoners (Crofts *et al.*, 1996; Dolan, 1993), the average frequency of injecting is once or twice a month (Dolan *et al.*, 1996b; Turnbull *et al.*,1991). Few community-based methadone programs enrol IDUs who inject so infrequently. Nevertheless, there are aspects of prison life that may justify a departure from the standard entry criteria used in community-based methadone programs.

The main argument for providing methadone to prisoners on a maintenance basis is reducing transmission of blood-borne infections among inmates (Hall *et al.*, 1993; Dolan *et al.*, 1994b; Dolan *et al.*, 1995). Most prison systems differ from their surrounding communities in several ways. First, syringe sharing in prison is similar to the risk of syringe sharing in a shooting gallery. In both locations, large numbers of strangers engage in very risky behaviour with extremely high rates of partner change (Dolan *et al.*, 1996b). Therefore, each episode of syringe sharing in prison involves a much greater risk than an episode of sharing in community settings where sterile injecting equipment is usually accessible and the few needle contacts are usually sex partners and close friends rather than strangers.

Secondly, despite HIV being prevalent among IDUs in many

countries, few HIV prevention programs have been implemented in prison systems (Harding & Schaller, 1992). In particular, one of the most effective measures against HIV transmission, namely, syringe exchange, has only been adopted in Switzerland and Germany (Nelles & Harding 1995; Heino pers. com., 1996) on a pilot basis and is unlikely to be implemented in more than a few prison systems around the world (Dolan *et al.,* 1996a). In countries, such as the UK and Australia, where there are very favourable experiences of community-based syringe exchange, such programs in prison have been explicitly ruled out (Groves, 1991; Debus, pers. com., 1996). In other countries, such as the US, the strong resistance to community-based syringe exchange schemes, suggests the possibility of prison-based syringe exchange schemes is very remote.

Thirdly, although bleach programs for inmates are provided in number of countries, recent evidence suggests these programs may be of only little value in preventing HIV transmission among incarcerated IDUs (Normand *et al.,* 1995). In addition, injecting equipment in prison has usually been extensively tampered with to aid in its concealment (Seamark & Gaughwin, 1994). These alterations often make effective cleaning of the injecting equipment more difficult than would otherwise be the case. Furthermore, two studies of prison-based bleach programs found that inmates still had difficulty in gaining access to bleach even after the program had operated for a few years (Dolan *et al.,* 1994a; Dolan *et al.,* 1996b). This suggests that even if effective disinfectants and cleaning methods were formulated, prison-based bleach programs may still be ineffective. Methadone maintenance treatment becomes more important in prison because other HIV prevention measures are unlikely to be implemented or, if implemented, to be successful.

Fourthly, the substantial decreases in the level of syringe sharing by IDUs observed in most community settings over the last decade have not been reported in prisons (Dolan, 1993; Crofts *et al.,* 1996). In one study, IDUs with a recent history of prison were at significantly more risk in prison than in the community because sharing had become so rare in the community (Dolan *et al.,* 1996d).

All these arguments are based on the underlying assumption that a sufficient level of transmission of blood-borne viral infections (such as hepatitis B and C and HIV) occurs in prison, and that methadone maintenance treatment can reduce transmission within prisons. Six cohort studies of HIV transmission among prisoners have detected few cases (Brewer *et al.,* 1988; Castro *et al.,* 1991; Mutter *et al.,* 1994;

Centers for Disease Control, 1986; Kelley *et al.*,1986; Horsburgh *et al.*, 1990). Long-term prisoners (serving sentences greater than one year) are probably at lower risk of infection than short-term prisoners as they reside in high-security prisons where there is little opportunity to engage in risk behaviour and become infected (Dye & Issacs 1991).

Evidence is now beginning to appear that HIV transmission may not be as rare as previously thought. A study of prisoners in Glasgow (Taylor *et al.*, 1995) detected a high incidence of HIV infection. Estimates that included inmates (151) who declined to participate in the study, concluded that between three and five times the number of inmates initially detected may have been infected within a six-month period (Scottish Affairs Committee, 1994). A network of HIV infection has also been reported among Australian inmates (Dolan *et al.*, 1996c). In that study, it was difficult to prove conclusively that infection had occurred in prison because of the very considerable inmate movement. These two studies illustrate how the dynamic nature of prison populations can facilitate rapid dissemination of infections while complicating accurate monitoring of transmission.

Although evidence documenting HIV transmission in prison is limited, most prison systems have all the elements necessary for substantial transmission. Prison populations contain a large concentration of IDUs and therefore HIV prevalence is generally higher than in surrounding communities. Injecting is widespread in prison. A review of nine studies of IDUs in England and Australia found that between one-quarter and one-half reported injecting when last in prison (Gaughwin *et al.*, 1991). However, the frequency of injecting was low in prison, with injecting generally occurring once or twice a month (Dolan *et al.*, 1996d; Shewan *et al.*,1994; Turnbull *et al.*,1991). Despite the low frequency, injecting in prison invariably involves syringe sharing with a large number of strangers in an almost random manner of mixing (Turnbull *et al.*, 1991; Dolan *et al.*, 1996b). Random mixing of partners (needle and sexual) produces the worst possible scenario for HIV transmission (Kaplan & Heimer, 1992).

HOW DO PRISON METHADONE PROGRAMS OPERATE?

A survey of countries believed to provide methadone in prison was carried out in 1995 (Dolan & Wodak, 1996). Experts from fourteen countries responded to the survey with basic details of their prison methadone programs. Use of methadone to detoxify prison entrants were reported from eight countries (see Table 15.2). The duration of detoxification ranged from 12 weeks (in one Australian state) to one week (in England, Wales and Ireland). Six of these countries provide methadone on a maintenance basis to prisoners under certain conditions.

Table 15.2
Provision of methadone detoxification in prison

Location	weeks of detoxification	Maintenance Exceptions	Reference
Australia			
South Australia	12	a,b,c	Liew
Victoria	10	b,c	Hearn
Queensland	10	b	
Scotland	4		Shewan
New Zealand	3	b,d	Edwards
Sweden	2-3	e	Klang
Portugal	2#		Keating
England & Wales	1	b	Wool
Ireland	2*	b	Dooley
Netherlands	5 mg/day	d	de Jong

only in one of 48 prisons
* up to 7 weeks if HIV positive
Maintenance Exceptions
a) HIV infected, b) pregnant, c) serving short sentences, d) at doctor's discretion, e) AIDS

Table 15.3
Methadone maintenance programs in prison

Location	Daily census	Inmates on methadone	% of inmates on methadone	Mean dose
1. USA, New York	14,500	400	3	35
2. Australia, NSW	6,400	800	13	80
3. Spain, Catalunya	2,000	100	5	60
4. Switzerland, Basel	?	180	?	?
5. Denmark	3,574	201	?	?
6. France, Paris	54,000	<50	3	50
7. Germany	55,657	?	?	?

Sources (pers. com.):
1. Magura, 1994; 2. Jefferies, 1996; 3. Ministerio, 1993; 4. Federal Office, 1993; 5. Schioler, 1996; 6. Fournier, 1995 and 7. Federal Ministry of Justice, 1995

A small number of prison methadone programs operate in Europe. A relatively large program operates in Modelo prison in Spain (Ministerio de Justicia e Interior, 1993). That program was originally restricted to HIV-positive inmates but now HIV-negative inmates are also considered. In Basel, Switzerland, all prison entrants who were in methadone treatment prior to prison can continue treatment if they wish (Herzog *et al.,* 1993). There is a small pilot study where inmates receive heroin in one Swiss prison (Uchtenhagen, pers. com., 1996), which is in line with similar service provision in the community (Uchtenhagen pers. com., 1996). In France, approximately 50 inmates out of a national total of 54,000 are maintained on methadone at an average dose of 50 mg (Fournier, pers. com., 1995). Although, no central data on prisoners on methadone are collected in Germany, apparently some inmates continue and even commence methadone treatment while in prison. Table 15.3 summarises prison methadone maintenance programs known to exist.

Prison methadone maintenance programs operate in seven countries. Most programs cater for less than 10 percent of inmates even though, as noted earlier, approximately 20 to 50 percent of prisoners are IDUs. The only prison methadone programs to have been well documented are at Riker's Island, New York (Magura *et al.,* 1993) and in New South Wales, Australia (Hall *et al.,* 1993). Both programs were established in 1986 as time-limited treatments. The Riker's Island program was a detoxification program and the New South Wales program was a pre-release program.

HOW SUCCESSFUL ARE PRISON METHADONE MAINTENANCE PROGRAMS ?

Prison methadone maintenance programs should be assessed in relation to their stated aims. Only the programs at Riker's Island and in New South Wales have clearly defined and documented aims. The aims and therefore the operation of these programs have varied over time in ways that complicate any evaluation of the programs. A number of studies of these two programs have been completed.

Eleven studies of the New South Wales prison methadone program were carried out between 1986 and 1991 by the Department of Corrective Services (Gorta, 1992). In general, the program in New South Wales appears to have benefited some inmates who reported a lower frequency of drug use in prison and less involvement in the prison drug trade (Wale & Gorta, 1987). These reports were supported by urinalysis tests which showed decreased use of heroin and other drugs. Methadone diversion was found to be uncommon among methadone clients in prison as very few urine samples contained no methadone (Gorta, 1987a; Bertram, 1991).

The prison methadone programs in New South Wales and Riker's Island both aimed to reduce criminal recidivism. No differences in recidivism was found among prisoners who had been on the methadone program compared with a matched group of untreated prisoners (Hume & Gorta, 1989). However, as the program targeted (and achieved) an over-representation of disadvantaged IDUs, it is inappropriate to compare the results with prisoners who were less disadvantaged. Not surprisingly, many custodial staff believed that the New South Wales program was unsuccessful in reducing recidivism (Hume & Gorta 1988). Substantial evidence from studies in community settings clearly indicates that methadone maintenance treatment reduces criminality (Ward *et al.*, 1992), particularly among newly released prisoners (Dole *et al.*, 1969).

Methadone treatment is an attractive form of treatment to IDUs. Virtually all (95%) prisoners at Riker's Island who were offered a place in the methadone program accepted (Magura *et al.*, 1993). IDUs maintained on methadone in prison were more likely to present for treatment after release than IDUs who only underwent detoxification in prison (Magura *et al.*, 1993). Retention in community-based methadone programs was low after one year for clients in the New South Wales prison methadone program (Ward *et al.*, 1992; Gorta, 1987b) and in the New York program (Magura *et al.*, 1993).

There is no clear evidence at present that prison-based methadone programs prevent blood-borne viral infections, yet many staff of the New South Wales program believe this to be the case (Hume & Gorta, 1988). The National Drug and Alcohol Research Centre studied 185 IDUs recently released from prison in 1993. Approximately one-third of respondents had received no methadone treatment, one-third had received partial treatment and one-third had received methadone maintenance treatment (dosages in excess of 60 mgs and for the duration of imprisonment) (Dolan *et al.*, 1996e). The three groups were similar in terms of age of first injection, age daily injecting commenced, age first imprisoned and the number of treatment episodes. IDUs who received methadone maintenance reported a significantly lower level of risk behaviour in prison than untreated inmates. Also inmates who received partial treatment (i.e., either sub-optimal doses or limited duration) were similar to the untreated IDUs in terms of risk behaviour (Dolan *et al.*, 1996d). This finding may have implications for the treatment of IDUs in the community. In general, IDUs who inject infrequently are excluded from methadone treatment programs. The finding that methadone treatment can reduce injecting even when IDUs inject infrequently suggests that non-dependent IDUs in the community may benefit from methadone treatment, provided there are the resources to provide it.

WHAT ARE THE OBJECTIONS TO METHADONE PROGRAMS IN PRISON ?

A number of arguments against provision of methadone to prisoners have been raised including decreasing motivation to accept non-drug treatment (Wool, 1991) and reducing the likelihood that IDUs who become abstinent in prison will remain drug free after release (Wool, 1991). Methadone has high retention rates, and it has been demonstrated to be the most effective treatment for heroin-dependent persons (Ward *et al.*, 1992). The resumption of injecting soon after prison release is almost inevitable (Turnbull *et al.*, 1991; Dolan *et al.*, 1990; Dolan, 1993).

Other objections to the provision of methadone to prisoners include a conflict with the aim of keeping prisons drug-free, operational difficulties of dispensing methadone in prison environments (McLeod, 1991; Hume & Gorta, 1988) and the possibility of creating methadone-dependent prisoners from non-dependent inmates. Providing prisoners with mood altering substances is strongly opposed by many prison guards. However, most correctional services have found with experience that it is virtually impossible to keep drugs out of prison and that the operational difficulties of providing a methadone service within a correctional facility can be overcome. Experience also shows that while most IDUs lose their tolerance and dependence in prison, a relapse to dependence soon after release is extremely common.

The basis of much opposition to the provision of methadone to prisoners is the conflicting aims of custodial and health staff (McLeod, 1991). There have been reports that methadone programs can suffer if operated by correctional staff rather than independent health staff (Herzog *et al.*, 1993). Independence of health staff from custodial staff has been recommended to avoid a conflict of interest (Commonwealth of Australia, 1988).

HOW SHOULD METHADONE PROGRAMS BE STUDIED IN PRISON?

The same high standards applied to the evaluation of methadone programs in the community should be applied in prison settings. Researchers need to be independent from the methadone program. The ideal study of methadone in prison would be a randomised controlled trial. This would be ethical (Oakley, 1990) given the lack of evidence that methadone treatment is as effective in prison as in the community. Particular attention would need to be paid to short-term prisoners who are probably at higher risk of becoming infected in prison. The ideal outcome measures would be objective data collected prospectively. Examples of such measures include serological testing for new viral infections and hair testing for the use of illicit drugs while in prison. The first randomised controlled trial (n=300) of methadone maintenance in prison will be conducted between 1996 and 1998 by the authors of this chapter.

DISCUSSION

There is reasonable justification for providing methadone to IDUs on prison entry, nearing release and during the entire period of incarceration. Although few supporting data exist, this should not be misinterpreted to mean that prison methadone programs are unwarranted. Recent studies suggest that HIV transmission in prison is not rare, although transmission in prison is difficult to document for largely logistical reasons (Dolan *et al.*, 1996c; Dolan *et al.*, 1995).

Prison methadone programs operate in few countries. The programs that exist have limited capacity in comparison with the potential demand for treatment. When information is available, demand for methadone treatment in prison far out-strips supply (Herzog *et al.*, 1993; Jefferies, pers. com., 1996). When treatment is offered, it is almost always accepted (Magura *et al.*, 1993). The two major prison methadone programs in the world, at Riker's Island and in New South Wales, have been modified extensively over the years. While modifications are common in newly established health services, they invariably complicate evaluation.

The level of knowledge of community-based methadone programs should be drawn upon when implementing methadone programs in prison. Given the strong emphasis on cost-effectiveness these days, it is surprising that an effective treatment such as methadone is rarely provided in an environment where the concentration of IDUs is so high. If prison methadone programs conform to community standards, then it is likely that they will achieve a similar degree of success in reducing HIV infection. As few alternative HIV prevention measures exist for inmates, methadone programs may be even more important in prison settings than in community settings.

Methadone programs can only treat individuals who inject heroin or other opiates. A wide variety of drugs are injected in prison (Dolan *et al.*, 1996b) as they are in the community. Therefore other forms of treatment are required for injectors of non-opiate drugs. Because of the resistance to, and problems associated with, conducting innovative research in prisons, these alternative treatment programs need to be first developed in community settings.

The provision of methadone in prison may be best facilitated by commencing treatment for inmates at entry and prior to release from prison. If these limited methadone programs can be implemented reasonably well, then a progression to providing methadone on a maintenance basis throughout sentence should be considered. As some IDUs report commencing injecting in prison (Dolan *et al.*, 1996b; Taylor *et al.*, 1995) maintenance programs will also need to cater for inmates who apply for treatment during their sentence. Evidence of the spread of blood-borne viral infections among prisoners may need to be collected before prison authorities are convinced that methadone maintenance programs are warranted.

SUMMARY

The provision of methadone within prison settings can be justified for limited periods and on a maintenance basis throughout the sentence. Methadone provision to prisoners on entry can alleviate heroin (and methadone) withdrawal symptoms. Provision prior to release from prison may reduce the risk of overdose or a return to crime following return to the community. The major rationale for the provision of methadone on a maintenance basis during incarceration is to reduce injecting and subsequent transmission of hepatitis B and C and HIV.

Although the arguments for prison methadone programs appear valid there are few such programs in the world. Methadone is used to detoxify inmates in eight countries and a small proportion of inmates are maintained on methadone in seven countries. The limited research that has been conducted on prison-based methadone programs has focused generally on operational aspects rather than HIV transmission. Methadone programs have been implemented successfully in prisons and appear to be beneficial. There is much less evidence to support the effectiveness of methadone maintenance treatment in prison compared with community settings because so much less research has been conducted in prison. It is likely that methadone maintenance in prison will have similar results to those in the community.

Prison methadone programs differ from those in the community in terms of entry criteria, aims and operational aspects. Prison methadone programs are relatively new. Therefore the aims and details of service delivery are still evolving. The continuing development of prison methadone programs complicates evaluation. Prison-based methadone programs need to be subjected to rigorous evaluations. The ideal study of methadone in prison would be a randomised controlled trial where objective outcome measures are collected prospectively.

REFERENCES

Advisory Council on the Misuse of Drugs (1993). *AIDS and drug misuse update.* London HMSO.

Anonymous (1992). The crisis in Correctional Health Care: The impact of the National Drug Control Strategy on Correctional Health Services. American College of Physicians, National Commission on Correctional Health Care and American Correctional Health Services Association. *Annals of Internal Medicine, 117,* 71-7.

Bertram, S. (1991). *Results of gaols urinalyses update: July - December 1989. Evaluation of New South Wales Department of Corrective Services pre-release methadone program study no 10.* Sydney, Australia: Research and Statistics Division, New South Wales Department of Corrective Services.

Brewer, T.F., Vlahov, D., Taylor, E., Hall, D., Munoz, A., & Polk, F. (1988). Transmission of HIV-1 within a statewide prison system. *AIDS,*

2, 363-367.

Castro, K., Shansky, R., Scardino, V., Narkunas, J., Coe, J., & Hammett, T. (1991). HIV transmission in correctional facilities. Paper presented at the VII International Conference on AIDS, Florence, 16-21 June.

Centers for Disease Control (1986). Acquired Immunodeficiency Syndrome in correctional facilities: A report of the National Institute of Justice and the American Correctional Association. *Morbidity and Mortality Weekly Report,* 35(12), 195-199.

Commonwealth of Australia. (1988). *National Methadone Guidelines.* Canberra, Australia: Australian Government Publishing Service.

Crofts, N., Webb-Pullman, J., & Dolan, K. (1996). *An analysis of trends over time in social and behavioural factors related to the transmission of HIV among IDUs and prison inmates.* Canberra, Australia: Australian Government Publishing Service.

Crofts, N., Stewart, T., Hearne, P., Ping, X.Y., Breschkin, A.M., & Locarnini, S.A. (1995). Spread of blood-borne viruses among Australian prison entrants. *British Medical Journal,* 310, 285-88.

Darke, S., Ross, J., Cohen, J., & Hall, W. (1994). *Context and correlates of non-fatal overdose among heroin users in Sydney.* NDARC Monograph No 20. Sydney, Australia: National Drug and Alcohol Research Centre.

Department of Corrective Services (1994). *Annual Report 1993-1994.* Sydney, Australia: New South Wales Government.

Dolan, K. (1993). Drug injectors in prison and the community in England. *International Journal of Drug Policy,* 4, 179-183.

Dolan, K.A., Donoghoe, M., & Stimson, G. (1990). Drug injecting and syringe sharing in custody and in the community: An exploratory survey of HIV risk behaviour. *Howard Journal,* 29, 177-186.

Dolan, K., Hall, W., & Wodak, A. (1994a). *Bleach availability and risk behaviour in prison in New South Wales.* Technical Report No 22. Sydney, Australia: National Drug and Alcohol Research Centre.

Dolan, K., Hall, W., & Wodak, A. (1996e). Methadone maintenance reduces injecting in prison *British Medical Journal,* 312, 1162.

Dolan, K., Hall, W., Wodak, A., & Gaughwin, M. (1994b). Evidence of HIV transmission in an Australian prison. *Medical Journal of Australia,* 160, 734.

Dolan, K., Rutter, S., Wodak, A., Hall, W., Maher L., & Dixon D. (1996a). Is syringe exchange feasible in a prison setting? *Medical Journal of Australia,* 164, 508.

Dolan K., Shearer J., Hall, W., & Wodak, A. (1996b). *Bleach is easier to obtain but inmates are still at risk infection in New South Wales prisons.* Technical Report 25. Sydney, Australia: National Drug and Alcohol Research Centre.

Dolan, K., & Wodak A. (1996). An international review of methadone provision in prisons. *Addiction Research,* 4, 85-97.

Dolan, K., Wodak, A., Hall, W., Gaughwin, M., & Rae F. (1996d). HIV risk behaviour before, during and after imprisonment in New South Wales. *Addiction Research, 4,* 151-160

Dolan, K., Wodak A., & Penny, R. (1995). AIDS behind bars: Preventing HIV spread among incarcerated drug injectors. *AIDS, 9,* 825-32.

Dolan, K., Wodak, A., Saksena, N., Dwyer, D., & Sorrell, T. (1996c). *A network of HIV infection among Australian inmates.* XI International AIDS Conference. Vancouver. Abstract no.6594.

Dole, V.P., Robinson, J.W., Orraca, J., Towns, E., Searcy, P., & Caine, E. (1969). Methadone treatment of randomly selected criminal addicts. *New England Journal of Medicine,* **280,** 1372-1375.

Dye, S., & Isaacs, C. (1991). Intravenous drug misuse among prison inmates: Implications for spread of HIV. *British Medical Journal,* **302,** 1506.

Gaughwin, M.D., Douglas, R.M., & Wodak, A.D. (1991). Behind bars - risk behaviours for HIV transmission in prisons, a review. In J. Norberry, S.A. Gerull, & M.D. Gaughwin (Eds.), *HIV/AIDS and Prisons.* Canberra, Australia: Australian Institute of Criminology.

General Accounting Office (1994). *Bureau of prisons health care: Inmates' access to health care is limited by lack of clinical staff.* Report by United States General Accounting Office, February, GAO/HEHS-94-36.

Glaser, J.B., & Greifinger, R.B. (1993). Correctional health care: A public health opportunity. *Annals of Internal Medicine,* **118,** 139-145

Gore, S.M., Bird, A.G., Burns, S.M., Goldberg, D.J., Ross, A.J., & Macgregor, J. (1995). Drug injection and HIV prevalence in inmates of Glenochil prison. *British Medical Journal,* **310,** 293-296.

Gorta, A. (1992). *Monitoring the New South Wales prison methadone program: A review of the research 1986-1991.* Research Publication New South Wales Department of Corrective Services Publication no. 25. Sydney, Australia: New South Wales Department of Corrective Services.

Gorta A (1987a). *Results of gaol urinalyses January - June 1987. Process evaluation of New South Wales Department of Corrective Services prison methadone program study no 4.* Sydney, Australia: Research and Statistics Division, New South Wales Department of Corrective Services.

Gorta A (1987b). *Process evaluation of New South Wales Department of Corrective Services prison methadone program study no 3.* Sydney, Australia: Research and Statistics Division, New South Wales Department of Corrective Services.

Grönbladh, L., Ohlund, L.S., & Gunne, L.M. (1990). Mortality in heroin addiction: Impact of methadone treatment. *Acta Psychiatrica Scandinavia,* **82,** 223-227.

Groves, T. (1991). Prison policies on HIV under review. *British Medical Journal,* **303,** 1354.

Hall, W., Ward, J., & Mattick, R. (1993). Methadone maintenance treatment in prisons: The New South Wales experience. *Drug and*

Alcohol Review, **12**, 193-203.

Harding, T., & Schaller, G. (1992). *HIV/AIDS and prisons: Update and policy review June 1992.* Unpublished manuscript, University Institute of Legal Medicine, Geneva.

Herzog, C., Fasnacht, M., Stohler, R., Ladewig, D. (1993). Methadone substitution as an AIDS-preventive measure in the prison environment. Paper presented at the European Symposium on Drug Addiction & AIDS, Siena, Italy, October 4-6.

Horsburgh, C.R., Jarvis, J.Q., McArthur, T., Ignacio, T., & Stock, P. (1990). Seroconversion to Human Immunodeficiency Virus in prison inmates. *American Journal of Public Health,* **80**, 209-10.

Hume, S., & Gorta, A. (1989). The effects of the New South Wales prison methadone program on criminal recidivism and retention in methadone treatment. *Process evaluation of New South Wales Department of Corrective Services prison methadone program study no 7.* Sydney, Australia: Research and Statistics Division, New South Wales Department of Corrective Services.

Hume, S., & Gorta, A. (1988). *Views of key personnel involved with the administration of the prison methadone program. Process evaluation of New South Wales Department of Corrective Services prison methadone program study no 5.* Sydney, Australia: Research and Statistics Division, New South Wales Department of Corrective Services.

Jeanmonod, R., Harding, T., & Staub, C. (1991). Treatment of opiate withdrawal on entry to prison. *British Journal of Addiction,* **86**, 457-463.

Kaplan, E., & Heimer, R. (1992). A model-based estimate of HIV infectivity via needle sharing. *Journal of Acquired Immune Deficiency Syndromes,* **5**, 1116-1118.

Kelley, P.W., Redfield, R.R., Ward, D.L., Burke, D.S., & Miller, R.N. (1986). Prevalence and incidence of HTLV-111 infection in a prison. *Journal of the American Medical Association,* **256**, 2198-99.

Maden, A., Swinton, M., & Gunn, J. (1992). A survey of pre-arrest drug use in sentenced prisoners. *British Journal of Addiction,* **87**, 27-33.

Magura, S., Rosenblum, A., Lewis, C., & Joseph, H. (1993). The effectiveness of in-jail methadone maintenance. *Journal of Drug Issues,* **23**, 75-99.

Mattick, R.P., & Hall, W. (1996). Is detoxification effective ? *Lancet,* **347**, 97-100.

Mauer, M. (1995). Russia, United States World Leaders in incarceration. *Overcrowded Times: Solving the prison problem,* **5**(5) 1,9.

McLeod, F. (1991). Methadone, prisons and AIDS. In J. Norberry, M. Gaughwin and S.A. Gerull (Eds.), *HIV/AIDS and prison.* Canberra, Australia: Australian Institute of Criminology.

Metzger, D. S., Woody, G. E., McLellan, A. T., O'Brien, C. P., Druley, P., Navaline, H., DePhilippis, D., Stolley, P., & Abrutyn, E. (1993).

Human Immunodeficiency Virus seroconversion among intravenous drug users in- and out-of-treatment: An 18-month prospective follow-up. *Journal of Acquired Immune Deficiency Syndromes,* **6,** 1049-1055.

Ministerio De Justicia e Interior. (1993). Memoria. Delegacion del Gobierno para el Plan nacional sobre Droras, Madrid.

Mutter, R.C., Grimes, R.M., & Labarthe, D. (1994). Evidence of intraprison spread of HIV infection. *Archives of Internal Medicine,* **154,** 793-795.

National Institute on Drug Abuse (1992). *Drug Abuse treatment in prison and jails.* Washington, DC: US Government Printing Office.

Nelles, J., & Harding, T. (1995). Preventing HIV transmission in prison: A tale of medical disobedience and Swiss pragmatism. *Lancet,* **346,** 1507-08.

Normand, J., Vlahov, D., & Moses L. (1995). *Preventing HIV transmission. The role of sterile needles and bleach.* Washington, DC: National Academy Press.

Oakley, A. (1990). Who's afraid of the randomised controlled trial ? Some dilemmas of the scientific method and "good" research practice. *Women & Health,* **15**(4), 25-59.

Seamark, R., & Gaughwin, M. (1994). Jabs in the dark: Injecting equipment found in prisons, and the risks of viral transmission. *Australian Journal of Public Health,* **18,** 113-116.

Scottish Affairs Committee (1994). *Drug abuse in Scotland, report.* London: HMSO.

Shewan, D., Macpherson, S., Reid, M., & Davies, J.B. (1994). *Evaluation of the Saughton drug reduction programme. Main Report.* Edinburgh: Central Research Unit.

Taylor, A., Goldberg, D., Emslie, J., Wrench, J., Gruer, L., Cameron, S., Black, J., Davis, B., McGregor, J., Follett, E., Harvey, J., Basson, J., & McGavigan, J. (1995). Outbreak of HIV infection in a Scottish prison. *British Medical Journal,* **310,** 289-292.

Turnbull, P.J., Dolan, K.A., & Stimson, G.V. (1991). *Prisons, HIV and AIDS: Risks and experiences in custodial care.* Horsham, UK: Avert.

Wale, S., & Gorta, A. (1987). *Views of inmates participating in the pilot pre-release methadone program. Process evaluation of New South Wales Department of Corrective Services pre-release methadone program study no. 2.* Sydney, Australia: Research and Statistics Division, New South Wales Department of Corrective Services.

Walker, J., Hallinan, J., & Dagger, D. (1992). Australian prisoners 1992. Results of the National Prison Census 30 June 1992. Canberra, Australia: Australian Institute of Criminology.

Ward, J., Mattick, R., & Hall, W. (1992). *Key issues in methadone maintenance treatment.* Sydney, Australia: New South Wales Univeristy Press.

Wodak, A. (1991). Behind bars: HIV risk taking behaviour of Sydney male IDUs injectors while in prison. In J. Norberry, M. Gaughwin and S.A. Gerull (Eds.), *HIV/AIDS and prison.* Canberra, Australia: Australian Institute of Criminology.

Wool, R. (1991). *Caring for drug misusers.* London: Directorate of Health Care, Prison Service Library, Abel House.

World Health Organization (1993). *WHO guidelines on HIV infection and AIDS in prisons.* Geneva: WHO.

World Health Organization. (1994). *Multi-city study on drug injecting and risk of HIV infection.* Geneva: WHO.

Zador, D. Sunjic, S., & Darke, S. (1995). *Toxicological findings and circumstances of heroin caused deaths in New South Wales.* NDARC Monograph No. 22. Sydney, Australia: National Drug and Alcohol Research Centre.

16

METHADONE MAINTENANCE DURING PREGNANCY

JEFF WARD, RICHARD P. MATTICK
AND WAYNE HALL

INTRODUCTION

As heroin dependence became increasingly more widespread during the 1960s, it was inevitable that pregnant women in this predicament would present for care. At first, neither drug treatment clinics nor maternity wards knew how to deal with the serious complications that arose in these women and their infants (Suffet & Brotman, 1984). For example, in the early 1970s, the Food and Drug Administration in the USA recommended 21-day methadone detoxification programs as the treatment of choice for the pregnant addict. However, reports of an association between withdrawal and still birth, as well as a range of other complications, led to this recommendation being dropped (Chavkin, 1990). Since then, the treatment of choice for the opioid-dependent pregnant woman has been methadone maintenance throughout pregnancy (Finnegan, 1983; Finnegan, 1991; Kaltenbach et al., 1993).

In this chapter we examine the rationale and evidence for the use of methadone maintenance as a treatment for opioid-dependent pregnant women and provide an overview of the clinical issues involved in caring for these women and their potential offspring. Important clinical issues in methadone maintenance for this population include selecting an appropriate methadone dose, providing appropriate antenatal care, making counselling available during treatment, and managing the abstinence syndrome in the neonate. The focus of this review is restricted to the care of pregnant women in methadone programs and the immediate impact that methadone maintenance has on their newborn children. Previous reviews in this area have been relied upon (e.g., Finnegan, 1983; Householder *et al.,* 1982) because of the extent and variety of material that is relevant to this topic. Finnegan (1980, 1991) has provided comprehensive accounts of the clinical issues. We would refer the reader to her work for further detail concerning obstetric and medical care.

RATIONALE AND EVIDENCE FOR THE USE OF METHADONE MAINTENANCE DURING PREGNANCY

The Opioid-Dependent Pregnant Woman

A woman dependent on illicit opioids must be considered medically to be in a high-risk category when she is pregnant. Such a woman is at risk for the usual health-related problems found among injecting drug users (e.g., hepatitis, HIV infection, endocarditis, etc.), as well as anaemia, cystitis and a variety of problems specifically related to pregnancy, including premature labour and abruption of the placenta which may result in the death of both woman and foetus (see Finnegan, 1983, 1991 for more details). During pregnancy, these women often do not have the benefit of the three important conditions for a healthy pregnancy: adequate rest, nutrition and antenatal care (Finnegan, 1988). As well as being at risk medically, opioid-dependent pregnant women also suffer from a range of other problems (Finnegan *et al.,* 1991; Waldby, 1988). These include various psychological (low self-esteem, depression, anxiety states) and social problems (poverty, homelessness, legal crises, domestic violence). Many of these women have lost children to child welfare agencies in the past and, as a consequence, feel reluctant to contact health care agencies and remain suspicious when they do. They are well aware that they belong to one of the most highly stigmatised groups of women in society (Jessup, 1990; Waldby, 1988).

It is not surprising that the foetus of a drug-dependent woman does not always fare well in its deprived environment. Besides the impediment of lack of adequate nutrition, rest and antenatal care, the foetus has to contend with problems created by the cycle of withdrawal and intoxication associated with the mother's dependent opioid use. Intoxication and withdrawal both place stress upon the foetus. Opioid withdrawal during pregnancy is dangerous and has been associated with foetal death; this is especially the case if the woman is experiencing withdrawal while she is in labour (Finnegan, 1983). According to Hoegerman *et al.* (1990), of even greater concern is the uncertainty about adulterants with which illicit drugs may have been cut in moving down the distribution network. Some of the contaminants found in black market heroin may be teratogenic (i.e., exposure causes morphological changes in the developing foetus). However, opioids themselves have no known teratogenic effects on the human foetus (Finnegan, 1983).

Many heroin-dependent women present late for care, because they often misinterpret the signs and symptoms of their pregnancy. Menstrual problems, especially amenorrhoea, are common in this population (Finnegan, 1980). After entering methadone maintenance, menstruation usually returns to normal within six to 12 months. According to Kreek (1996), this is due to the stabilising effect of the chronic administration of a long-acting opioid agonist as opposed to the intermittent administration of a shorter acting opioid such as heroin which reduces the release of luteinising hormone from the hypothalamus in humans, thereby preventing ovulation and disrupting menstruation. The concomitant nutritional deficiencies, infections (e.g., hepatitis, pelvic infections) and psychosocial stresses of illicit drug use may also contribute to amenorrhoea. The high incidence of menstrual abnormalities among these women has given rise to one of the perennial mythologies of the heroin subculture – that a woman is unlikely to become pregnant while she is using heroin (Waldby, 1988). This mythology, in turn, is in part responsible for a neglect of contraception as a safeguard against unwanted pregnancy. When heroin-using women do become pregnant, it is often unexpected and the early signs and symptoms (nausea, headaches, fatigue, etc.) may be mistaken for withdrawal symptoms or the effects of "dirty drugs" (i.e., harmful contaminants). This means that they often do not become aware that they are pregnant and hence do not present for treatment until relatively late.

The Rationale for Methadone Maintenance During Pregnancy

The rationale for the use of methadone maintenance for pregnant women who are opioid dependent has two main components (Mackie-Ramos & Rice, 1988): methadone replaces illicit opioids of uncertain composition and dose with a pure substitute at a stable dose; and enrolment in a methadone maintenance program allows the woman to receive the antenatal care and advice necessary for a successful pregnancy. Detoxification from all drugs is unrealistic for most of this population and often results in the mother experiencing an abstinence syndrome leading to foetal distress, which is more harmful than a medically supervised methadone dependence (Finnegan, 1991). Pregnant women who are maintained on methadone have no need to engage in drug-related crime or prostitution, usually improve their nutritional intake, reduce their risk for HIV and hepatitis infections, are more willing to attend for antenatal care, and can spend more time preparing for birth and becoming a parent because they are relieved of the burden of drug seeking.

The Effectiveness of Methadone Maintenance During Pregnancy

Research evidence has consistently shown that methadone maintenance produces superior outcomes compared to not being in treatment for this population. As well as a reduction in drug use and crime, methadone maintenance retains patients in treatment, providing them with sufficient antenatal care to achieve as successful a birth as possible given the circumstances. The gains to be expected are comparative: better outcomes are expected than if these women remained heroin dependent and received little or no antenatal care. When assessed in this way, properly delivered methadone maintenance is a highly successful intervention for opioid-dependent pregnant women.

Most of the problems experienced by infants born to opioid-dependent mothers are due to premature birth and being small for gestational age (Ellwood *et al.*, 1987; Finnegan, 1983; 1991). The evidence clearly and consistently shows that infants born to methadone-maintained mothers are born later and are larger for gestational age than those born to opioid-dependent women who are not in treatment (Finnegan, 1980; Giles *et al.*, 1989; Householder *et al.*, 1982). Pregnant women in methadone maintenance programs attend for more antenatal care than do women out of treatment (Finnegan, 1983; Giles *et al.,* 1989; Soepatmi, 1994). Both attendance at antenatal care and the improved outcomes mentioned above are related to time spent in methadone maintenance (Doberczak *et al.,* 1987; Ellwood *et al.,* 1987; Suffet & Brotman, 1984). The amount of antenatal care received is an important predictor of outcome for both mother and foetus (Suffet & Brotman, 1984; Wilson, 1989).

Although some of the problems experienced by infants born to opioid-dependent mothers are drug related (e.g., neonatal abstinence syndrome), most of the morbidity and mortality for these newborns is due to the harm associated with a heroin-using lifestyle. The specific effects of opioids such as heroin on the neonate are difficult to specify due to insurmountable methodological problems in carrying out research in this area. The effects of heroin are confounded by the harm associated with the lifestyle (intoxication–withdrawal cycle, drug contaminants, infections, poverty, etc.), the difficulty in specifying and quantifying drugs taken, and the influence of inadequate care (Deren, 1986; Hoegerman *et al.,* 1990; Householder *et al.,* 1982; Kaltenbach & Finnegan, 1989; Kreek, 1983a; Kaltenbach, 1994). For example, the almost universal incidence of cigarette smoking among opioid-dependent women must decrease birth weight (Doberczak *et al.,* 1987; Ellwood *et al.,* 1987; Giles *et al.,* 1989). According to Wilson (1989), studies on the subsequent intellectual development of infants exposed to heroin *in utero* suggest that inadequate antenatal care is common for children who turn out to be severely impaired. There have been no demonstrated long-term disadvantages for infants born to methadone-maintained women when lifestyle factors are taken into account (e.g., Lifschitz *et al.,* 1985).

In any discussion of the efficacy of methadone maintenance for pregnant women, it has to be kept in mind that it is not so long ago that infants born to heroin-dependent mothers had little chance of survival (Finnegan, 1988). The dramatic increase in survival and reduction in morbidity in this group is due to developments that have taken place in the capacity to successfully care for high-risk neonates. These developments and the use of methadone maintenance in combination with good antenatal care means that many of these women will give birth to infants at term. For example, Finnegan (1988) reports that of 196 admissions to her program 72% of women gave birth to infants at term, 12% were born prematurely, 8% suffered medical complications, and 8% died *in utero.*

PREGNANCY AND METHADONE DOSAGE

In order to limit foetal exposure to all drugs to a minimum, it would at first glance seem that the ideal use of methadone for the heroin-dependent pregnant woman would be to stabilise her on a low dose of methadone (<40 mg) early in her pregnancy, to slowly reduce the methadone dose (5 mg per fortnight) between the 14th and 32nd weeks, and for mother and infant to be drug-free at birth (Finnegan, 1980, 1991, 1983; Gerada *et al.,* 1990; Kaltenbach *et al.* 1993). If required or desired, withdrawal is best carried out during this period because the process may induce abortion before the 14th week and premature labour or withdrawal-induced foetal stress after the 32nd week. Where detoxification is the only practical alternative, or in cases where a patient insists on detoxification, the withdrawal regimen mentioned above of dose decreases of 5 mg every two weeks is recommended. Such detoxification is ideally conducted under the supervision of a perinatal specialist experienced in the management of drug dependence and should be halted if either foetal distress or premature labour eventuates.

Nevertheless, detoxification is an unrealistic option for most heroin-dependent women and pregnancy does not significantly alter this. Most women on a methadone withdrawal regimen such as the one described above would quickly relapse to heroin use, which is far more dangerous than a medically supervised methadone maintenance regimen (Finnegan, 1980). Finnegan (1991), who has extensive experience with this population, reports a 100% failure to achieve abstinence in her program in Philadelphia, either because patients were unable to bear the diminishing doses of methadone, or could not proceed due to the likely onset of premature labour. Tranquillisers, such as diazepam, are contraindicated for the relief of withdrawal symptoms for pregnant women undergoing detoxification because of possible negative effects on the foetus. If a patient is unable to continue with withdrawal, then her methadone dose should be readjusted upwards in slow increments until she reaches a level she feels comfortable with.

Methadone Dose and Neonatal Withdrawal

If withdrawal is not possible, then the next most desirable option, according to some authors, is maintenance on as low a dose of methadone as possible (Batey *et al.,* 1990; Gerada *et al.,* 1990; Suffet

& Brotman, 1984). There are two reasons put forward for this recommendation: the lowest dose of methadone will have the least negative effects upon the foetus; and the lower the dose of methadone, the less withdrawal distress will be experienced by the newborn infant. However, neither of these two reasons bear a simple relationship to the research evidence when other outcomes are taken into account. For example, in the case of the effect of high doses of methadone on the foetus, Doberczak *et al.* (1987) found that higher doses of methadone were associated with greater increases in maternal weight during pregnancy. As Kreek (1983b) has pointed out, it is not clear from the evidence what the effects of different methadone dosage regimens are on the developing foetus and the evidence will not be clear until studies are done on opioid-dependent women who do not use alcohol, nicotine or other drugs during their pregnancy. Further, the risks associated with relapse to heroin use or substitution with other drugs such as benzodiazepines, which might complicate withdrawal in the neonate, have to be considered. When factors like these are taken into account, it would seem advisable to adopt the principle of providing sufficient methadone to meet the needs of the mother, based on the more general principle that what is good for the mother is generally good for the foetus. Finnegan (1991) points out that it is counter-productive to treat mother and foetus as if they were 'separate and competing entities'. In any case, there is no evidence to suggest that either pregnancy or outcome for the neonate is related to methadone dose with doses up to 100 mg daily (Finnegan, 1980, 1991; Thakur *et al.,* 1990).

Although some studies have found an association between maternal methadone dose and severity of neonatal withdrawal (e.g., Collins, 1990, 1992; Suffet & Brotman, 1984), this relationship has not been consistently observed (e.g., Mack *et al.,* 1991; Finnegan, 1991). However, a recent study reported by (Doberczak *et al.,* 1993), has found maternal methadone dose at birth to be associated with plasma levels in both the mother and the neonate, suggesting that there is some consistency between the oral dose ingested by the mother and the level of exposure and presumably dependence in the neonate. However, when considering the neonatal abstinence syndrome, it has to be kept in mind that this syndrome is a relatively benign and treatable manifestation in comparison to the complications that often arise when a heroin-dependent or poly-drug abusing woman has received insufficient antenatal care (Finnegan cited in Gastel & Collins, 1983). Although some authors have recently revived the debate by advocating a reduction in maternal methadone doses in order to reduce neonatal withdrawal (Malpas *et al.,* 1995; Jarvis & Schnoll, 1994; Doberczak *et al.,* 1993), it would seem inadvisable to restrict methadone doses without taking into account the attendant risks associated with the onset of withdrawal in the expectant mother and the likelihood of relapse that follows as a consequence.

Assessment and Initial Methadone Dose

Under no circumstances should a pregnant woman be administered naloxone to diagnose opioid dependence because of the hazards involved for both woman and foetus of rapidly inducing a state of severe withdrawal (Finnegan, 1991; Kaltenbach *et al.,* 1993). Assessment should be based on the taking of a careful history and a physical examination. Finnegan (1991) recommends the following procedure for commencing methadone maintenance in a hospital setting. As soon as the beginning of withdrawal is apparent, 10 mg of methadone is administered, followed by 5 mg every four to six hours until the symptoms are alleviated. The next day, the previous day's total dose is administered and again supplemented as needed. Most patients can be adequately stabilised on 20 to 35 mg, though increases may be necessary after discharge from hospital. An adequate maintenance dose will depend on length of dependence, mode of administration, how long the patient has been on methadone maintenance, and the concurrent prescription of other drugs known to enhance the metabolism of methadone (e.g., phenytoin – see Chapter 9 for a discussion of this phenomenon). The dose of methadone administered should be increased in small increments if there is relapse to heroin use, ongoing illicit drug use or indications of increased methadone metabolism in the third trimester.

As already noted, the effects of opioids on the woman will also affect the foetus and both withdrawal and intoxication may lead to serious complications. For these reasons, initial stabilisation on methadone has often taken place during a short period of hospitalisation, so that the patient can be closely observed and have her physical condition assessed (e.g., Ellwood *et al.,* 1987; Finnegan, 1991), especially if she has presented late in her pregnancy (Gerada *et al.,* 1990). However, methadone maintenance can be commenced on an outpatient basis (Giles *et al.,* 1989; Batey *et al.,* 1990). When a woman is inducted as an outpatient, Batey *et al.* (1990) recommend an initial methadone dose of 20 to 40 mg (depending upon assessment) because rapid stabilisation is necessary to promptly halt illicit opioid use. Patients on this intake regimen are then closely monitored on a daily basis to ensure a quick response in cases where dosage adjustments are necessary.

Methadone Metabolism in the Pregnant Woman

Pregnancy is one of a number of factors known to induce the metabolism of methadone in human beings (Finnegan, 1983; Kreek, 1983a, 1983b; Pond *et al.,* 1985) (see Chapter 9 for a discussion of other factors). Pond *et al.* (1985), in a study of nine pregnant women, found that for all the subjects the concentration of methadone in plasma at its lowest point during the 24-hour dosing cycle (trough plasma level) was lower, when adjusted for dose, than what it was when measured post-partum. Three of these nine women experienced withdrawal symptoms towards the end of their pregnancies and these symptoms were associated with significant differences in trough plasma levels pre- and post-partum. These differences in methadone plasma levels were greater than could be expected when changes in dose and increases in body weight and fluid were taken into account.

The authors hypothesised that towards the end of pregnancy the foetus begins to metabolise methadone and that this accounts for the drop in plasma levels, although this has yet to be demonstrated (see Finnegan, 1983). Kreek (1996) has suggested that a more likely explanation for the drop in methadone plasma levels during the third trimester is the high level of progestogens in late pregnancy which are known to induce the metabolism of a number of drugs in the liver. Whatever the cause may be, the observation of decreased plasma levels and unexpected withdrawal symptoms in some women during the third trimester is a consistent one (Finnegan, 1983; Kreek, 1983a, 1983b). This phenomenon is arguably responsible, in part, for the high level of relapse observed during the third trimester.

Two solutions have been proposed for the woman who begins to experience withdrawal in the third trimester: split-dosing and an increase in dose. Split-dosing has been recommended as a way in which to maintain plasma levels at a more steady level and has been found to be satisfactory in achieving this goal in some cases (Hoegerman *et al.,* 1990; Pond *et al.,* 1985; Sutton & Hinderliter, 1990; Wittmann & Segal, 1991). Wittmann & Segal (1991), in a study of seven women whose methadone dose was inadequate during the third trimester, found through the use of ultrasound that the foetus in such cases became agitated by the end of the usual 24-hour dosing cycle and showed restricted movement after the woman had been dosed. They found that split-dosing reduced these fluctuations in foetal movement. If split-dosing were to be considered seriously as an option, then allowing these women to take at least one of their doses home with them would also have to be taken into consideration.

GROUP THERAPY FOR METHADONE-MAINTAINED PREGNANT WOMEN

Although the rate of attendance at general or specific purpose groups (educational, psychotherapeutic, etc.) is usually low or non-existent among the general methadone maintenance patient population, in the case of pregnant women such groups are desirable and, under the right circumstances, reasonably well attended (Batey *et al.,* 1990; Finnegan, 1991; Finnegan *et al.,* 1991; Holmes, 1989; Mackie-Ramos & Rice, 1988). Mackie-Ramos and Rice (1988) point out that these women have two things in common: they are drug dependent and they are pregnant. Attending a group allows them to discuss their problems and become informed about pregnancy, birth and parenting with women who share their own experience. Attendance at groups may remain quite low, however, if no incentive is provided. At a specialist Drugs in Pregnancy Service at a Sydney hospital, the provision of incentives and clever scheduling has been successful in encouraging attendance. An effective formula has been to schedule the group between morning dosing time and an afternoon antenatal clinic held for the patients, and to provide lunch and child care while the group is meeting (Holmes, pers. com., 15 October, 1991).

As well as offering antenatal education and parenting skills training, groups for drug-dependent women also need to address specific issues pertinent to their situation. Concerns about the effect of past drug use, methadone and past and current infections (e.g., hepatitis) upon their future child are very common. Batey *et al.* (1990) suggest that many of these women may have a range of unresolved psychological problems arising out of family experiences and at the hands of the legal and welfare systems. Other current psychological problems (e.g., anxiety and depression) are also likely. In this sense, then, groups for these women may need to be more like group therapy sessions than the usual antenatal classes. This does not preclude or replace the need for individual counselling where necessary.

Finnegan *et al.* (1991) do not recommend mixed-sex groups. Many drug-dependent women have been sexually or physically abused at some time in their lives and may not feel free to communicate in the presence of males. In a group restricted to women, group members are able to express themselves freely without fearing male censure. The issue of group composition is a specific component of the more general issue of whether male partners should be treated in the same methadone maintenance program. Finnegan (1991) and Batey *et al.* (1990) recommend that partners be enrolled in the same program. Finnegan prefers a family-oriented treatment approach, while Batey *et al.* suggest that having the partner in the same methadone maintenance reduces conflict. Conflict with regard to access to methadone maintenance does appear to be a serious problem for these couples. Waldby (1988) documents several case histories where the basis of a couple's relationship (drug-dependent lifestyle) was threatened by the woman's entry to methadone maintenance. It is common for pregnant women to have priority access to methadone maintenance in many places throughout the world. This quick access to treatment often leaves the couple in a situation in which the woman is trying to abstain from illicit drug use while her partner continues his use because he cannot find a program that will accept him. A family-oriented treatment approach obviates this difficulty by treating both the woman and her partner.

The issue of involving partners in treatment in specialist programs for pregnant women, however, does not meet with consensus from workers in the field. The high incidence of domestic violence in this population has led some workers to see the need for the methadone maintenance unit to function as a safe place for women, a role that may at times be difficult to fulfil if the unit is also dispensing to the partner concerned (Holmes, pers. com., 15 October, 1991).

ANTENATAL CARE

Two of the reasons why drug-dependent women reportedly do not seek out antenatal care is that they expect a negative reaction from clinic staff and fear that their child might be removed from their care by child welfare authorities (Gerada *et al.,* 1990). It is important, therefore, that such women are treated in a non-judgemental fashion (Finnegan, 1980). It must be remembered in this regard that health care workers ignorant of the research concerning the positive role of methadone in the management of opioid dependence may regard methadone as no different from heroin. For these reasons, the ideal situation is where a methadone maintenance unit specialising in the care of pregnant women works with an antenatal care unit. It has been found in the past that women in methadone maintenance attend for more antenatal visits than heroin-dependent women out of treatment, but that they still do not attend as regularly as women who are not drug dependent. Giles *et al.* (1989) have suggested scheduling more frequent visits for drug-dependent women, both in and out of methadone maintenance treatment, as a way of making up for low attendance rates. The importance of this aspect of care cannot be overemphasised given the consistent observation that amount of antenatal care is associated with fewer complications and a number of measures of positive outcome.

BIRTH AND THE POSTNATAL PERIOD

Analgesia and Anaesthesia During Labour and Birth

Methadone-maintained women should be given standard analgesia when required during labour (Batey *et al.*, 1990; Gerada *et al.*, 1990). Kreek (1996) recommends doses towards the upper end of the normal range and, if necessary, shorter dosing intervals. Methadone as taken during methadone maintenance does not provide pain relief. This remains true even if the woman needs to receive her daily dose of methadone during labour. However, according to Collins and Capus (1991), opioids for pain relief should be avoided where possible during labour because they may increase the opioid load on the infant at birth. Other interventions, such as the use of nitrous oxide and non-opioid epidural anaesthesia, are preferable, because they should not affect the infant. Increasing the opioid load on the infant during labour may lead to a sedated neonate which in turn may lead to the administration of naloxone, the usual procedure for dealing with this condition. The use of naloxone with infants born to opioid-dependent women (methadone or heroin) may precipitate an acute neonatal abstinence syndrome and should be administered only under the supervision of medical staff who have experience with this procedure in this population. Once the woman has given birth, the use of opioids for pain relief is again indicated.

The Neonatal Abstinence Syndrome

Description

Finnegan (cited in Gastel & Collins, 1983) has pointed out that the withdrawal syndrome observed in infants born to methadone-maintained women has to be viewed within an appropriate context. Compared to the problems observed in the neonates of heroin-dependent women out of treatment, the condition is relatively benign and responds readily to appropriate treatment. The neonatal abstinence syndrome has been described by Finnegan (1983) as:

> ...a generalized disorder characterized by signs and symptoms of central nervous system hyperirritability, gastrointestinal dysfunction, and respiratory distress, and by vague autonomic symptoms that include yawning, sneezing, mottling, and fever. Initially, the infants appear only to be restless. Tremors begin when the infants are disturbed and progress to the point where they occur when the infants are not disturbed. High-pitched cry, increased muscle tone, and further irritability develop. When examined, the infants have deep tendon reflexes and an exaggerated Moro reflex. The rooting reflex is increased, and the infants are frequently seen sucking their fists or thumbs, yet when fed the infants have extreme difficulty and regurgitate frequently because of uncoordinated and ineffectual sucking and swallowing reflexes. Because of loose stools, decreased intake, and regurgitation, the infants are susceptible to dehydration and electrolyte imbalance (p. 410).

This syndrome usually begins within 72 hours, but may appear up to two weeks after birth. The timing of onset is influenced by many factors including the drug(s) used by the mother, the dose taken, when the drug(s) was last taken in relation to birth, the nature of labour, anaesthesia and analgesia used during labour, the gestational age of the infant, nutritional factors, and the presence of disease in the infant. Many patterns of symptoms are also observed, from the mild through to the severe, and from the transient through to the more longer lasting (Finnegan, 1983). As we have seen, some reports suggest that the neonatal abstinence syndrome is more likely as maternal methadone dose increases (e.g., Collins, 1992; Suffet & Brotman, 1984). Approximately 30% of infants recently born to methadone-maintained women at one Sydney specialist program required pharmacotherapy for the syndrome after birth (Collins & Capus, 1991).

A recent case report by Sutton and Hinderliter (1990) describes a protracted withdrawal syndrome in two infants born to methadone-maintained women who were taking large doses of illicit diazepam regularly. The two infants experienced a withdrawal syndrome typical for methadone abstinence, which was successfully dealt with by paregoric (camphorated tincture of opium), but at one week the symptoms reappeared despite this medication. The authors attributed this phenomenon to diazepam withdrawal. Diazepam passes through the placenta and accumulates in the foetus. Its half-life is longer in the infant than the adult and this reappearance of withdrawal, they argue, is consistent with a second abstinence syndrome due to another drug. The observations made in these two cases are consistent with the discussion of these issues by Finnegan (1980) and highlight the necessity of knowing the drug history of the woman concerned so that the appropriate pharmacological intervention can be used. As Kreek (1996) points out, an apparent neonatal methadone abstinence syndrome may be the result of the mother's use of alcohol or drugs other than methadone.

Treatment

It is important that all neonates at risk for withdrawal are assessed systematically with a scoring chart designed for this purpose (Batey *et al.*, 1990; Finnegan, 1983; see Finnegan, 1980 for such a chart). According to the instructions for the assessment instrument in use, once treatment is warranted (as indicated by a consistently high score above a certain level on a specified number of occasions), it should begin immediately. The treatment of choice is pharmacotherapy and the most commonly used drugs are paregoric and phenobarbitone (Finnegan 1983). Although once used, diazepam is no longer recommended (Finnegan, 1980; 1988). Two specialist programs treating pregnant women recommend either the use of phenobarbitone for all cases (Batey *et al.*, 1990), or an orally administered solution of morphine for opioid withdrawal and the use of phenobarbitone for benzodiazepine, barbiturate and alcohol withdrawal (Collins, 1992). Hoegerman *et al.* (1990) recommend methadone 1 mg to 2 mg twice daily. In the case of the opioid agonists, initial dosing is carried out to achieve prompt relief and then subsequently the dose is tapered slowly to achieve detoxification while causing as little distress as possible.

Finnegan (1980; Finnegan *et al.*, 1991) recommends involving mothers in the treatment of their babies' withdrawal to promote mother-infant attachment and to help the mother alleviate her guilt feelings and develop her self-efficacy. In cases of less severe withdrawal (abstinence syndrome scores less than critical level for pharmacological intervention), simple measures may be shown to the mother such as reducing stimuli, swaddling and the provision of a pacifier. In other cases where a course of pharmacotherapy is indicated, treatment on an outpatient basis is possible, with the mother administering the medication to her child (Collins, 1992). More generally, Finnegan *et al.* (1991) point out that teaching these women to care for their babies involves:

> ...educating the mother about her infant's needs and by teaching comforting techniques and how to interact with her infant in a positive, responsive manner. This intervention is essential because infants exposed to drugs *in utero* tend to be difficult to feed, have poor sucking reflex and are often irritable and difficult to console... Without intervention, mothers with limited care-giving skills and resources attempt to parent infants difficult to care for and who provide little positive reinforcement (p. 236).

It is not uncommon for hospital staff who lack experience with drug-dependent women to become angry when an infant experiences discomfort after birth as a result of the mother's drug use or treatment in the case of methadone maintenance. Methadone unit staff can function as a source of support and advocacy in these situations.

Methadone Maintenance and Breastfeeding

Breastfeeding is recommended for the infants of methadone-maintained women (Batey *et al.*, 1990; Finnegan, 1980; Kaltenbach *et al.*, 1993). According to Finnegan (1980), breastfeeding contributes to the development of mother-infant attachment, provides the infant with maternal antibodies, is nutritionally tailored to the infant and is thought by some to assist in reducing the severity of the neonatal abstinence syndrome because of the small amount of methadone that is contained in the milk (e.g., Hoegerman *et al.*, 1990; Mack *et al.*, 1991). However, Pond *et al.* (1985) found only very low levels of methadone in breast milk, even at high maintenance doses. They found that the highest dose an infant would receive via breast milk would be approximately 0.01 mg to 0.03 mg of methadone in a day. Doses this low would not be expected to have any clinical effects (Kreek, 1996). However, Finnegan (1980) suggests that this may change by three to six months of age due to the volume of milk consumed and therefore recommends that the infant should be weaned at this stage. Breastfeeding is, however, contraindicated in cases where the mother continues to use alcohol or other drugs at hazardous levels, because her breast milk would pass on these substances to her child (Kaltenbach *et al.,* 1993). Similarly, when women are HIV positive or are chronic carriers of hepatitis B, breastfeeding is contraindicated (Finnegan, 1991). The position with regard to hepatitis C remains unclear at the time of writing (MacDonald *et al.,* 1996). While no clear cases of transmission by breastfeeding have been reported, current draft National Health and Medical Research Council (1996) guidelines in Australia recommend breastfeeding for hepatitis C antibody women, unless they have a cracked or bleeding nipple, in which case milk from that breast should be expressed and discarded. However, in cases where the woman tests positive for the presence of hepatitis C RNA, more care may be warranted.

CONCLUSION

While for some methadone maintenance for pregnant women is a controversial intervention, the evidence clearly suggests that for many opioid-dependent women it is less harmful than continued heroin use or detoxification. Methadone programs for pregnant women have much in common with the usual methadone maintenance program and in this regard, unless otherwise indicated, the principles of patient management outlined in the rest of this book also apply.

Finnegan (1980, 1991) has consistently argued that methadone by itself is not a sufficient intervention for the dependent pregnant woman to successfully give birth. The evidence and clinical opinion cited in this chapter supports this proposition. It is the combination of methadone maintenance, specialised antenatal care, education and counselling that keeps these women in treatment and makes possible a maximum number of trouble-free births. Although apparently an expensive option, as Ellwood *et al.* (1987) have pointed out, when the substantial cost of neonatal intensive care for infants born to drug-dependent women not in treatment is taken into account, comprehensive methadone maintenance programs for this population begin to look not only effective as an intervention but cost-effective as well.

SUMMARY

Opioid-dependent pregnant women are a high-risk group. As pregnant women, they do not usually have access to the usual conditions for a successful pregnancy, namely adequate nutrition, rest or antenatal care. The daily use of illicit opioids (such as heroin) expose the woman and her foetus to dangerous fluctuations in blood heroin levels, a range of unknown drugs and contaminants, and a range of infections associated with injecting drug use, including hepatitis and HIV. Opioid-dependent women not in treatment usually give birth prematurely and their babies are small for their gestational age. These children suffer from a variety of complications due to their prematurity and until relatively recently many of them died soon after birth. Developments over the past few decades in the ability to care for neonates at risk has decreased the mortality rate among infants born to heroin-dependent mothers.

Methadone maintenance replaces an illicit drug of dependence of unknown quality and uncertain supply with a pure opioid that is administered under medical supervision. Providing a pregnant woman with a daily dose of methadone means that she and her foetus are no longer subject to the peaks and troughs of heroin blood levels, nor to an unknown range of contaminants, some of which may be teratogenic. Enrolment in a methadone maintenance program also allows the delivery of adequate antenatal care. Research evidence to date unconditionally supports comprehensive methadone maintenance programs for opioid-dependent pregnant women. When compared to such women out of treatment, women in methadone maintenance programs have longer pregnancies, have fewer complications at birth and have infants who are larger for their gestational age.

In order to minimise exposure to all drugs, the ideal treatment course for an opioid-dependent pregnant woman would be to initiate low dose methadone maintenance and then to withdraw her during the safest period for detoxification (14 to 32 weeks) so that she would be drug-free at birth. Few such women, however, can achieve total abstinence without relapse or obstetrical complications intervening. Therefore, the treatment of choice for most opioid-dependent women is methadone maintenance throughout their pregnancy. Similarly, although it has been argued that the maternal methadone dose should be kept as low as possible in the interests of preventing an unnecessary withdrawal in the neonate, the best clinical principle to follow is that what is in the best interest of the mother will, in the end, be best for the foetus. Therefore, issues concerning methadone dosing have to be viewed in the light of the risks posed by relapse and the obstetrical complications associated with withdrawal symptoms. Pregnancy may affect the metabolism of methadone, especially during the third trimester when lower than expected levels of methadone in blood plasma may be observed. Some women report the onset of unexpected withdrawal symptoms during this period that may need to be dealt with by splitting or increasing the daily methadone dose.

Group sessions for pregnant women in methadone maintenance are both feasible and desirable. Such groups may function as antenatal and parenting classes, as well as an opportunity to discuss issues of relevance, such as drug use and other specific concerns that opioid-dependent women may have. These groups are most successful when they are restricted to women only.

Antenatal care for women in methadone maintenance should be delivered in a non-judgmental fashion. Where possible, special clinic times specifically for methadone maintenance patients should be scheduled and operated by staff experienced in working with this population. Women on methadone maintenance should not be denied analgesia or anaesthesia during labour or birth. Opioids should be avoided during labour but are indicated after the woman has given birth. In such cases, the adult analgesic dose should be administered in addition to the usual daily methadone.

Many infants born to methadone-maintained women will exhibit an abstinence syndrome, usually within 72 hours of being born. The severity of the neonatal abstinence syndrome should be assessed using an instrument designed for this purpose. The syndrome responds well to paregoric, morphine, methadone or phenobarbitone. Breastfeeding is not contraindicated for women on methadone maintenance. The amount of methadone present in breast milk is minute and unlikely to harm an infant in the first six months of life. Breast milk provides the infant with maternal antibodies and breastfeeding encourages mother-infant attachment.

REFERENCES

Batey, R. G., Patterson, T., & Sanders, F. (1990). Practical issues in the methadone management of pregnant heroin users. *Drug and Alcohol Review,* **9,** 303-310.

Chavkin, W. (1990). Drug addiction and pregnancy: Policy crossroads. *American Journal of Public Health,* **80,** 483-487.

Collins, E. (1990). Outcomes for the children of mothers who used heroin/ methadone during pregnancy. Paper presented to National Methadone Conference, Sydney, Australia.

Collins, E. (1992). Pregnancy. Paper presented to 1992 National Methadone Conference, Sydney, Australia.

Collins, E., & Capus, C. (1991). Human immunodeficiency virus (HIV) & hepatitis status of pregnant drug dependent women. Paper presented at 9th Australian Perinatal Society Annual Congress, Melbourne, Australia.

Deren, S. (1986). Children of substance abusers: A review of the literature. *Journal of Substance Abuse Treatment,* **3,** 77-94.

Doberczak, T. M., Kandall, S. R., & Friedmann, P. (1993). Relationships between maternal methadone dosage, maternal-neonatal methadone levels, and neonatal withdrawal. *Obstetrics & Gynecology,* **81,** 936-940.

Doberczak, T. M., Thornton, J. C., Bernstein, J., & Kandall, S. R. (1987). Impact of maternal drug dependency on birth weight and head circumference of offspring. *American Journal of Diseases of Children,* **141,** 1163-1167.

Ellwood, D. A., Sutherland, P., Kent, C., & O'Connor, M. (1987). Maternal narcotic addiction: Pregnancy outcome in patients managed by a specialized drug-dependency antenatal clinic. *Australian and New Zealand Journal of Obstetrics and Gynaecology,* **27,** 92-98.

Finnegan, L. P. (Ed.). (1980). *Drug dependence in pregnancy: Clinical management of mother and child.* London: Castle House.

Finnegan, L. P. (1983). Clinical perinatal and development effects of methadone. In J. R. Cooper, F. Altman, B. S. Brown, & D. Czechowicz (Eds.), *Research on the treatment of narcotic addiction: State of the art* (pp. 392-443). Rockville, MD: National Institute on Drug Abuse.

Finnegan, L. P. (1988). *Drug addiction and pregnancy: The newborn drugs, alcohol, pregnancy and parenting.* London: Kluwer.

Finnegan, L. P. (1991). Treatment issues for opioid-dependent women during the perinatal period. *Journal of Psychoactive Drugs,* **23,** 191-201.

Finnegan, L. P., Hagan, T., & Kaltenbach, K. A. (1991). Scientific foundation of clinical practice: Opiate use in pregnant women. *Bulletin of the New York Academy of Medicine,* **67,** 223-239.

Gastel, B., & Collins, T. E. (1983). Discussion summary [of L.P. Finnegan, Clinical perinatal and development effects of methadone.]. In J. R. Cooper, F. Altman, B. S. Brown, & D. Czechowicz (Eds.), *Research on the treatment of narcotic addiction: State of the art* (p. 454-455). Rockville, MD: National Institute on Drug Abuse.

Gerada, C., Dawe, S., & Farrell, M. (1990). Management of the pregnant opiate user. *British Journal of Hospital Medicine,* **43,** 138-141.

Giles, W., Patterson, T., Sanders, F., Batey, R., Thomas, D., & Collins, J.

(1989). Outpatient methadone programme for pregnant heroin using women. *Australian and New Zealand Journal of Obstetrics and Gynaecology, 29*, 225-229.

Hoegerman, G., Wilson, C. A., Thurmond, E., & Schnoll, S. H. (1990). Drug-exposed neonates. *Western Journal of Medicine, 152*, 559-564.

Holmes, J. (1989). Women, narcotics, pregnancy. Paper presented at The Women, Alcohol and Other Drugs Conference, Adelaide, Australia.

Householder, J., Hatcher, R., Burns, W., & Chasnoff, I. (1982). Infants born to narcotic-addicted mothers. *Psychological Bulletin, 92*, 453-468.

Jarvis, M. A. E., & Schnoll, S. H. (1994). Methadone treatment during pregnancy. *Journal of Psychoactive Drugs, 26*, 155-161.

Jessup, M. (1990). The treatment of perinatal addiction: Identification, intervention, and advocacy. *Western Journal of Medicine, 152*, 553-558.

Kaltenbach, K., & Finnegan, L. P. (1989). Children exposed to methadone in utero: Assessment of developmental and cognitive ability. *Annals of the New York Academy of Sciences, 562*, 360-362.

Kaltenbach, K., Silverman, N., & Wapner, R. (1993). Methadone maintenance during pregnancy. In M. W. Parrino (Ed.), *State methadone treatment guidelines* (pp. 85-93). Rockville, MD: Center for Substance Abuse Treatment, U.S. Department of Health and Human Services.

Kaltenbach, K. A. (1994). Effects of in-utero opiate exposure: New paradigms for old questions. *Drug and Alcohol Dependence, 36*, 83-87.

Kreek, M. J. (1983a). Critique [of L.P. Finnegan, Clinical perinatal and development effects of methadone.]. In J. R. Cooper, F. Altman, B. S. Brown, & D. Czechowicz (Eds.), *Research on the treatment of narcotic addiction: State of the art* (444-453). Rockville, MD: National Institute on Drug Abuse.

Kreek, M. J. (1983b). Factors modifying the pharmacological effectiveness of methadone. In J. R. Cooper, F. Altman, B. S. Brown, & D. Czechowicz (Eds.), *Research on the treatment of narcotic addiction: State of the art* (pp. 95-114). Rockville, MD: National Institute on Drug Abuse.

Kreek, M. J. (1996). Long-term pharmacotherapy for opiate (primarily heroin) addiction: Opioid agonists. In C. R. Schuster & M. J. Kuhar (Eds.), *Pharmacological aspects of drug dependence: Toward an integrated neurobehavioral approach* (pp. 487-562). Berlin: Springer.

Lifschitz, M. H., Wilson, G. S., Smith, E. O., & Desmond, M. M. (1985). Factors affecting head growth and intellectual function in children of drug addicts. *Pediatrics, 75*, 269-274.

MacDonald, M., Crofts, N., & Kaldor, J. (1996). Transmission of HCV: Rates, routes and cofactors. Unpublished manuscript, National Centre in HIV Epidemiology and Clinical Research, University of New South Wales, Australia.

Mack, G., Thomas, D., Giles, W., & Buchanan, N. (1991). Methadone levels and neonatal withdrawal. *Journal of Paediatrics and Child Health,*

27, 96-100.

Mackie-Ramos, R.-L., & Rice, J.-M. (1988). Group psychotherapy with methadone-maintained pregnant women. *Journal of Substance Abuse Treatment,* 5, 151-161.

Malpas, T. J., Darlow, B. A., Lennox, R., & Horwood, L. J. (1995). Maternal methadone dosage and neonatal withdrawal. *Australian and New Zealand Journal of Obstetrics and Gynaecology,* 35, 175-177.

National Health and Medical Research Council. (1996). *Draft report on a strategy for the detection and management of hepatitis C in Australia.* Canberra, Australia: National Health and Medical Research Council.

Pond, S. M., Kreek, M. J., Tong, T. G., Raghunath, J., & Benowitz, N. L. (1985). Altered methadone pharmacokinetics in methadone-maintained pregnant women. *Journal of Pharmacology and Experimental Therapeutics,* 233, 1-6.

Soepatmi, S. (1994). Developmental outcomes of children of mothers dependent on heroin or heroin/methadone during pregnancy. *Acta Paediatrica Supplement,* 404, 36-39.

Suffet, F., & Brotman, R. (1984). A comprehensive care program for pregnant addicts: Obstetrical, neonatal, and child development outcomes. *International Journal of the Addictions,* 19, 199-219.

Sutton, L. R., & Hinderliter, S. A. (1990). Diazepam abuse in pregnant women on methadone maintenance: Implications for the neonate. *Clinical Pediatrics,* 29, 108-111.

Thakur, N., Kaltenbach, K., Peacock, J., Weiner, S., & Finnegan, L. (1990). The relationship between maternal methadone dose during pregnancy and infant outcome. *Pediatric Research,* 27, 227a.

Waldby, C. (1988). *Mothering and addiction: Women with children in methadone programs.* National Campaign Against Drug Abuse Monograph Series 4. Canberra, Australia: Australian Government Publishing Service.

Wilson, G. S. (1989). Clinical studies of infants and children exposed prenatally to heroin. *Annals of the New York Academy of Sciences,* 562, 183-194.

Wittmann, B. K., & Segal, S. (1991). A comparison of the effects of single- and split-dose methadone administration on the fetus: Ultrasound evaluation. *International Journal of the Addictions,* 26, 213-218.

17

PSYCHIATRIC COMORBIDITY AMONG THE OPIOID DEPENDENT

JEFF WARD, RICHARD P. MATTICK
AND WAYNE HALL

INTRODUCTION

Opioid abuse/dependence is classified as a psychiatric disorder by the two major diagnostic systems employed within psychiatry, the ICD-10 (WHO, 1992) and the DSM-IV (American Psychiatric Association, 1994). Accepting that this is the case, in this chapter we review the literature on the prevalence of psychiatric disorders among opioid users and refer to these as comorbid conditions in the restricted sense that these disorders co-occur with opioid abuse/dependence. As one of us has observed elsewhere, in accepting the classification of opioid abuse/dependence as a psychiatric disorder, we make no substantive assumption about the status of opioid use as a "psychiatric" or "mental" disorder (Hall, 1996).

As will be seen below, it has been a consistent finding from studies of the prevalence of psychiatric disorders among opioid users that the rates of a number of these disorders are higher than their estimated occurrence in the general population. The disorders that are more common are the depressive disorders, the anxiety disorders, personality disorders, and alcohol abuse/dependence. In the sections that follow, we first briefly review what population surveys have revealed about the prevalence of psychiatric disorders in the general population, and we then discuss in detail those disorders which are most common among opioid users and the implications of their occurrence for patient management. We then examine the variation of the rates of these disorders according to gender. In the final section, we explore what the likely nature of the relationship between opioid dependence and psychiatric comorbidity might be in the light of the few studies which have attempted to examine this issue.

POPULATION SURVEYS

In this section we briefly review the results of two large population surveys of psychiatric disorders conducted in the USA, the Epidemiologic Catchment Area (ECA) study (Robins & Regier, 1991) and the National Comorbidity Survey (NCS) (Kessler *et al.*, 1994; see Hall, 1996 for a fuller discussion of the relevance of these studies). For the purposes of the present discussion, these studies are important because they provide estimates of the prevalence of specific psychiatric disorders for the general US population which can be used as base rates with which to compare prevalence data for samples of in- and out-of-treatment opioid-dependent individuals (Regier *et al.*, 1990). Without estimates for the general population, it is difficult to assess just how elevated the apparently high rates of psychiatric disorders among opioid users are. The fact that much of the research on opioid users that will be discussed in this chapter has been carried out in the USA makes the findings of the ECA and the NCS especially useful for this purpose.

Table 17.1 summarises the ECA and NCS estimates of the lifetime prevalence of psychiatric disorders that are common among opioid users, along with the results of similar surveys of in- and out-of-treatment samples of the opioid using population. As can be seen from Table 17.1, in the general population the lifetime prevalence for any psychiatric disorder was estimated to be 32% in the ECA and 48% in the NCS. The major reasons for the discrepancy in the proportion afflicted have been attributed to: the fact that the NCS sample was younger, and hence contained more people with mental disorders that generally commence in early adult life; the NCS estimates were corrected for non-response which increased overall rates; and a number of differences in the criteria used to assess phobias and depressive disorders in the NCS which were likely to increase the rate of reporting (Hall, 1996). The latter point is borne out by the discrepancy of approximately 10% in the estimates of anxiety and depressive disorders, with the ECA and NCS estimates for these two classes of disorders being 6% versus 17% and 15% versus 25% respectively (Kessler *et al.*, 1994; Regier *et al.*, 1990). A similar discrepancy was observed for any alcohol use disorder with an estimate of 14% in the ECA study and 24% in the NCS study. The estimates for antisocial personality disorder (ASPD) were similar in the two studies (3% versus 4%).

Both the ECA and the NCS studies screened their respective samples for opioid use disorders. In the ECA study, 0.7% of the study participants were diagnosed with an opioid use disorder (Regier *et al.*, 1990). When compared with members of the sample not diagnosed with an opioid use disorder, the odds of opioid users being diagnosed with another psychiatric disorder were estimated to be seven times more likely (odds ratio = 6.7; Regier *et al.*, 1990). When relationships between specific disorders were examined, opioid users were found to be nine times more likely to be diagnosed with schizophrenia (odds ratio = 8.8), although when Table 17.1 is examined this elevated rate of schizophrenia, although compatible with rates found in Dutch studies of opioid users (Hendriks, 1990; Limbeek *et al.*, 1992), is not consistent with other US studies which have specifically sampled opioid users (Khantzian & Treece, 1985; Rounsaville *et al.*, 1982a; Strain *et al.*, 1991a). Opioid users also had elevated rates for affective disorders (odds ratio = 5.0), anxiety disorders (odds ratio = 2.8), ASPD (odds ratio = 24.3), and alcohol use disorders (odds ratio = 12.8). Unlike schizophrenia, these latter findings of substantial comorbidity between opioid use and the other major categories of psychiatric disorders have been confirmed in studies that have specifically sampled opioid users. In the next section, we examine the findings of these studies in detail.

SURVEYS OF OPIOID USERS

As well as setting out the findings of the ECA and NCS studies, Table 17.1 sets out the results of surveys that have been conducted of psychiatric disorders among opioid users. In interpreting the findings of these surveys, a number of factors have to be kept in mind to ensure that the derived estimates are placed within the correct context. First of all, when comparing the estimates of these surveys with population surveys such as the ECA and the NCS, it has to be recognised that

Table 17.1

Estimates of the lifetime prevalence of psychiatric disorders among opioid users and the general population

Authors	Sample and country of origin (n)	Diagnostic criteria	Any non-substance abuse psychiatric diagnosis %	Schizo-phrenia %	Major depressive disorder %	Anxiety disorder %	Alcohol dependence %	Antisocial personality disorder
Rounsaville et al. (1982a)	Opioid users in treatment - USA (533)	RDC	87[a]	1	54	16	35	27
Khantzian & Treece (1985)	Opioid users in and out of treatment - USA (133)	DSM-III	93[a]	0	56	11	14	35
Woody et al. (1985)	Methadone patients - USA (110)	DSM-III	-	-	35	20	19	45
Hendriks (1990)	Opioid and cocaine users seeking treatment - The Netherlands (152)	DSM-III	83	4	37	41	52	60
Regier et al. (1990)	Opioid users in community - USA (142)	DSM-III	65[b]	11	31[c]	32	66[d]	37
Strain et al. (1991a)	Methadone patients - USA (66)	DSM-III-R	47	0	20	2	26	30
Limbeek et al. (1992)	Opioid addicts seeking treatment - The Netherlands (203)	DSM-III	70	5	23	38	63[d]	59
Mattick et al. (1993b)	Methadone patients - Australia (271)	DSM-III-R	-	2	30	>40%	-	42
Milby et al. (1996)	Current and discharged methadone-maintained war veterans (102)	DSM-III-R	-	12	32	55	-	-
Regier et al. (1990) & Robins & Regier (1991)	General population sample - USA (20,291)	DSM-III	32[b]	1	6	15	8 (Males = 14)	3 (Males = 5)
Kessler et al. (1994)	General population sample - USA (8,098)	DSM-III-R	48[b]	1	17	25	14 (Males = 20)	4 (Males = 6)

Notes. RDC = Research Diagnostic Criteria. [a]Includes personality disorders other than antisocial personality disorder. [b]Includes alcohol and substance use disorders. [c]Includes any affective disorder. [d]Includes alcohol abuse as well as dependence.

opioid users are more likely to be male and are more likely to fall within the 20 to 40 age category (Anthony & Helzer, 1995). Therefore estimates of comorbid relationships between opioid use and other disorders will be affected if the distribution of the comorbid disorder varies by sex and age.

A second major issue for interpreting these surveys is whether the study participants were sampled from treatment settings or not. Opioid users in treatment have been found to have elevated rates of psychiatric disorders in comparison to those who do not seek treatment (Rounsaville & Kleber, 1985), and this reflects the broader tendency found in the ECA study for individuals diagnosed with a drug (other than alcohol) use disorder who were in treatment to have significantly higher rates of other psychiatric disorders than those who were not in treatment (Regier *et al.*, 1990). While this reflects the increased likelihood of a disorder being detected because the individual concerned can seek treatment for either of them (the phenomenon known as Berkson's bias) it also reflects, at least in the case of drug use, an extra motivating factor in influencing the decision whether to seek treatment or not (Galbaud du Fort *et al.*, 1993). This is borne out by the findings of Rounsaville and Kleber (1985) who reported that in their comparison of opioid users in and out of treatment, they found differences in rates of depression, legal difficulties and poorer social functioning but not in estimates of drug consumption. This suggests that it is not heavy drug use alone that motivates opioid users to seek out treatment but personal difficulties, such as depression and legal and social problems. Although this implies that estimates of the prevalence of psychiatric disorders among treatment samples are likely to be overestimates of the true rate of these disorders among all opioid users, it is irrelevant for the present discussion because we are interested in the rates of these disorders among clinical populations.

A number of other factors are also likely to influence the rates of some disorders. The diagnostic system used, as we have seen for the rates derived for the ECA and the NCS studies, may influence the rates (Anthony & Helzer, 1995; Weiss *et al.*, 1992b). As we shall see below for depressive disorders, it is also important, when assessing surveys of methadone patients, to take into account when the patients were interviewed (Weiss *et al.*, 1992b). Most opioid users present for treatment in a distressed state, often exhibiting symptoms of anxiety and depression that may resolve within a couple of weeks of commencing treatment.

It is not surprising when we look at the rates in Table 17.1 that there is considerable variation in some of the estimates. However, the general pattern of the results is clear and suggests elevated rates for depression, alcoholism and antisocial personality disorder. The anxiety disorders present a more mixed picture. These findings of elevated rates of psychiatric morbidity are supported by a number of studies that have found clinically significant psychological morbidity as assessed by the General Health Questionnaire among approximately 60% of patients attending for methadone treatment (Darke *et al.*, 1994b; Darke *et al.*, 1992; Hartgers *et al.*, 1992; Swift *et al.*, 1990). The specific findings and implications for treatment for each of the major categories of disorders are discussed in separate sections below. While each of the disorders is discussed as a separate entity, it should be remembered that among both the general population (Hall, 1996) and samples of opioid users (Hendriks, 1990; Limbeek *et al.*, 1992; Milby *et al.*, 1996), comorbidity is common whether or not a substance use disorder is present. This is especially true of anxiety and depressive disorders where the likelihood of being diagnosed with one is considerably enhanced if the other is also present (Kessler, 1995a).

Depressive Disorders

By far the most common and consistently reported example of elevated psychiatric comorbidity among opioid users is depression (see Table 17.1). As already noted, the ECA study found that people diagnosed with an opioid use disorder were five times more likely to have had a depressive disorder than those not so diagnosed (Regier *et al.*, 1990). However, when the rates for ever having experienced a major depressive disorder as listed in Table 17.1 are examined, a considerable range is revealed for opioid users, ranging from as low as 20% to those as high as 56%. This suggests that up to one-half of patients in opioid replacement therapy may have suffered a major depressive episode at some time in their lives.

Consistent with what is known about other populations, opioid users in treatment are more likely to be diagnosed with depression than their counterparts who have not sought treatment (Lipsitz *et al.*, 1994; Rounsaville & Kleber, 1985). Depression is more commonly diagnosed among female methadone patients (Croughan *et al.*, 1982; Lipsitz *et al.*, 1994; Rounsaville *et al.*, 1982a; Strain *et al.*, 1991a), as is true of the general population (Hall, 1996). A diagnosis of depression has been found to predict poorer psychosocial functioning and to increase the risk of relapse to heroin use in the event of life crises among methadone maintenance patients (Rounsaville *et al.,* 1986), suggesting that such patients might warrant special attention.

The relationship between having a depressive disorder and being in methadone maintenance treatment has to be considered along with studies that have found a decline in the incidence of depression over time in samples of methadone maintenance patients assessed at entry to treatment and periodically thereafter (Dorus & Senay, 1980; Magruder-Habib *et al.,* 1992; Steer & Kotzker, 1980; Strain *et al.,* 1991b). This is also true for other substance dependence problems (Bryant *et al.,* 1992) and for alcohol dependence (Mattick *et al.,* 1993a). As has already been noted, it is well known that some form of crisis often precipitates a decision to seek out treatment, and it may be the case that studies that assess patients on entry to treatment may overestimate the relationship between being in treatment and being depressed. The stabilisation that being in methadone maintenance brings to a person's life may be enough in many cases to eliminate depressive disorders that are reactions to stressful situations associated with a heroin-using lifestyle (e.g., housing, legal, relationship problems). Patients who remain depressed after stabilisation on methadone may need specialist treatment.

Anxiety Disorders

In the DSM classification system the class known as the anxiety disorders consists of panic disorder, phobic disorders, obsessive-compulsive disorder, generalised anxiety disorder and post-traumatic stress disorder (American Psychiatric Association, 1994). As can be seen from Table 17.1, the rates for anxiety disorders taken as a class appear not to be elevated in all but one of the samples of opioid users from the US when compared with the general population estimates from the ECA and the NCS studies. The exception to this observation is to be found in the sample reported on by Milby *et al.* (1996) which consisted exclusively of war veterans who suffered from very high rates of post-traumatic stress disorder. Other than the Milby *et al.* study, four studies included in Table 17.1 have reported elevated rates for anxiety disorders: the ECA study (Regier *et al.,* 1990); two studies carried out in The Netherlands (Hendriks, 1990; Limbeek *et al.,* 1992); and one study carried out in Australia (Mattick *et al.,* 1993b).

An examination of the findings of the studies included in Table 17.1 for each of the anxiety disorders surveyed shows that some disorders are consistently elevated. For example, four studies found elevated rates for panic disorder (Hendriks, 1990; Limbeek *et al.*, 1992; Mattick *et al.*, 1993b; Milby *et al.*, 1996), three found the same for social phobia (Hendriks, 1990; Mattick *et al.*, 1993b; Milby *et al.*, 1996), and four the same for generalised anxiety disorder (Mattick *et al.*, 1993b; Milby *et al.*, 1996; Rounsaville *et al.*, 1982a; Woody *et al.*, 1985). Similarly, two studies found elevated rates for agoraphobia (Hendriks, 1990; Milby *et al.*, 1996), two found phobias in general to be elevated (Limbeek *et al.*, 1992; Rounsaville *et al.*, 1982a) and one study found an excess of obsessive-compulsive disorder (Limbeek *et al.*, 1992). These findings suggest that anxiety disorders may be elevated in clinical populations in Australia (Mattick *et al.*, 1993b), The Netherlands (Hendriks, 1990; Limbeek *et al.*, 1992), and for some disorders (generalised anxiety disorders, phobias) in the USA (Milby *et al.*, 1996; Rounsaville *et al.*, 1982a; Woody *et al.*, 1985).

Two studies have also suggested that post-traumatic stress disorder may be more common among opioid users, although, as already mentioned, one of them, the study by Milby and colleagues (1996), was carried out in a methadone clinic for war veterans who would be expected to have a higher rate of post-traumatic stress disorder. The other study (Cottler *et al.*, 1992), which was an analysis of a subset of the ECA data for cocaine and opioid users combined, found that in comparison to participants who were not drug users, cocaine/opioid users were more likely to have been exposed to a traumatic event (43% versus 13% of controls), that this was most often a physical attack, and that they were more likely to be diagnosed with post-traumatic stress disorder than people who did not use cocaine or opioids (8% versus 0.3%). These findings support the hypothesis that illicit opioid and cocaine use increases the risk of exposure to traumatic events, particularly physical attack, and to the subsequent development of post-traumatic stress disorder.

Alcohol Use Disorders

Alcohol abuse and dependence has consistently been shown in population surveys to be one of the most common psychiatric diagnoses along with phobias and major depression (Hall, 1996). Another consistent finding of these surveys is that males are more likely to be diagnosed with alcohol abuse and/or dependence than are females. While the rates of alcohol dependence for the general population were estimated to be 8% in the ECA and 14% in the NCS studies overall, the rates for males were 14% and 20% respectively. Even taking the rate for males in order to adjust for the excess of males in the samples of opioid users, it is clear from the table that in the majority of studies there are very high rates of alcohol dependence. This is consistent with opioid users being estimated to be 13 times more likely to also be diagnosed with an alcohol use disorder in the ECA sample (Regier *et al.*, 1990). The significance of these high rates of alcoholism among opioid users has been highlighted by studies that have shown alcohol abuse and dependence to be significant predictors of mortality in both in- and out-of-treatment samples (Mattick & Hall, 1993).

Antisocial Personality Disorder

According to Robins *et al.* (Robins *et al.*, 1991):

> Antisocial personality is a disorder that begins in childhood with a variety of behavior problems at home and in school and continues into adult life with failure to conform to social norms in many areas including work, family, and other interpersonal relationships. Persons with the disorder tend to be aggressive and impulsive and are thought to lack normal capacities for love, guilt, and cooperation with authority figures. Many of them come into conflict with the legal system (p. 258).

The ECA population estimate for the lifetime prevalence of ASPD is 2.6% (Regier *et al.*, 1990), which is similar to the more recent NCS estimate of 3.5% (Kessler *et al.*, 1994). In both the ECA and NCS studies, men (4.5% and 5.8%) were far more likely than women (0.8% and 1.2%) to have had this disorder at some time in their lives. As already noted above, in the ECA study, individuals diagnosed with an opioid use disorder were found to be 24 times more likely to be diagnosed with ASPD than their non-opioid using counterparts (Regier *et al.*, 1990). These differences between men and women and the high rates for opioid users have been consistently found in studies of drug users.

As can be seen from Table 17.1, consistently high rates of ASPD have been found in opioid-dependent samples. Other studies have found rates as high as 55% (e.g., (Kosten *et al.*, 1982), suggesting that there may be some variability in the application of diagnostic criteria.

Rounsaville *et al.* (1982a) demonstrated that this was the case when they diagnosed ASPD using two different sets of criteria and found a marked difference in rate. When DSM-III criteria were used, 54% of the sample was diagnosed with ASPD, but when the Research Diagnostic Criteria were used only 27% were so diagnosed. Two main reasons have been suggested for this difference. The first is that the DSM-III criteria (and this is also true of the DSM-III-R and the DSM-IV) include many items that describe the typical dependent heroin user's lifestyle (theft, unemployment, defaulting on debts, recklessness, irresponsibility) which may, in many cases, be a function of opioid dependence rather than any underlying personality disorder (American Psychiatric Association, 1987; American Psychiatric Association, 1994). However, the necessity for there to be evidence of a conduct disorder with onset before the age of 15 should, to some extent, obviate this confusion. As Weiss *et al.* (1992b) point out, according to the Research Diagnostic Criteria, a diagnosis of ASPD is not made if some of the symptoms are clearly attributable to the substance abuse itself.

A second criticism that has been made of the DSM criteria is that they focus on overt behaviour and do not include enough items that have been traditionally labelled psychopathic traits, such as the inability to experience love and guilt (Gerstley *et al.*, 1990). It should also be noted that there is a much larger debate about the usefulness of the diagnosis, and whether it is justifiable to infer that there is an underlying psychiatric disorder from criminal, deviant and antisocial behaviour. This debate has waxed and waned since the first use of diagnostic labels such as 'psychopath' and 'sociopath' which began early this century (Blackburn, 1988; Courtwright, 1982; Robins *et al.*, 1991).

Despite the controversy surrounding the diagnosis, there has been considerable research interest in recent years in ASPD and its correlates. As Darke notes in Chapter 4 of this volume, ASPD is associated with increased HIV risk-taking behaviour and consequently with high rates of HIV infection among opioid users (Brooner *et al.*, 1990; Brooner *et al.*, 1993a). While Hesselbrock *et al.* (1992) suggest that a diagnosis of ASPD might result in an earlier onset of dependence and poor response to treatment as it does with alcoholics, the evidence in both regards is less than clear. For example, in the NCS study the likelihood of progressing from a conduct disorder in childhood to ASPD is more likely in the presence of a substance use disorder than any other diagnosis (Kessler, 1995b). Although methadone patients with a diagnosis of ASPD appear not to respond to psychotherapy unless they are also depressed (Woody *et al.*, 1985), they appear to respond to methadone treatment as well as other patients (Darke *et al.*, 1994a; Gill *et al.*, 1992; Rousar *et al.*, 1994; Rutherford *et al.*, 1994). As Darke has suggested in Chapter 4, this research suggests that the diagnosis of ASPD is perhaps best seen simply as an indicator of an individual who is more at risk than others.

Other Personality Disorders

As well as ASPD, the DSM-IV lists ten other personality disorders: paranoid, schizoid, shizotypal, borderline, histrionic, narcissistic, avoidant, dependent, obsessive-compulsive and personality disorder not otherwise specified (see American Psychiatric Association, 1994 for a full description of these disorders). According to the DSM-IV, a personality disorder is described as follows:

> Personality traits are enduring patterns of perceiving, relating to, and thinking about the environment and oneself that are exhibited in a wide range of social and personal contexts. Only when personality traits are inflexible and maladaptive and cause significant functional impairment or subjective distress do they constitute Personality Disorders. The essential feature of a Personality Disorder is an enduring pattern of inner experience and behavior that deviates markedly from the expectations of the individual's culture and is manifested in at least two of the following areas: cognition, affectivity, interpersonal functioning, or impulse control. (p. 630)

Additionally, this pattern of experience and behaviour must have developed in adolescence or early adulthood, must persist across a variety of situations and circumstances and cannot be accounted for by another mental disorder, physiological condition or the use of drugs.

A number of studies have found very high rates of personality disorders other than ASPD among opioid users and methadone patients in comparison to those found in the general population. Estimates for the prevalence of personality disorders among the general population are based on a limited number of studies but suggest that around 10% of the population meet criteria for these disorders (including ASPD; Lyons, 1995). By way of contrast, of the six surveys of methadone patients, four have found a prevalence of any personality disorder (including ASPD) to be approximately 65% (range 63-73%; Khantzian & Treece, 1985; Kosten *et al.,* 1982; Musselman & Kell, 1995; Rutherford *et al.,* 1994), while the two remaining studies have found prevalences of 37% (Brooner *et al.,* 1993b) and 40% (Rousar *et al.,* 1994). An examination of the four surveys of methadone patients which allow separation of ASPD from other personality disorders reveals a prevalence of personality disorders other than antisocial of approximately 30% (range 28-32%) in three studies (Khantzian & Treece, 1985; Kosten *et al.,* 1982; Rutherford *et al.,* 1994) and of 15% in another study (Rousar *et al.,* 1994).

The most common distinct personality disorder after ASPD is borderline personality disorder, with an estimated prevalence of between 8% and 12% in four studies (Brooner *et al.,* 1993b; Kosten *et al.,* 1982; Rousar *et al.,* 1994; Rutherford *et al.,* 1994), although Khantzian and Treece (1985) found only 4% of their sample met criteria for this disorder. This represents an elevated rate for a majority of studies in comparison to the general population estimate of 3% (Lyons, 1995). This result was confirmed using a slightly different diagnostic system by Musselman & Kell (1995) who compared rates for this and other disorders for a sample of methadone patients to the published norms for the general population on the Millon Clinical Multiaxial Inventory. However, these elevated rates as seen in methadone patients are typical for clinical samples (e.g., psychiatric, primary health care) because aspects of the disorder increase the likelihood of seeking help when compared to other personality disorders. People with borderline personality disorder are characterised by "a pervasive pattern of instability of interpersonal relationships, self-image, and affects, and marked impulsivity that begins by early adulthood and is present in a variety of contexts." (American Psychiatric Association, 1994, p. 650). Other features of the disorder are frantic efforts to avoid abandonment, recurrent suicidal behaviour, inappropriate outbursts of anger and, at times, paranoid ideation in response to stress.

While personality disorders other than antisocial may be common among methadone maintenance patient populations, this is also true of other clinical settings. Furthermore, although the outcomes of treatments for other psychiatric disorders (e.g., depressive and anxiety disorders) is negatively affected by the presence of a comorbid personality disorder (Reich & Green, 1991), this does not appear to be true for the typical outcomes of methadone treatment in the two studies that have examined this issue (Cacciola *et al.,* 1996; Kosten *et al.,* 1989). However, individuals who meet the criteria for borderline personality disorder are more depressed and more likely to be alcoholic than their peers, suggesting that this particular group may be more at risk (Cacciola *et al.,* 1996; Kosten *et al.,* 1989).

Overall, the most important implication of the high rates of both antisocial and other personality disorders among methadone patients is that it makes the day-to-day task of managing these patients difficult and thought should be given to ensuring that the clinic is a safe, therapeutic environment for the practice of treatment to take place (see Chapter 7). However, because of difficulties in the assessment of personality disorders (Lyons, 1995; Perry, 1992) and the limited options for treating them (Quality Assurance Project, 1991a; Quality Assurance Project, 1991b), it is not recommended at this time that staff in methadone clinics be overly concerned about formally diagnosing these conditions.

SEX DIFFERENCES IN RATES OF PSYCHIATRIC DISORDERS

Both the ECA and the NCS studies found similar patterns in the distribution of psychiatric disorders across the two sexes. There was a male excess for substance use disorders and ASPD and a female excess in depressive and anxiety disorders (Hall, 1996). However, while both studies found an equal prevalence rate for any psychiatric disorder in the past year for women and men (20% for both sexes in the ECA and 31% versus 28% in the NCS), there was an excess of lifetime prevalence among men (36%) compared with women (30%) in the ECA study which was not as apparent in the NCS (47% for women versus 49% for men – Kessler *et al.,* 1994; Robins & Regier, 1991). When investigated, it was found that the main reason for the excess of lifetime psychiatric disorder among men in the ECA study was that men made up such a large proportion of alcohol disorder diagnoses.

The differences between men and women in the general population are mirrored in the findings of studies carried out with opioid-dependent populations. Women have been found to suffer from more anxiety disorders (Rounsaville *et al.,* 1982a) and more depressive disorders than men (Calsyn *et al.,* 1996; Croughan *et al.,* 1982; Khantzian & Treece, 1985; Magruder-Habib *et al.,* 1992; Rounsaville *et al.,* 1982a; Strain *et al.,* 1991a), whereas men tend to be more likely to be diagnosed with ASPD (Croughan *et al.,* 1982; Khantzian & Treece, 1985; Rounsaville *et al.,* 1982a) and alcohol use disorders (Rounsaville *et al.,* 1982). These data are consistent with the findings of surveys using the General Health Questionnaire (Darke *et al.,* 1994b; Darke *et al.,* 1992; Hartgers *et al.,* 1992; Swift *et al.,* 1990) which have found that women have significantly higher levels on this global measure of psychopathology than men. These findings suggest that male and female methadone patients present with different patterns of comorbid psychiatric disorders.

RELATIONSHIP BETWEEN OPIOID DEPENDENCE AND OTHER PSYCHIATRIC DISORDERS

In the previous sections, we have seen that there is a high level of psychiatric comorbidity associated with a diagnosis of opioid dependence. In this section, we consider in what way opioid dependence and these comorbid disorders might be related to each other. Meyer (1986) describes a number of possibilities. Certain conditions (e.g., ASPD or depression): (a) may lead to drug dependence; (b) may facilitate its onset and course; (c) may arise as a result of drug dependence; (d) may simply be associated with drug dependence (both being caused by some other factor); or (e) the two disorders may simply occur together by chance and may not be related in any meaningful way at all. The evidence reviewed above suggests that opioid dependence often occurs together with other psychiatric disorders and the example of depression will be used to illustrate each of options outlined by Meyer (1986). For example, depression: (a) may lead to opioid use as an attempt at self-medication; (b) may lead to a more severe dependence than is seen in non-depressed individuals; (c) may arise as a result of being opioid dependent and the lifestyle associated with it; (d) may be the result of factors common to the genesis of both opioid dependence and depression (e.g., poverty, lack of social support, and chronic unemployment); or (e) may be the result of a neurochemical imbalance that has nothing to do with opioid dependence and is only more common among a given sample of opioid users as a result of chance.

The most important distinction, in terms of treatment options, is whether a given psychiatric disorder is an antecedent or consequence of opioid dependence. Taking depression again as an example, it is sometimes argued that depression is a consequence of the stressors associated with an opioid dependent lifestyle. If this is the case then the successful treatment of the dependence should, in time, lead to the resolution of the symptoms of depression. The evidence described above concerning the relationship between time in methadone maintenance and a decline in depressive symptoms supports this argument for some patients. However, it does not necessarily follow that depression which develops as a consequence of an opioid-dependent lifestyle will remit simply as a result of methadone treatment. Depressive disorders that arise as a result of stressful life events may develop a dynamic of their own and become chronic without treatment. According to the opposite viewpoint – that drug dependence is a consequence of pre-existing depression (often known as the self-medication hypothesis) – the successful treatment of opioid dependence would necessitate treating the underlying psychopathology (Khantzian, 1985).

There are few studies that have tried to disentangle the nature of the relationship between opioid dependence and other, comorbid psychiatric disorders, but each of them suggest that the nature of this relationship most probably varies across individuals. Data collected for the ECA study have been analysed to try to disentangle the temporal sequence of the onset of drug abuse and other non-substance related psychiatric disorders. In this analysis, Christie *et al.* (1988) found that among young adults aged 18 to 30 years, a pre-existing anxiety or depressive disorder doubled the risk of the later development of drug abuse disorders (excluding alcohol). Another study carried out in Canada on a sample of people presenting for a range of alcohol and drug problems found some variation across disorders and across individuals in the sequencing of onset for drug problems and other psychiatric disorders (Ross *et al.,* 1988). For anxiety and depressive disorders, it was less likely that the psychiatric disorder preceded drug abuse problems, although it should be noted that a substantial proportion (23–40%) reported the reverse relationship.

Looking more specifically at the onset of opioid dependence and its relationship with comorbid conditions, Rounsaville *et al.* (1982b) found three different pathways to opioid dependence among a sample of opioid users presenting for treatment. The first group, consistent with the self-medication hypothesis, was found to have suffered significant childhood disruption and trauma and, as a consequence, their personality development and psychological health were affected.

Thirty-one percent of the sample fell into this category. A second group was identified that was characterised by an early onset of delinquency prior to the onset of opioid use and dependence. Just under one-quarter (24%) of the sample fell into this category. A third group was identified that was characterised by the absence of serious psychiatric comorbidity or pre-opioid use delinquency. This group, a majority in the sample (45%), appear to have become addicted to opioids primarily through the use of the drugs themselves, as no predisposing factors could be identified. However, this group had suffered serious disruption to their lives as a result of their addiction.

Finally, in a study designed specifically to examine the self-medication hypothesis among a sample of admissions for opioid or cocaine abuse/dependence, Weiss *et al.* (1992a) found that two-thirds of the respondents reported using drugs to deal with feelings of depression. The authors observed that self-medication may occur in response to a depressed mood without there being any diagnosable major depressive disorder, although this appeared to differ between the sexes. While women reported that they self-medicated for depression regardless of whether they were suffering from a major depressive disorder, men only reported self-medication if they suffered from a major depressive disorder.

CONCLUSION

The evidence reviewed in this chapter suggests that patients attending for opioid replacement therapy have elevated rates of psychiatric comorbidity. Furthermore, although specific diagnoses may not be associated with a poorer response to opioid replacement therapy, as Darke has concluded in this volume, the overall severity of their psychiatric problems has been found to be so related. While some of this morbidity appears to remit purely as a consequence of the general stabilisation that occurs as a result of opioid replacement therapy, in at least a proportion of cases this will not be the case. As some of this morbidity is treatable (e.g., depression and the anxiety disorders), we would suggest that after stabilisation on the substitute opioid has been achieved that all patients should be screened using appropriate self-completion questionnaires, such as the Beck Depression and Anxiety Inventories (Beck & Steer, 1987, 1990). Patients with high scores on screening instruments such as these could then be referred for specialist assessment and treatment.

The high levels of psychiatric comorbidity among patients attending for opioid replacement also have implications for day-to-day management. While specific comorbid conditions each have their own difficulties associated with them, a high load of such patients often leave clinical staff feeling hopeless and angry, which often results in them attributing blame to patients for their own situation. As O'Neill (1993) has pointed out, some of this shifting of blame is a result of the stigmatisation of psychiatric disorders and drug use which pervade the community within which clinicians live and to which they are not immune, and some of it is a result of the special difficulties associated with managing specific disorders (e.g., the hopelessness associated with depression and the uncontrolled outbursts of anger which are aspects of some personality disorders).

SUMMARY

Opioid dependent individuals suffer depressive disorders, anxiety disorders, personality disorders and alcohol abuse/dependence at much higher rates than occur in the general community. The sex differences in the occurrence of these disorders that are apparent in the general community are also apparent among the opioid dependent. Depression and anxiety disorders are more common among women and ASPD and alcohol abuse/dependence are more common among men.

One of the most common psychiatric conditions among opioid users is depression. However, there is some evidence that a proportion of this morbidity remits in response to opioid replacement therapy, suggesting that it might be the result of the life crises associated with an opioid dependent lifestyle. Patients who remain depressed after stabilisation on a replacement opioid are likely to need specialist assessment and treatment. Many methadone maintenance patients when assessed are diagnosed with ASPD, with the majority by far being men. There is controversy over the usefulness of this diagnosis in general and, specifically, in its application to opioid-dependent individuals.

The nature of the relationship between opioid dependence and other psychopathology is not clear. There is evidence that some disorders, such as depression, precede drug use and may predispose its sufferers to self-medicating drug use. Other evidence suggests that other cases of disorders such as depression may be due to the stresses and chaotic lifestyle associated with being dependent on illicit drugs.

The evidence concerning psychiatric comorbidity among methadone maintenance patients suggests that patients accepted for treatment should be assessed with a screening instrument for remediable psychiatric disorders once they have been stabilised on methadone and referred for specialist assessment where indicated.

REFERENCES

American Psychiatric Association. (1987). *Diagnostic and Statistical Manual of Mental Disorders (DSM-III-R)*. (3rd Edition, Revised). Washington, DC: American Psychiatric Association.

American Psychiatric Association. (1994). *Diagnostic and Statistical Manual of Mental Disorders (DSM-IV)*. (4th Edition). Washington, DC: American Psychiatric Association.

Anthony, J. C., & Helzer, J. E. (1995). Epidemiology of drug dependence. In M. T. Tsuang, M. Tohen, & G. E. Zahner (Eds.), *Textbook in psychiatric epidemiology* (pp. 361-406). New York: Wiley-Liss.

Beck, A. T., & Steer, R. A. (1987). *Beck depression inventory: Manual.* USA: Harcourt, Brace & Jovanovich.

Beck, A. T., & Steer, R. A. (1990). *Beck anxiety inventory: Manual.* USA: Harcourt, Brace & Jovanovich.

Blackburn, R. (1988). On moral judgements and personality disorders: The myth of psychopathic personality revisited. *British Journal of Psychiatry,* **153**, 505-512.

Brooner, R. K., Bigelow, G. E., Strain, E., & Schmidt, C. W. (1990). Intravenous drug abusers with antisocial personality disorder: Increased HIV risk behavior. *Drug and Alcohol Dependence, 26*, 39-44.

Brooner, R. K., Greenfield, L., Schmidt, C. W., & Bigelow, G. E. (1993a). Antisocial personality disorder and HIV infection among intravenous drug abusers. *American Journal of Psychiatry, 150*, 53-58.

Brooner, R. K., Herbst, J. H., Schmidt, C. W., Bigelow, G. E., & Costa, P. T. (1993b). Antisocial personality disorder among drug abusers: Relations to other personality diagnoses and the five-factor model of personality. *Journal of Nervous and Mental Disease, 181*, 313-319.

Bryant, K. J., Rounsaville, B., Spitzer, R. L., & Williams, J. B. W. (1992). Reliability of dual diagnosis: Substance dependence and psychiatric disorders. *Journal of Nervous and Mental Disease, 180*, 251-257.

Cacciola, J. S., Rutherford, M. J., Alterman, A. I., McKay, J. R., & Snider, E. (1996). Personality disorders and treatment outcome in methadone maintenance patients. *Journal of Nervous and Mental Disease, 184*, 234-239.

Calsyn, D. A., Fleming, C., Wells, E. A., & Saxon, A. J. (1996). Personality disorder subtypes among opiate addicts in methadone maintenance. *Psychology of Addictive Behaviors, 10*, 3-8.

Christie, K. A., Burke Jr., J. D., Regier, D. A., Rae, D. S., Boyd, J. H., & Locke, B. Z. (1988). Epidemiologic evidence for early onset of mental disorders and higher risk of drug abuse in young adults. *American Journal of Psychiatry,* 145, 971-975.

Cottler, L. B., Compton III, W. M., Mager, D., Spitznagel, E. L., & Janca, A. (1992). Posttraumatic stress disorder among substance users from the general population. *American Journal of Psychiatry,* 149, 664-670.

Courtwright, D. T. (1982). *Dark paradise: Opiate addiction in America before 1940.* Cambidge, Mass.: Harvard University Press.

Croughan, J. L., Miller, J. P., Wagelin, D., & Whitman, B. Y. (1982). Psychiatric illnesses in male and female narcotic addicts. *Journal of Clinical Psychiatry,* 43, 225-228.

Darke, S., Hall, W., & Swift, W. (1994a). Prevalence, symptoms and correlates of anti-social personality disorder among methadone maintenance clients. *Drug and Alcohol Dependence,* 34, 253-257.

Darke, S., Swift, W., & Hall, W. (1994b). Prevalence, severity and correlates of psycho-logical morbidity among methadone maintenance clients. *Addiction,* 89, 211-217.

Darke, S., Wodak, A., Hall, W., Heather, N., & Ward, J. (1992). Prevalence and predictors of psychopathology among opioid users. *British Journal of Addiction,* 87, 771-776.

Dorus, W., & Senay, E. C. (1980). Depression, demographic dimensions, and drug abuse. *American Journal of Psychiatry,* 137, 699-704.

Galbaud du Fort, G., Newman, S. C., & Bland, R. C. (1993). Psychiatric comorbidity and treatment seeking: Sources of selection bias in the study of clinical populations. *Journal of Nervous and Mental Disease,* 181, 467-474.

Gerstley, L. J., Alterman, A. I., McLellan, A. T., & Woody, G. E. (1990). Antisocial personality disorder in patients with substance abuse disorders: A problematic diagnosis. *American Journal of Psychiatry,* 147, 173-178.

Gill, K., Nolimal, D., & Crowley, T. J. (1992). Antisocial personality disorder, HIV risk behavior and retention in methadone maintenance therapy. *Drug and Alcohol Dependence,* 30, 247-252.

Hall, W. (1996). What have population surveys revealed about substance use disorders and their co-morbidity with other mental disorders? *Drug and Alcohol Review,* 15, 157-170.

Hartgers, C., Van Den Hoek, J. A. R., Coutinho, R. A., & Van Der Pligt, J. (1992). Psychopathology, stress and HIV-risk injecting behaviour among drug users. *British Journal of Addiction,* 87, 857-865.

Hendriks, V. M. (1990). Psychiatric disorders in a Dutch addict population: Rates and correlates of DSM-III diagnosis. *Journal of Consulting and Clinical Psychology,* 58, 158-165.

Hesselbrock, V., Meyer, R., & Hesselbrock, M. (1992). Psychopathology and addictive disorders: The specific case of antisocial personality disorder. In

C. P. O'Brien & J. H. Jaffe (Eds.), *Addictive states* (pp. 179-191). New York: Raven.

Kessler, R. C. (1995a). Epidemiology of psychiatric comorbidity. In M. T. Tsuang, M. Tohen, & G. E. Zahner (Eds.), *Textbook in psychiatric epidemiology* (pp. 179-197). New York: Wiley-Liss.

Kessler, R. C. (1995b). The National Comorbidity Survey: Preliminary results and future directions. *International Journal of Methods in Psychiatric Research, 5*, 139-151.

Kessler, R. C., McGonagle, K. A., Zhao, S., Nelson, C. B., Hughes, M., Eshleman, S., Wittchen, H., & Kendler, K. S. (1994). Lifetime and 12-month prevalence of DSM-III-R psychiatric disorders in the United States: Results from the National Comorbidity Survey. *Archives of General Psychiatry, 51*, 8-19.

Khantzian, E. J. (1985). The self-medication hypothesis of addictive disorders: Focus on heroin and cocaine dependence. *American Journal of Psychiatry, 142*, 1259-1264.

Khantzian, E. J., & Treece, C. (1985). DSM-III psychiatric diagnosis of narcotic addicts: Recent findings. *Archives of General Psychiatry, 42*, 1067-1071.

Kosten, T. A., Kosten, T. R., & Rounsaville, B. J. (1989). Personality disorders in opiate addicts show prognostic specificity. *Journal of Substance Abuse Treatment, 6*, 163-168.

Kosten, T. R., Rounsaville, B. J., & Kleber, H. D. (1982). DSM-III personality disorders in opiate addicts. *Comprehensive Psychiatry, 23*, 572-581.

Limbeek, J. V., Wouters, L., Kaplan, C. D., Geerlings, P. J., & Alem, V. V. (1992). Prevalence of psychopathology in drug-addicted Dutch. *Journal of Substance Abuse Treatment, 9*, 43-52.

Lipsitz, J. D., Williams, J. B. W., Rabkin, J. G., Remien, R. H., Bradburn, M., Sadr, W. E., Goetz, R., Sorrell, S., & Gorman, J. M. (1994). Psychopathology in male and female intravenous drug users with and without HIV infection. *American Journal of Psychiatry, 151*, 1662-1668.

Lyons, M. J. (1995). Epidemiology of personality disorders. In M. T. Tsuang, M. Tohen, & G. E. Zahner (Eds.), *Textbook in psychiatric epidemiology* (pp. 407-436). New York: Wiley-Liss.

Magruder-Habib, K., Hubbard, R. L., & Ginzburg, H. M. (1992). Effects of drug misuse treatment on symptoms of depression and suicide. *International Journal of the Addictions, 27*, 1035-1065.

Mattick, R. P., Baillie, A., Grenyer, B., Hall, W., Jarvis, T., & Webster, P. (Eds.). (1993a). *An outline for the management of alcohol problems: Quality assurance project.* Canberra: Australian Government Publishing Service.

Mattick, R. P., Bell, J., & Hall, W. (1993b). Psychiatric morbidity, antisocial personality disorder, and treatment response in methadone patients.

Paper presented at the 55th Annual Scientific Meeting of the College on Problems of Drug Dependence, Toronto, Canada.

Mattick, R. P., & Hall, W. (Eds.). (1993). *A treatment outline for approaches to opioid dependence.* Canberra: Australian Government Publishing Service.

Meyer, R. E. (1986). How to understand the relationship between psychopathology and addictive disorders: Another example of the chicken and the egg. In R. E. Meyer (Ed.), *Psychopathology and addictive disorders* (pp. 3-16). U.S.A.: Guilford.

Milby, J. B., Sims, M. K., Khuder, S., Schumacher, J. E., Huggins, N., McLellan, A. T., Woody, G., & Haas, N. (1996). Psychiatric comorbidity: Prevalence in methadone maintenance treatment. *American Journal of Drug and Alcohol Abuse,* 22, 95-107.

Musselman, D. L., & Kell, M. J. (1995). Prevalence and improvement in psychopathology in opioid dependent patients participating in methadone maintenance. *Journal of Addictive Diseases,* 14, 67-82.

O'Neill, M. M. (1993). Countertransference and attitudes in the context of clinical work with dually diagnosed patients. In J. Solomon, S. Zimberg, & E. Shollar (Eds.), *Dual diagnosis: Evaluation, treatment, training, and program development* (pp. 127-146). New York: Plenum.

Perry, J. C. (1992). Problems and considerations in the valid assessment of personality disorders. *American Journal of Psychiatry,* 149, 1645-1653.

Quality Assurance Project. (1991a). Treatment outlines for antisocial personality disorder. *Australian and New Zealand Journal of Psychiatry,* 25, 541-547.

Quality Assurance Project. (1991b). Treatment outlines for borderline, narcissistic and histrionic personality disorders. The Quality Assurance Project. *Australian and New Zealand Journal of Psychiatry,* 25, 392-403.

Regier, D. A., Farmer, M. E., Rae, D. S., Locke, B. Z., Keith, S. J., Judd, L. L., & Goodwin, F. K. (1990). Comorbidity of mental disorders with alcohol and other drug abuse: Results from the Epidemiologic Catchment Area (ECA) study. *Journal of the American Medical Association,* 264, 2511-2518.

Reich, J. H., & Green, A. I. (1991). Effect of personality disorders on outcome of treatment. *Journal of Nervous and Mental Disease,* 179, 74-82.

Robins, L. N., & Regier, D. A. (Eds.). (1991). *Psychiatric disorders in America: The Epidemiologic Catchment Area study.* New York: Free Press.

Robins, L. N., Tipp, J., & Przybeck, T. (1991). Antisocial personality. In R. L.N. & D. A. Regier (Eds.), *Psychiatric disorders in America: The Epidemiologic Catchment Area study* (pp. 258-290). New York: The Free Press.

Ross, H. E., Glaser, F. B., & Germanson, T. (1988). The prevalence of psychiatric disorders in patients with alcohol and other drug problems. *Archives of General Psychiatry,* 45, 1023-1031.

Rounsaville, B. J., & Kleber, H. D. (1985). Untreated opiate addicts: How do they differ from those seeking treatment. *Archives of General Psychiatry,* **42,** 1072-1077.

Rounsaville, B. J., Kosten, T. R., Weissman, M. M., & Kleber, H. D. (1986). Prognostic significance of psychopathology in treated opiate addicts: A 2.5-year follow-up study. *Archives of General Psychiatry,* **43,** 739-745.

Rounsaville, B. J., Weissman, M. M., Kleber, H., & Wilber, C. (1982a). Heterogeneity of psychiatric diagnosis in treated opiate addicts. *Archives of General Psychiatry,* **39,** 161-166.

Rounsaville, B. J., Weissman, M. M., Wilber, C. H., & Kleber, H. D. (1982b). Pathways to opiate addiction: An evaluation of differing antecedents. *British Journal of Psychiatry,* **141,** 437-446.

Rousar, E., Brooner, R. K., Regier, M. W., & Bigelow, G. E. (1994). Psychiatric distress in antisocial drug abusers: Relation to other personality disorders. *Drug and Alcohol Dependence,* **34,** 149-54.

Rutherford, M. J., Cacciola, J. S., & Alterman, A. I. (1994). Relationships of personality disorders with problem severity in methadone patients. *Drug and Alcohol Dependence,* **35,** 69-76.

Steer, R. A., & Kotzker, E. (1980). Affective changes in male and female methadone patients. *Drug and Alcohol Dependence,* **5,** 115-122.

Strain, E. C., Brooner, R. K., & Bigelow, G. E. (1991a). Clustering of multiple substance use and psychiatric diagnoses in opiate addicts. *Drug and Alcohol Dependence,* **27,** 127-134.

Strain, E. C., Stitzer, M. L., & Bigelow, G. E. (1991b). Early treatment time course of dep-ressive symptoms in opiate addicts. *Journal of Nervous and Mental Disease,* **179,** 215-221.

Swift, W., Williams, G., Neill, O., & Grenyer, B. (1990). The prevalence of minor psycho-pathology in opioid users seeking treatment. *British Journal of Addiction,* **85,** 629-634.

Weiss, R. D., Griffin, M. L., & Mirin, S. M. (1992a). Drug abuse as self-medication for depression: An empirical study. *American Journal of Drug and Alcohol Abuse,* **18,** 121-129.

Weiss, R. D., Mirin, S. M., & Griffin, M. L. (1992b). Methodological considerations in the diagnosis of coexisting psychiatric disorders in substance abusers. *British Journal of Addiction,* **87,** 179-187.

WHO. (1992). *The ICD-10 classification of mental and behavioural disorders: Clinical descriptions and diagnostic guidelines.* Geneva: World Health Organisation.

Woody, G. E., McLellan, A. T., Luborsky, L., & O'Brien, C. P. (1985). Sociopathy and psychotherapy outcome. *Archives of General Psychiatry,* **42,** 1081-1086.

IV CONCLUSION

18

THE FUTURE OF OPIOID REPLACEMENT THERAPY

WAYNE HALL, JEFF WARD AND RICHARD P. MATTICK

When the first edition of this book was written, methadone maintenance was still a controversial treatment for opioid dependence in Australia. There was continuing debate about whether methadone treatment should be provided at all; the question of how best to deliver it was only beginning to be asked. This reflected opposition to methadone maintenance from clinicians in the drug and alcohol field, and public and political ambivalence about the long-term maintenance of opioid-dependent people on an opioid drug.

One consequence of this ambivalence was that many methadone maintenance programs provided what the research evidence indicated was sub-standard forms of treatment. Entry to treatment was made difficult for fear of creating iatrogenic dependence and, once in treatment, patients received the lowest possible doses of methadone for fear of prolonging their opioid dependence. Some programs also encouraged their patients to achieve abstinence within a year or two, and program staff regarded their inability to achieve this aim as evidence of the therapeutic failure of methadone maintenance treatment.

A major aim of the first edition of this book (Ward *et al.*, 1992) was to make clear that there was good evidence for the effectiveness of methadone treatment in reducing illicit heroin use and improving patient well-being when it was delivered as a form of maintenance treatment. A secondary aim was to identify the key features of effective methadone maintenance treatment as indicated by research. Among the features of effective treatment were providing an adequate methadone dose within a program whose staff had a maintenance orientation to treatment. We believe that our book played some role in changing thinking about methadone maintenance treatment among program staff and policy makers, even if largely by reinforcing and legitimising changes that were occurring for other reasons.

Our book was also written at a time when the funding of methadone maintenance treatment in Australia was less of an issue than it has since become. It was written in the middle of a ten-year period during which the Federal Government funded a continuous expansion of methadone maintenance treatment in Australia. The cost-effectiveness of methadone maintenance treatment was only briefly discussed in the concluding chapter of the previous edition, where we noted the need to consider research into the effectiveness and costs of different ways of funding and providing methadone maintenance treatment.

In the four years since the publication of the first edition, economic issues in the delivery of methadone maintenance treatment have come to the fore. Continuing demand for methadone maintenance treatment and increasing governmental demands for increased efficiency in health care delivery have produced major changes in the methods of delivering methadone maintenance treatment. A major change has been the increased involvement of the private medical sector in delivering methadone treatment. Specialist private methadone maintenance clinics have been developed and, more recently, there has been a rapid expansion of primary care methods of delivery which involve general practitioners prescribing, and pharmacists dispensing, methadone. The use of alternative opioid maintenance drugs has also been proposed, such as buprenorphine, naltrexone, LAAM, and injectable heroin, to provide increased patient choice and possibly to reduce costs of delivery.

In this concluding chapter, we identify some of the key issues for the future delivery of methadone maintenance treatment. These issues are priorities for research into improving the effectiveness and efficiency of delivery of methadone maintenance treatment. We will illustrate these issues by using Australian experience with which we are most familiar. We believe that these issues may have application in other countries, but this can best be judged by those familiar with the historical and cultural differences between countries in patterns of illicit opioid use and methods of health care delivery.

THE SUPPLY OF OPIOID SUBSTITUTION TREATMENT IN AUSTRALIA

The number of persons enrolled in methadone maintenance treatment in Australia has increased steadily over the past decade from approximately 4,446 in June 1987 to 14,996 in June 1994 (and an estimated 18,000 by June 1995). The participation rate per 100,000 of the population aged 15 to 44 has increased from 59 in June 1987 to 182 in June 1994 (Commonwealth Department of Human Services and Health, 1995).

In the past seven years, the largest increase in the supply of methadone maintenance treatment places has come from the expansion of treatment provided in the private sector, rather than from an expansion of publicly funded treatment programs (Commonwealth Department of Health and Human Services, 1995). That is, there has been a larger increase in persons receiving methadone treatment from private medical practitioners than from publicly funded treatment programs. Nationally, the number of clients enrolled in public methadone programs increased from 2,701 in June 1987 to 6,541 in June 1994 while over the same period the numbers enrolled in private programs increased from 1,745 to 8,449. The participation rates have increased over the same period from 36 to 79 per 100,000 for public methadone programs and from 23 to 102 per 100,000 for private programs (Commonwealth Department of Human Services and Health, 1995). The largest increases in private sector treatment places have been in New South Wales and Victoria (Commonwealth Department of Human Services and Health, 1995). In New South Wales the percentage of treatment places provided in private programs increased from 49% in June 1987 to 68% in June 1995 (New South Wales Drug and Alcohol Directorate, 1996).

Private methadone maintenance programs are run by general practitioners and psychiatrists who are licensed by the State governments to dispense methadone to opioid-dependent persons.

The direct medical costs of these programs are paid by the Commonwealth Government through Medicare (the Australian national health insurance scheme) in the form of bulk-billing for medical services and urinalysis. Patients also pay a dispensing fee which averages $40 to $50 a week. Private methadone maintenance programs differ from public programs in a number of respects (Bell *et al.*, 1995). They generally do not provide any formal counselling for clients although the prescribers regularly see their clients (three times a month on average) for which they receive a consultation fee that is paid in full by Medicare. Private programs typically give a higher average methadone dose (64 mg compared with 59 mg in public programs), and they have more liberal policies towards take-away methadone doses than public clinics (giving out an average of 16 per month as against less than three per month in public clinics) (Bell *et al.*, 1995).

In 1994, it cost approximately $2,662 per annum to provide methadone maintenance treatment in Australia in public programs. The direct costs of private methadone programs to government were considerably less: $552 per annum for programs run by general practitioners and $1,728 for those run by psychiatrists. These estimates do not include the direct costs paid by clients ($2,340 per annum at $45 per week over 52 weeks). When the clients' contribution is added, the average costs of methadone maintenance treatment provided in private programs ($2,892 for general practitioners and $4,068 for psychiatrists) were higher than methadone maintenance treatment provided in public programs. The costs of methadone maintenance treatment were considerably less than the estimated annual cost of $14,000 per client for treatment in residential treatment programs (Commonwealth Department of Human Services and Health, 1995). In 1993/94, it was estimated that the States and Commonwealth governments contributed $15.2m and $15.3m respectively to the costs of providing public and private methadone maintenance treatment in Australia (Commonwealth Department of Human Services and Health, 1995).

These data indicate that there has been a steady ten-year expansion in the number of treatment places in methadone maintenance in Australia, and a probable increase in the proportion of opioid-dependent persons who are receiving treatment. Most of this expansion has occurred in the private medical sector, in both specialist clinics and by general practitioner/pharmacist delivery. The expansion has been largely funded by the Commonwealth Government through the Medicare system, and by patients through the imposition of dispensing fees. The major concerns expressed about the expanded role of the private sector has been the loss of central control of treatment delivery, and the possibly adverse impact of the dispensing fee on retention in treatment and the impact of treatment on drug use and crime.

The annual costs of methadone maintenance treatment in public and private programs is modest by comparison with drug-free treatment alternatives, and one might add the estimated costs of imprisonment which is approximately $40,000 per annum in the state of New South Wales. Nevertheless, Commonwealth and State governments have become concerned at the prospect of funding an indefinite expansion of methadone treatment places in the face of a shrinking revenue base and cost pressures in health care more generally. These factors are operating to prevent further increase in expansion and to reduce the cost of delivering methadone treatment precisely when there are indications of continuing recruitment to heroin use, if not an increased rate of recruitment.

THE DEMAND FOR METHADONE MAINTENANCE TREATMENT IN AUSTRALIA

The best estimate derived from a series of individually imperfect estimates is that there were approximately 59,000 dependent heroin users in Australia in 1991 (Hall, 1995). The range of the estimates was between 36,000 and 120,000 (Hall, 1995), indicating the degree of uncertainty of the estimates. Comparison with similarly derived estimates in the mid-1980s (34,000) suggested that the number of dependent heroin users had increased over the past decade (Hall, 1995).

The expansion of methadone maintenance treatment places over the period 1987-1995 has exceeded the likely increase in numbers of dependent heroin users. In 1987, approximately 17% of the estimated number of opioid-dependent persons (34,000) were enrolled in methadone maintenance treatment. This increased to 30% of the estimated number of dependent heroin users in 1995. Although the proportion of regular heroin users enrolled in methadone maintenance has substantially increased over the past five years, this comprises less than half of the estimated dependent heroin users in Australia.

Nonetheless it would be unwise to assume that the potential demand for methadone treatment is an additional 41,000 places – the discrepancy between the estimated number of regular heroin users in the population (59,000) and the number currently enrolled in methadone maintenance treatment (18,000). First, the size of the heroin using population is probably not stable. There are a number of soft indicators that the rate of recruitment to heroin use may also have increased recently. There has probably been an increase in the availability of cheaper and purer heroin in Australia in the past several years (Australian Bureau of Criminal Intelligence, 1996). There have been increasing numbers of seizures at the customs barrier, a small but steady increase in number of arrests for heroin offences, and a dramatic increase in the number of heroin overdose deaths. There are also indications that a new cohort of younger Indo-Chinese heroin users are being recruited in South Western Sydney (Maher, 1996). Recent research conducted by the National Drug and Alcohol Research Centre also suggests that some of the amphetamine injectors who initiated use in the mid-1980s are now becoming regular heroin users.

Second, not all dependent heroin users are interested in drug treatment in general, or in methadone maintenance treatment in particular. An unknown but probably substantial minority become abstinent without seeking professional assistance (Biernacki, 1986), and a substantial proportion of those who enrol in drug treatment, including methadone maintenance treatment, drop out. Studies of street heroin users have identified heroin users who actively avoid methadone maintenance treatment (Beschner & Walters, 1985; Hunt *et al.*, 1986).

Factors Influencing Demand for Methadone Maintenance Treatment

The demand for methadone maintenance treatment is dynamic. It will be affected by the balance of the benefits and costs of the heroin-using lifestyle. The benefits of heroin use are the euphoric effects of heroin and the excitement of the heroin-using subculture, compared with the humdrum tedium of lowly paid and unskilled work, if available. The costs of heroin use include the necessity to generate large amounts of cash (or to actively engage in drug distribution) to finance drug use; the risks of violence associated with drug dealing; the risks of arrest and imprisonment for property and drug offences; the risks of experiencing a drug overdose or contracting infectious diseases from needle sharing; and the risk of sexually transmitted diseases among women and men engaged in sex work. Heroin users who tire of these aspects of their lives may consider entering methadone maintenance treatment. Whether they do so will depend upon the availability and attractiveness of such treatment.

Among the factors pushing dependent heroin users into treatment was the advent of HIV/AIDS among injecting drug users a decade ago. The threat of potentially fatal and chronic infectious diseases has been accentuated by the recent recognition of the high prevalence and incidence of hepatitis C infection among Australian injecting drug users (Bell *et al.,* 1990). Another factor pushing dependent heroin users into treatment may be the impact of law enforcement strategies on reducing the availability, increasing the price and reducing the purity of heroin. For example, arrests of street heroin dealers may interrupt drug distribution, much of which is controlled by user-dealers financing their own drug use. Interruptions at this level of the distribution system may make it harder to sustain dependent heroin use by increasing search time. More generally, the uncertain availability, high cost and variable quality of street heroin may influence users to cease heroin use. These disadvantages are heightened by the rigours of the criminal lifestyle, such as the violence used to enforce compliance in drug dealing and to "rip off" low-level drug dealers.

Very little research has been conducted on why dependent heroin users decide to cease their heroin use and why they seek treatment to do so. Joe *et al.* (1990) report the reasons given by 372 daily heroin users for deciding to abstain at their last episode of abstinence. The most commonly cited reasons were feeling "tired of the hustle" involved in maintaining daily heroin use (83%), and the feeling that the individual had "hit bottom" and needed to make a dramatic change in their lives (82%). The next most common reasons were having experienced a major personal or special life event, such as entering a new relationship or having children (66%), fearing being gaoled (57%) and having family responsibilities (56%). Specific aspects of heroin using life style that were lower down the list included: the high cost (40%) and the poor quality of heroin (36%), being tired of having no money (34%), fearing a drug overdose (31%), and being sent to gaol (30%).

Once a dependent heroin user decides to become abstinent, it is unclear what factors will influence whether or not treatment is sought and, if so, what type of treatment is selected. It is likely that a major factor will be the attractiveness of different forms of treatment to users. We know from the 12-year follow-up of the DARP cohort in the USA that methadone maintenance treatment attracted the largest proportion of dependent heroin users (Marsh *et al.*, 1990). If this finding is applicable to Australia, then the increased availability of methadone maintenance over the past decade has probably contributed to an increased uptake of this form of treatment. Evidence from both Australia (Bell *et al.*, 1994) and the US (Woody *et al.*, 1975) also suggests that reducing the barriers to entering methadone maintenance treatment (by providing rapid assessment and intake) increases its attractiveness and treatment retention.

Some changes in the method of delivering methadone maintenance treatment in Australia over the past decade have probably also increased demand for this treatment. One of these has been more liberal policies towards continuing heroin use while in treatment, a policy change made in response to the advent of HIV. Another factor has been the more liberal provision of take-away doses, especially in private treatment programs, since daily dosing is one of the least liked aspects of methadone maintenance treatment (Beschner & Walters, 1985; Hunt *et al.*, 1986). The adoption of higher methadone doses and a maintenance approach to treatment in many Australian programs have been shown to increase retention in methadone maintenance treatment (Caplehorn & Bell, 1991; Caplehorn *et al.*, 1993).

Other changes in method of delivery may have reduced demand. One of these has been the imposition of direct dispensing charges in many private and in some public methadone maintenance programs. Given that many patients derive their income from social welfare (e.g., sickness and unemployment benefits) (Bell *et al.*, 1995), the payment of a $40-$50 a week dispensing fee represents a substantial part of their income. It has been suggested that this money may be raised by selling take-away methadone doses, or by continued involvement in property crime or drug dealing, even if at a lower level than before entry to treatment. Research on the impact of dispensing fees is a priority given the increasing reliance upon the private sector to deliver methadone maintenance treatment in Australia.

The net effects of these factors has probably been to increase demand for methadone maintenance treatment in Australia. The question is: Could demand and uptake of methadone treatment be increased (assuming that this is a desirable thing from a public health and public policy point of view)? The options available to do so are limited. These are briefly discussed below.

INCREASING THE UPTAKE OF OPIOID MAINTENANCE TREATMENT

Increasing the Push into Treatment

Not all of the factors that can influence demand for methadone maintenance treatment are easily manipulated by policy. In the case of law enforcement, for example, recent research suggests that the ability of police activity to produce short-term fluctuations in the market price and purity of heroin appears to be limited (Weatherburn & Lind, 1995). Increased attention to street level dealing may increase the inconvenience of being a regular heroin user, thereby encouraging more dependent heroin users to seek treatment. It remains to be seen, however, whether short-term increases in the intensity of street level law enforcement have any enduring effects on entry to treatment and, if so, whether these benefits are purchased at the price of adverse effects on public health, such as increasing unsafe and risky patterns of drug use (Maher, 1996).

One modifiable factor that has been underused in Australia is providing drug treatment during imprisonment. Imprisonment is one of the most common "interventions" received by many dependent heroin users who are imprisoned for property or drug offences at some time in their heroin-using careers. Yet few receive any drug treatment while they are imprisoned, even though this is an ideal opportunity to intervene with a captive population for whom drug treatment may provide a welcome respite from the tedium of prison life. It is a missed opportunity since there is evidence that some forms of prison-based drug treatment reduce drug use and recidivism after release (Gerstein & Harwood, 1990). This includes evidence from the first randomised controlled trial of methadone maintenance treatment conducted by Dole *et al.* (1969).

The Role of Treatment Coercion

A popular proposal for increasing the number of dependent heroin users in treatment is to divert more of them from the criminal justice system into drug treatment under legal coercion. This option may be especially appropriate for the most criminally involved heroin-dependent offenders who some studies suggest may actively avoid treatment (Beschner & Walters, 1985).

The arguments in favour of providing treatment under coercion, and the evidence of its effectiveness, have been reviewed in detail elsewhere (Hall, in press). The conclusions of that review were that the most ethically defensible form of legally coerced drug treatment was that in which offenders had a choice as to whether they accept treatment or imprisonment. If they choose to be treated, they should have a choice of treatment options, rather than being compelled to enter a particular form of drug treatment.

The evidence from American studies, such as DARP and TOPS, suggests that coercion does not impair the effectiveness of treatment, provided that the threat of return to the criminal justice system remains credible (Anglin, 1988; Gerstein & Harwood, 1990; Hubbard *et al.,* 1988; Simpson & Friend, 1988). This suggests that drug treatment under coercion is an effective way of increasing the number of dependent heroin users in methadone maintenance treatment and other forms of drug treatment (Hall, in press).

Nonetheless, there are reasons for cautioning against an overly enthusiastic embrace of treatment under coercion. First, funding would be needed for additional places in existing treatment services. The failure to do so would place an undue burden on existing community-based treatment services and deprive those who voluntarily seek treatment from receiving it. Second, there is a need to evaluate the effectiveness and cost-effectiveness of drug treatment under coercion. This is to ensure that we are not wasting scarce treatment resources on unsuitable clients, that the programs provide effective and humane treatment, and that they provide a credible alternative to imprisonment rather than being seen by offenders and correctional staff as a "soft option" to be exploited by those who wish to evade imprisonment (Gerstein & Harwood, 1990).

Increasing the Attractiveness of Opioid Replacement Therapy

Methadone maintenance treatment can be made more attractive by being made more readily available to those who request it. This is shown by the steady growth in the number of methadone patients in Australia over the past decade. Even so there are limits on the number of treatment places that can be provided. Scarce resources limit the preparedness of government (either Federal or State) to fund an increasing number of methadone maintenance places. Sooner or later limits will be imposed on funding for such treatment and demands will be made to find more efficient and less expensive ways of delivering opioid maintenance treatment. Some of these may coincidentally be more attractive to dependent heroin users than the current methods of delivery.

One approach to improving the efficiency of methadone maintenance treatment delivery is to experiment with general practitioners as prescribers and community pharmacists as dispensers of methadone. The much more expensive multi-disciplinary public methadone maintenance clinics, and the specialist private methadone programs, might be restricted to the role of stabilising new clients and to dealing with more complex and difficult clients. Community-based general practitioner and pharmacy based treatment may be more attractive to many dependent heroin users than the large, highly visible and more controlling specialist clinics. The mainstreaming of methadone maintenance treatment in primary health services may also increase treatment uptake by reducing the stigma of being a patient in a large and publicly conspicuous clinic.

Another approach to increasing treatment efficiency may be to use longer acting opioid maintenance drugs, such as buprenorphine and LAAM. Because these drugs have a longer half-life than methadone, the frequency of dosing could be three times a week rather than daily, reducing the costs of maintaining an opioid-dependent person, and the necessity for irksome and disruptive daily attendance for patients. Buprenorphine is a mixed agonist-antagonist opioid which has the additional advantages of a lower risk of overdose and an easier withdrawal process than methadone. These are substantial advantages. Methadone has a bad (if not always deserved) reputation for greater addictiveness, side-effects and overdose risk than heroin among heroin users in the United States (Beschner & Walters, 1985; Hunt *et al.,* 1986; Rosenblum *et al.,* 1991). There is anecdotal evidence of similar views among heroin users in Australia but no research has been done on the issue.

We could possibly increase the number of methadone maintenance treatment spaces by providing better assistance to stabilised methadone maintenance treatment patients who want to withdraw from methadone. This should be done in such a way that it does not place undue pressure on clients to become abstinent. It should be the choice of the client to stop, not the result of imposing an arbitrary time limit, such as two years, on enrolment in treatment. It may be achieved by improving relationships between methadone maintenance treatment and drug-free treatment services, or it may require the development of organised aftercare and support services in some methadone maintenance treatment programs.

The attractiveness of methadone maintenance treatment to heroin users can be increased by making various changes in program policies and philosophies. These include: increasing average methadone doses, being more tolerant of intermittent heroin use, especially earlier in treatment, and by adopting more liberal policies on take-away doses of methadone. "Streaming" may also be introduced into some methadone maintenance treatment programs. This involves providing low threshold programs that have a less onerous assessment process and that make fewer demands upon patients to change drug use or behaviour. Some of these changes have been made in Australian methadone maintenance treatment programs in response to HIV/ AIDS, and they probably partly explain the steady increase in the numbers of heroin users seeking methadone maintenance treatment.

Even if public funds were inexhaustible, there are limits on community tolerance of new methadone clinics being opened within residential areas (Senay, 1988). There may also be limits on public tolerance of certain program policies. Reductions in the therapeutic demands made on methadone clients to reduce their opioid drug use, for example, risks blurring an important distinction between drug substitution for therapeutic purposes and the simple provision of socially sanctioned opioids under medical supervision. Increasing the number of take-away doses may also have adverse effects, such as increasing diversion of methadone to finance methadone maintenance treatment and heroin use. Increased methadone diversion may, in turn, lead to increased methadone overdose deaths, including deaths among heroin users who are not enrolled in methadone maintenance treatment, and it may also encourage the injection of oral methadone syrup with adverse health consequences for the individuals involved in this practice (Darke *et al.*, 1995).

These program changes may also impair the effectiveness of methadone maintenance treatment in reducing heroin use and crime.

It may be argued that, even so, this produces larger public health gains since methadone maintenance treatment which is delivered to more dependent heroin users will produce larger aggregate public health benefits, even if the average benefit derived by individuals is lower. This type of argument, however, may not convince the general public.

Should We Consider Injectable Heroin Maintenance?

One way of attracting more heroin users into drug treatment may be to offer injectable heroin maintenance treatment. This is a plausible option given the success of methadone maintenance treatment in reducing heroin use and crime, and the safety of administering pharmaceutically pure heroin under medical supervision. Its principal attraction is that it may increase the number of heroin users who are attracted into and retained in treatment by providing them with their preferred drug, heroin, by their preferred route of administration, injection.

There are reports of successful clinical experience using this form of maintenance treatment (e.g., Marks, 1987). The opportunity to prescribe injectable heroin has been part of the so-called "British system" since 1926, although it has only rarely been used (Strang & Gossop, 1994). Heroin maintenance treatment is also currently undergoing a controlled observational trial in a number of sites in Switzerland (Rihs, 1994; Uchtenhagen *et al.*, 1994), and a similar trial has been proposed in Australia (Bammer, 1995).

Some advocates of heroin maintenance treatment have created unrealistic expectations about its likely impact on heroin use and heroin-related crime. Even if we assume that heroin maintenance treatment, like methadone maintenance treatment, reduces illicit heroin use and crime among those receiving it, the impact at a population level is likely to be small. The major reason is that heroin maintenance treatment is unlikely to reach as large a minority of the heroin using population as that achieved by the steady expansion of methadone maintenance treatment over the past decade (Hall, 1995).

The major restraint upon the expansion of heroin maintenance treatment is societal concern about providing injectable heroin, even when it is restricted to dependent heroin users who receive it under medical supervision. These concerns take various forms (Bammer, 1995). Some community members have strong moral objections to providing any drug of dependence, whether it be heroin or methadone, to dependent drug users; for them abstinence is the only acceptable treatment aim and outcome. Parents of adolescents worry about sending the "wrong" message to youth about heroin and other drug use. Residents of localities that provide heroin maintenance treatment are concerned that there will be a "honey-pot" effect attracting even more heroin users into their communities. Treatment personnel may fear that heroin maintenance treatment will create an incentive for heroin users to become heroin dependent, that prescribed heroin will be diverted from dependent to non-dependent heroin users, and that heroin maintenance will adversely affect recruitment of dependent heroin users into less attractive forms of drug treatment.

The main consequence of these anxieties about heroin maintenance treatment will be to discourage its use on the scale necessary for it to reach a large number of heroin users. As was the case with the introduction of methadone maintenance treatment, these concerns are most likely to be addressed by restricting heroin maintenance treatment to dependent heroin users who have failed at other forms of drug treatment. This has been the Swiss practice, and it seems the most likely option for the proposed Australian Capital Territory heroin trial.

Even if there was stronger public support for heroin maintenance treatment, the costs of providing it mean that the scale of its provision would be modest. The costs of heroin maintenance are of the order of two to three times those of providing methadone maintenance (Rihs-Middle, pers. comm., 1995). The Swiss report that there were unanticipated costs in producing pharmaceutical quality heroin for injection. They also found it costly to provide the security to ensure the integrity of the drug at source, and to prevent its diversion in transit between factory and clinic. The logistics of delivering an injectable drug that is self-administered under medical supervision up to three times a day requires more staff and longer opening hours than oral methadone that is administered under supervision once a day.

If we assume a rough equivalence between heroin and methadone maintenance in their impact on heroin use and crime (Hartnoll *et al.*, 1980) then, on the grounds of cost-effectiveness, methadone would be preferable to heroin as a substitution therapy. That is, we would be able to attract more users into drug substitution by using methadone rather than heroin, even if the latter was more attractive than the former, because we could treat many more with methadone than we could with heroin. Heroin maintenance would have to produce substantially greater benefits for each participant than methadone maintenance to make it competitive.

A further restraint on the population impact of heroin maintenance is its unattractiveness to the heroin-using population. The assumption is that heroin maintenance will be much more attractive to heroin users than methadone maintenance, because it provides them with their preferred opioid drug by their preferred route of administration. This assumption ignores the stigma that may attach to receiving medically prescribed heroin and the restrictive circumstances under which it will be provided. Bammer and colleagues have found polarised views among heroin users (both in and out of treatment) about the desirability of providing heroin maintenance treatment (Bammer, 1995). Clinical experience in Britain and Switzerland has been that heroin users who receive prescribed heroin are stigmatised by their peers as "hopeless" cases. This perception will be reinforced if heroin maintenance is restricted to treatment failures. Those users who are attracted into heroin maintenance may also find the restrictions on the timing and place of heroin administration that are required to minimise diversion irksome, as do some methadone maintenance clients. They would make it difficult to sustain full-time paid employment, and they would present problems for women with dependent children.

All considered, there may be a case for cautious trial and evaluation of heroin maintenance treatment but only as an additional option for opioid-dependent persons. Expectations of this form of maintenance treatment need to be more realistic than has been the case in some media discussions. Heroin maintenance may provide an additional option for those dependent users who have failed to respond to other forms of treatment, including methadone maintenance treatment. It may also have benefits for the larger community if it reduces the criminal activity of a small group of criminally active dependent users, and if it reduces their risks of contracting or transmitting HIV and other infectious diseases. It will be much more expensive to provide heroin maintenance than methadone maintenance. Given the cost of its provision, it will not replace existing forms of treatment, nor will it provide a solution to all the problems that have been attributed to the failures of heroin prohibition. At most, heroin maintenance may provide a useful but modest addition to our ability to ameliorate some of the health and social problems that injecting opioid use produces in our community.

Ethical Issues in Expanding Methadone Maintenance Treatment

Any expansion of methadone maintenance treatment (or of opioid substitution treatment more generally), especially if undertaken to reduce drug-related crime, must strike a balance between benefiting heroin users and the wider community. An over-reliance upon legal coercion and punitive law enforcement policies to drive dependent heroin users into treatment runs the risk that methadone maintenance will become primarily a form of social control, rather than a therapeutic alternative to imprisonment. If this were to happen, methadone maintenance programs would become progressively more punitive and less attractive to users, and the staff who work in them. The high rates of patient and staff turnover would impair the effectiveness of methadone maintenance in reducing heroin use and crime, and the net effect of these policies would be to put public support for methadone maintenance treatment at risk.

Conversely, an over-reliance on providing maximally user-friendly methadone maintenance treatment programs could produce an expensive form of state-subsidised opioid distribution which has minimal therapeutic benefits to dependent heroin users. It would also be achieved at considerable social cost: the increased economic costs of providing methadone maintenance treatment, the costs of the methadone diversion, and perhaps, an increase in methadone overdose deaths, including deaths among individuals who were not enrolled in methadone maintenance treatment programs. These outcomes would also reduce public support for methadone maintenance treatment programs.

Regulating the Methadone Treatment System

A major threat to public support for the methadone treatment system comes from the possibility of illegal conduct by either medical and nursing staff, or patients, or both. This behaviour need not be widespread to have an adverse effect, given the public ambivalence about methadone maintenance treatment and the stigmatisation of methadone patients and the staff who treat them. A small number of well-publicised cases of medical malpractice or patient fraud could undermine public and political support for methadone maintenance treatment, thereby reducing funding.

Among these threats are the following: doctors could sell methadone to clients; they could enrol non-existent patients, especially under a capitation system; unscrupulous medical practitioners could register non-existent patients or collude with real patients to sell excess methadone. Methadone diversion, whether by program staff or patients, could lead to community criticism of the program. If these concerns are realised they may encourage more centralised systems of regulation and monitoring of methadone maintenance treatment. The administrative goal in regulating methadone maintenance treatment must be to minimise the risk of occurrence and to maximise the chance of detecting any such misconduct by staff or patients, without producing a bureaucratic system of control that interferes with good clinical practice. This will be a major challenge when economic pressures are pushing the models of provision towards the private sector, and towards decentralised systems involving general practitioners and private pharmacists.

Advocates of methadone maintenance treatment will need to place these problems in perspective. There is a downside to any treatment system, especially one with a criminally involved clientele. Just as motor vehicle fatalities and serious injuries are the price that our community is prepared to pay for the convenience of the motor vehicle as a form of transport, so too are there costs in having a methadone treatment system. The trick is to maximise its benefits and limit its harms, while acknowledging that it is not possible to have a system that has no negatives in it. In a sense, this means choosing between problems rather than solutions: a large group of opioid-dependent persons who obtain their drugs from an unregulated black market and pay for their drugs by dealing in drugs or engaging in predatory property crime; and reducing these societal costs by providing oral long-acting opioids to a substantial proportion of opioid-dependent people to improve their health and to reduce their adverse impact on the communities within which they live.

REFERENCES

Anglin, M.D. (1988). The efficacy of civil commitment in treating narcotic drug addiction. In C.G. Leukefeld, & F.M. Tims (Eds.), *Compulsory treatment of drug abuse: Research and clinical practice* (NIDA Monograph No 86, pp. 8-34). Rockville, MD: National Institute on Drug Abuse.
Anglin, M.D. and Hser, Y-I. (1990). Treatment of drug abuse. In M. Tonry and J.Q. Wilson (Eds.), *Drugs and crime: A review of research* (pp. 393-

460). Chicago: University of Chicago Press.

Australian Bureau of Criminal Intelligence. (1996) *Australian illicit drug report 1995-96.* Canberra: Commonwealth of Australia.

Bammer, G. (1995). *Report and recommendations of stage 2 feasibility research into the controlled availability of opioids.* Canberra, Australia: National Centre for Epidemiology and Population Health and Australian Institute of Criminology.

Bell, J., Batey, R.G., Farrell, G.C., Crewe, E.B., Cunningham, A.L., & Byth, K. (1990). Hepatitis C in intravenous drug users, *Medical Journal of Australia,* **153**, 274-276.

Bell, J., Caplehorn, J., & McNeil, D. (1994). The effect of intake procedures on performance in methadone maintenance. *Addiction,* **89**, 463-471.

Bell, J., Ward, J., Mattick, R.P., Hay, A., Chan, J., & Hall, W. (1995). *An evaluation of private methadone clinics* (National Drug Strategy Report Series No. 4). Canberrra, Australia: Australian Government Publishing Service.

Beschner, G.M., & Walters, J.M. (1985). Just another habit? the heroin users' perspective on treatment. In B. Hanson, G. Beschner, J.M. Walters and E. Bovelle (Eds.), *Life with heroin: Voices from the inner city* (pp. 75-107). Lexington, MA: Lexington Books.

Biernacki, P. (1986). *Pathways from heroin addiction: Recovery without treatment.* Philadelphia: Temple University Press.

Caplehorn, J.R.M. and Bell, J. (1991). Methadone dosage and retention of patients in maintenance treatment. *Medical Journal of Australia,* **154**, 195-199.

Caplehorn, J., McNeil, D., & Kleinbaum, D.G. (1993). Clinic policy and retention in methadone maintenance. *International Journal of the Addictions,* **28**, 73-89.

Commonwealth Department of Human Services and Health (1995). *Review of methadone treatment in Australia.* Canberra, Australia: Commonwealth Department of Human Services and Health.

D'Aunno, T., & Vaughn, T.E. (1992). Variations in methadone treatment practices: Results from a national study. *Journal of the American Medical Association,* 1992, **267**, 253-258.

Darke, S., Ross, J., & Hall. W. (1995). *The injection of methadone syrup in Sydney, Australia,* (NDARC Technical Report No.23). Sydney, Australia: National Drug and Alcohol Research Centre.

Dole, V.P., Robinson, J.W., Orraca, J., Towns, E., Searcy, P., and Caine, E. (1969). Methadone treatment of randomly selected criminal addicts. *New England Journal of Medicine,* **280**, 1372-1375.

Gerstein, D.R., & Harwood, H.J. (1990). *Treating drug problems Volume 1: A study of effectiveness and financing of public and private drug treatment systems.* Washington, DC: National Academy Press.

Hall, W. (1995). *The demand for methadone maintenance treatment in Australia.* (NDARC Technical Report No. 28). Sydney, Australia: National Drug and Alcohol Research Centre

Hall, W. (in press). The role of legal coercion in the treatment of offenders with alcohol and drug problems. *Australian and New Zealand Journal of Criminology.*

Hartnoll, R., Mitcheson, M.C., Battersby, A., Brown, G., Ellis, M., Fleming, P., & Hedley, N. (1980). Evaluation of heroin maintenance in controlled trial. *Archives of General Psychiatry,* **37,** 877-884.

Hubbard, R.L., Collins, J.J., Rachal, J.V., & Cavanaugh, E.R. (1988). The criminal justice client in drug abuse treatment. In C.G. Leukefeld, & F.M. Tims (Eds.), *Compulsory treatment of drug abuse: Research and clinical practice* (NIDA Monograph No 86, pp. 57-80). Rockville, MD: National Institute on Drug Abuse.

Hubbard, R.L., Marsden, M.E., Rachal, J.V., Harwood, H.J., Cavanaugh, E.R., & Ginzburg, H.M. (1989). *Drug abuse treatment: A national study of effectiveness.* Chapel Hill, NC: University of North Carolina Press.

Hunt, D.E., Lipton, D.S., Goldsmith, D.S., Strug, D.L., Spunt, B. (1986). "It takes your heart": The image of methadone maintenance in the addict world and its effect on recruitment into treatment. *International Journal of the Addictions,* 1986, **20,** 1751-1771.

Joe, G.W., Chastain, R.L., & Simpson, B.B. (1990). Reasons for addiction stages. In D.D. Simpson, & S.B. Sells (Eds.), *Opioid addiction and treatment: A 12-year follow-up.* Malabar, Fl: Robert E. Krieger.

Maher, L. (1996). Age, culture and risk: Contextualizing high-risk practices among new injectors in South West Sydney. Paper presented at the Seventh International Conference on the Reduction of Drug-related Harm, Hobart, Australia.

Marks, J. (1987). Management of drug addicts: Hostility, humanism and pragmatism. *The Lancet,* **I,** 1068-1069.

Marsh, K.L., Joe, G.W., Simpson, D.D., & Lehman, W.E.K. (1990). Treatment History. In D.D. Simpson, & S.B. Sells (Eds.), *Opioid addiction and treatment: A 12-year follow-up.* Malabar, Fl: Robert E. Krieger.

New South Wales Drug and Alcohol Directorate (1996). *Methadone program 1994/95 annual statistical report.* Sydney, Australia: Drug and Alcohol Directorate, New South Wales Department of Health.

Newman, R.G., & Whitehill, W.B. (1979). Double-blind comparison of methadone and placebo maintenance treatments of narcotic addicts in Hong Kong. *Lancet,* September **8,** 485-488.

Rosenblum, A., Magura, S., & Joseph, H. (1991). Ambivalence towards methadone treatment among intravenous drug users. *Journal of Psychoactive Drugs,* **23,** 21-27.

Rihs, M. (1994). The prescription of narcotics under medical supervision and research relating to drugs at the Federal Office of Public Health. Bern: The Swiss Federal Office of Public Health.

Senay, E. (1988). Methadone and public policy. *British Journal of Addiction*, **83**, 257-263.

Simpson, D.S., & Friend, H.J. (1988). Legal status and long-term outcomes for addicts in the DARP Followup Project. In C.G. Leukefeld, & F.M. Tims (Eds.), *Compulsory treatment of drug abuse: Research and clinical practice* (NIDA Monograph No 86, pp. 81-98). Rockville, MD: National Institute on Drug Abuse.

Strang, J, & Gossop, M. (Eds.). (1994). *Heroin addiction and drug policy: The British system.* New York: Oxford University Press.

Uchtenhagen, A., Dobler-Miklos, A., & Gutzwiller, F. (1994). Medically controlled prescription of narcotics: Fundamentals, research plan, first experiences. Unpublished manuscript.

Ward, J., Mattick, R. and Hall, W. (1992). *Key issues in methadone maintenance.* Sydney, Australia: New South Wales University Press.

Weatherburn, D., & Lind, B. (1995). *Drug law enforcement policy and its impact on the heroin market.* Sydney, Australia: New South Wales Bureau of Crime Statistics and Research.

Woody, G., O'Hare, K., Mints, J., & O'Brien, C. (1975). Rapid intake: A method for increasing retention rate of heroin addicts seeking methadone treatment. *Comprehensive Psychiatry*, **16**, 165-169.

INDEX

After a page number, 't' indicates a table.